'Lucy Upton's expert guidance makes fee[...] achievable and enjoyable. This book is [...] looking to nurture happy, healthy eate[...]

Annabel Karmel, number one bestselling children's cookery author

'With so much misinformation and nutrition noise online, it's refreshing to find a resource that covers it all while remaining fully evidence-based and grounded in science . . . empowering you to make informed decisions and give your children the best possible start to their healthy eating journey . . . This book truly is the ultimate guide to children's nutrition.'

Dr Chintal Patel, NHS GP and author of *Dr Chintal's Kitchen: Quick, Easy, Healthy Meals the Whole Family will Love*

'A truly comprehensive guide covering everything from milk, weaning, fussy eating and allergies. This book will give you so much more confidence when navigating what and how to feed your young children . . . I wish I had it at the start of my feeding journey, but it will now be a much-used companion when raising my little ones.'

Kate Lancaster, author of *Feed your Family Dairy Free*

'This book is the ultimate manual for feeding kids that every parent needs – it's like having your own personal dietitian in your pocket! It is written with compassion and care, drawing on Lucy's many years of guiding and supporting families with their little ones' feeding and nutrition journeys . . . This book is going to help so many families.'

Paula Hallam, specialist paediatric dietitian and author of *Plant Powered Little People*

'This book is an invaluable guide, packed with evidence-based advice and practical reassurance to help parents confidently navigate the early years. Whether you're facing allergies, picky eating, or just the daily juggle of family mealtimes, Lucy Upton provides a clear, balanced and non-judgmental approach to nourishing your child for the best possible start in life.'
Nichola Ludlam-Raine, specialist dietitian and author of
How Not to Eat Ultra-Processed

'Lucy has been a massive support on our little one's food journey. This book is the perfect foundation for children's nutrition and a must-buy for any parent.'
James Wythe, food blogger, dad and author of *Healthy Living James*

'We all just want to feel best equipped to make the right choices for our children and Lucy has created an incredible resource . . . Lucy mixes years of expertise with friendly, actionable and non-judgmental guidance. She takes the time to explain why certain approaches to nutrition are important and gives suggestions that feel realistic for navigating the challenges along the way. I can't wait to dip back into it as my little ones grow!'
Sian Radford, author of *Moon and Rue: Baby-Led Weaning Made Easy*

The Ultimate Guide to Children's Nutrition

How to nurture happy, healthy eaters in the first five years

Lucy Upton, MNutr

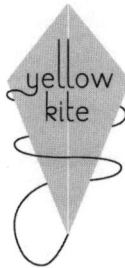

yellow kite

First published in Great Britain in 2025 by Yellow Kite
An imprint of Hodder & Stoughton Limited
An Hachette UK company

The authorised representative in the EEA is Hachette Ireland, 8 Castlecourt
Centre, Dublin 15, D15 XTP3, Ireland (email: info@hbgi.ie)

1

Diagrams by Jason Cox.

A CIP catalogue record for this title is available from the British Library

Trade Paperback ISBN 9781399740470
ebook ISBN 9781399740487

Typeset in Adobe Garamond Pro by Hewer Text UK Ltd, Edinburgh
Printed and bound in Great Britain by Clays Ltd, Elcograf S.p.A.

Hodder & Stoughton policy is to use papers that are natural, renewable
and recyclable products and made from wood grown in sustainable
forests. The logging and manufacturing processes are expected to
conform to the environmental regulations of the country of origin.

Hodder & Stoughton Limited
Carmelite House
50 Victoria Embankment
London EC4Y 0DZ

www.yellowkitebooks.co.uk

For my daughter Aurelia, Harry, my family and you – parents and caregivers everywhere.

I hope this book inspires you to approach your child's first five years of feeding and nutrition with confidence, curiosity and some joy (and, of course, peace of mind), knowing that you're building a foundation for a healthy, happy future.

Throughout this book we recognise that parenting and caregiving come in many forms, and that families are as diverse as the individuals who make them up. While we will use terms such as 'mother' and 'parent', we acknowledge that these roles and experiences are not defined by gender or biological sex. We respect and recognise all gender identities, expressions and feeding choices, including those who identify as fathers, non-binary parents, trans parents, and all other caregivers. This book primarily uses the term 'breastfeeding' but acknowledges and respects 'chest feeding' as an inclusive and valid expression for those who prefer or require it.

Contents

Foreword

Firstly, I am not surprised you have trusted Lucy's invaluable advice and bought this fantastic book!

Lucy has a wonderful way of breaking down the vast amount of information out there regarding child nutrition and presenting it in a way that is easy to follow and understand. As parents, all we want to do is make sure we are feeding our babies what they need and at the right time; Lucy's evidence-based advice helps parents to understand and feel confident in what to do, taking the worry out of feeding our families.

Lucy shares my view that food should be enjoyed. She highlights the importance of introducing food with flavour and making meal-times happy environments, to help parents reduce the understandable stress and confusion around feeding their family so they can enjoy this time with their children. We share the goal of helping parents begin their child's feeding journey with confidence and knowledge, to raise happy, healthy children.

In particular, I find Lucy's ability to cut through the jargon surrounding feeding children with allergies incredibly valuable. Through her work on social media especially, she helps an incredible number of parents to understand the 'what's and 'if's regarding feeding children with suspected or confirmed allergies and intolerances.

She shares vital, trustworthy information, in a way that is easy to process, with a sympathetic ear for those parents who may find this stage in parenting a little daunting or overwhelming.

In 2020 I wrote my first weaning and family-feeding cookbook, using my 'cook one meal for the whole family' approach to recipes. I entrusted Lucy to ensure all nutrition guidance was correct and the recipes were balanced and suitable for babies from 6 months old. That book was *my* baby and I needed to ensure that all of the information was 100 per cent up-to-date and accurate. To work with Lucy was and is a no-brainer; her dedication to knowledge- and evidence-based advice for child nutrition is second to none, so much so that we have since worked together on a further five cookbooks of mine.

This book encompasses all Lucy's expertise, evidence-based knowledge on all things nutrition-based for weaning and feeding children, broken down in an easy-to-digest format.

Once you've read this book, I guarantee you will feel empowered with knowledge and confidence to enter this exciting phase of parenting and bring joy into your family mealtimes.

Rebecca Wilson (What Mummy Makes)
Family feeding cookery author and expert

Why I Wrote This Book

There's famously no manual for the most demanding job out there – parenting. If there was, a big old chunk of it would be dedicated to feeding your tiny human. Despite the fact that eating is something that we all do every day, and is second nature to most of us, when you become a parent you suddenly view feeding, eating and nutrition through a whole new lens. Along with your beautiful new baby, you've also had thrust upon you the responsibility of nourishing and keeping them healthy and happy. And it can feel overwhelming. Questions about what to feed them, how much they should eat, how they are growing, the right balance of nutrients and so much more can take up some serious mental load, all while trying to navigate the ever-changing landscape of parenting.

Over the course of my career as a dietitian I've lost count of the number of times I've sat at the end of a busy clinic feeling the weight of parents' worries about nutrition and feeding, wondering why there isn't more easily accessible support and advice for parents on this topic. Feeding their children is something that countless parents have told me has been the hardest, most unpredictable, changeable, confusing or conflicting part of their parenting journey so far. It's also something that they don't get a day off from, and it is a deeply emotional subject. Children need good nutrition not just to survive but to thrive in their environment, and the early years are well recognised as the optimum time to 'get it right'.

There is also something interesting about feeding children, in that even before your baby is born your world can be filled with unsolicited advice, mixed messages and judgement about feeding choices, nutrition and more. Now, thanks to the surge of information that's accessible to everyone online, when you enter the world of parenting you're also inducted into an onslaught of parenting nutrition noise – a topic that battles sleep, toileting and behaviour for the top spot. My experience is that while some of this information is incredibly helpful, this noise really can deafen parents at a particularly vulnerable time, causing them to question their instincts, feel constantly conflicted or freeze in the overwhelm of deciding what's best for their new family.

This is one of the reasons why I started my social media page @childrensdietitian while I was still working full-time for the NHS and beginning my own nutrition business. I wanted a tiny corner of the internet where I could share information to help parents confidently feed their children. I was exasperated by the lack of evidence-based, non-judgemental, supportive and, most importantly, accurate and non-scaremongering advice about nutrition and feeding children.

Which brings me on to, well, me – and, more importantly, why I'm writing this book. While I don't much enjoy talking about myself, it's so important that you understand why on earth you should entrust me with writing a book that carries you through the first five vulnerable and immensely important years of feeding your child.

Firstly, I am a mum to an energetic little girl, Aurelia, which means that I'm experienced at riding this crazy parenting journey too. But, while being a parent has added a whole new and invaluable dimension of experience to my work, it is <u>not</u> what gives me the credentials to write this book. I've spent over fourteen years so far as a Specialist Paediatric (Children's) Dietitian, working with well and unwell children and their families from all backgrounds and cultures, alongside industry professionals, public health organisations, the media and more. I translate science into practical, actionable advice, and because I'm a dietitian, I have the qualifications, legal accountability and ethical standards to guide parents with reliable and trustworthy information. I'm also a feeding therapist, and while this isn't a formalised title, it involves additional training and experience working with not just *what* to feed children, but the important link with *how* they are fed too.

This book is a blend of that science, alongside the lived experience I've had with thousands of families over the years – through mealtime tantrums, tears, joy and everything in between.

But this book isn't about me. It's about you, your family and helping you to feel confident feeding your child. And with this huge responsibility come a few promises from me to you:

✧ I promise the information shared here is science-backed and evidence-based, entwined with real-life and practical advice that I've used with families for years. I'll explain the 'why' behind my recommendations wherever possible – it's not just 'because I said so'.

✧ This book does not make food the enemy, quite the opposite. Food is one of the most influential things over which you have some control for your child's health, and while that in itself can feel intimidating, it's my hope that this book will give you all the information you need to feel empowered with the nutrition and feeding decisions you will make for your children. While I do talk about nutrients and focus on specifics in this book, for life and health span I always encourage parents to step back and look at the bigger picture – the whole diet, not just single foods or nutrients.

✧ As a busy parent I don't intend for you to read and digest this book all in one go. I wanted to write something that came with you through the first five years of your child's life, so it is designed to sit on your shelf and be within arm's reach for dipping in and out of during different ages as and when you reach them, but it's also for those SOS times when something is worrying you about your child's food, diet, feeding habits or health.

✧ This book is free of judgement. My goal is and always will be to empower parents to make informed decisions that work for their family. To do that, you need accurate information, presented clearly and fairly. I know feeding can feel like a loaded topic these days, but I want this book to be a source of clarity and calm – always honest, but without pressure. If you find your head is buzzing after reading certain sections of this book, do what I always recommend to parents and focus on one thing at a time.

I also wrote this book because the first five years of a child's life are the time when parents need the information that I'm sharing the most. While the years fly by, this period is foundational for a child's long-term health, and nutrition and feeding practices are riding up front as something that we, as parents, can use to harness our children's wellbeing not just for now, but for life. Within these five years also fall the well-known 'first 1,000 days', a golden period (from conception to two) recognised as *the* time to shape children's futures. I know this may feel a touch overwhelming, especially when you're exhausted and adjusting to life with your tiny human, but these early years are a powerful investment in your child's health. Experts across the board agree – getting nutrition and feeding relationships right in these years has lasting benefits. It's also a time of a whirlwind of changes – nutritionally, developmentally, emotionally – and understanding them, stage by stage, can make a huge difference.

So, welcome to the wild and wonderful world of feeding your baby and beyond! From now on, feeding will be one of those top-priority, can't-ignore puzzle pieces of parenting that you're navigating. Every feeding age and stage can bring its own mix of emotions, from excitement to nerves and, probably, 'what on earth am I doing?' moments. But don't worry, you're not alone!

This book is *my chapter* of that parenting manual that everyone needs. Packaging up everything you need to know about children's nutrition and feeding in the first five years into a clear, evidence-based guide that can come with you on this wild ride called parenting. I hope it's worn and well used by the time your child puts on their school uniform, and if it helps even one family to a healthier, happier start, I've done my job well.

1

Milk Matters

Nourishing baby's first months (and beyond): 0–6 months

Nutrition and feeding milestones in the first six months of life:

✧ By six months of age, your baby's weight will be double their birth weight or more, and their length will increase on average by 1.5–2.5cm per month.
✧ Your baby needs more energy (calories) per kilogram of body weight than at any other time in their life.
✧ Your baby's brain will reach around 50 per cent of its adult size by six months of age.
✧ Milk will be your baby's primary source of nutrition; breast milk and/or formula milk provides the unique nutrition that your baby needs to fuel their rapid growth.
✧ Breast milk contains additional factors that support the development of your baby's immune system, gut and more.
✧ Your baby will feed regularly and on their own schedule (including overnight) to help meet their high energy needs.
✧ Responsively feeding your baby and recognising their hunger and fullness cues will help establish a healthy feeding relationship.

✧ **Milk feeding falls within the first 1,000 days (a time when what and how babies and children are fed is known to be incredibly important).**

I can't start this book or section without saying congratulations on your baby's arrival or imminent arrival! You'll be fully aware that your life is shifting forever, and it's an exciting journey filled with moments of wonder and joy, but I also relate to the feeling of wanting somewhere to turn to with the constant questions, worries and advice that will be going through your mind during these vulnerable first few months as a parent.

Milk feeding marks your baby's first feeding milestone, supporting the rapid growth and development that you will witness, and deciding which milk to provide is a significant and personal choice for you and your family. As a new parent, you might feel overwhelmed by advice on this subject from family, friends, healthcare professionals and even strangers, and it can be challenging to sift through this abundance of opinions! Over the following pages, my aim is to provide you with evidence-based information and guidance to help you make informed decisions and understand the right option for you, acknowledging that every feeding method deserves support and respect while ensuring that both your own and your baby's physical and emotional needs are met.

As a book about nutrition, this first section covers everything from what's in breast and formula milk to how to understand when your baby is hungry and common milk feeding worries, but depending on how you feed your baby, feel free to skip to the section that feels relevant for you.

I also want to acknowledge that the subject of milk feeding is a whole book of its own. You'll appreciate that with five years of children's nutrition and feeding to cover, I won't be able to talk about everything, but I have made sure that I've included what I feel are the most helpful and relevant points for all new parents. I've linked some fantastic resources and individuals on pages 440–2 too, for more information.

What does milk need to provide for your newborn baby?

Your tiny baby has just arrived and over the next year it will be growing and developing faster than at any other time in their life. To keep up with this, the nutrition your baby gets in these early months needs to be specially designed to meet these needs, and helpfully this is packaged up in the options you have for milk feeding – breast milk, formula milk or a combination of both.

To help you visualise just how tailored these milks are for your baby, I can use energy as just one example. The amount of energy your small baby needs is around three to four times more per kilogram of body weight than we need as fully grown adults. The amounts and types of nutrients your baby needs are different from those of an adult. This includes differences in protein and fat requirements, as well as how much of certain vitamins and minerals are needed.

Put simply, nutrition for your baby has to be unique because their nutritional needs are like no other time in their life and in these first six months, breast milk and/or formula milk is the only form of nutrition that will do this job. To add to this, your baby's small stomach size and limited built-up stores of energy and nutrients mean that these milk feeds will be sought after multiple times each day and night to help meet these needs.

Breast or formula milk?

Breast and formula milk both provide the nutrition your baby needs, but there are differences between the two. This will become apparent when I talk about the nutrition and composition ('ingredients') of breast and formula milk, but I want to reinforce that there is no judgement playing into my discussion of these differences. I've aimed to cover the science, facts and information that parents look for, or that they may benefit from understanding.

Whether you decide to breastfeed/chest feed, formula feed or do a combination of both, the choice is yours to make. There are many factors that parents must add to the decision-making process individually. These can include everything from health considerations for mum to previous feeding experiences, working arrangements and more. Feeding decisions are never black and white: the best ones ensure a baby, their mother and their parents are healthy and happy.

You do not need to justify your feeding choices to others. Equally, I would ask that as you embark on your journey into the parenting world you offer the same respect and care for the decisions made by all other parents, whether they are the same as or different to yours. Milk feeding, in particular, can be a hugely emotive and therefore sensitive area of nutrition and feeding to discuss, but as a health professional who has supported probably thousands of families with feeding their babies and children, I see first-hand the negative repercussions of judgement, blame or berating about feeding at a highly vulnerable time for babies and parents.

Breast milk

Experts widely agree that breastfeeding is the optimal source of nutrition for a baby. Breast milk is truly a unique 'food' that stands apart from other forms of nutrition for many reasons – it is perfectly tailored for your baby's needs, not just exclusively for the first six months of life but also ongoing once you start solids and into the toddler years. The World Health Organization (WHO) recommends exclusive breastfeeding up to six months, with ongoing breastfeeding alongside solids (food) until two years of age and beyond.

Breast milk is high in energy and the nutrients needed to keep up with your baby's rapid growth and brain development. But it isn't just a 'meal'; breast milk contains numerous 'extras' designed to support and bolster your baby's health as it enters a high-risk world (outside the womb) with an immature immune system and gut. These extras support breast milk's nutrition, optimising growth and development while safeguarding your baby (and you) against illness now, while also paying benefits forward for many years to come.

Over the following pages I'm going to cover:

✧ **Breast milk nutrition 101**

✧ **Beyond the nutrition – what else is in breast milk, and why it's important**

✧ **Breast milk benefits for mum and baby**

✧ **Looking after yourself when breastfeeding**

✧ **Supplements for you and your breast-milk-fed baby**

✧ **Breastfeeding basics: your quick guide to some essentials**

✧ **SOS – Frequently asked questions or worries about breastfeeding**

Breast-milk nutrition 101

The nutritional content of breast milk isn't stable, meaning it's not the same every day; it changes and adapts to meet your baby's needs as they grow and develop.

In the first few days after birth, a mother's body produces colostrum (first breast milk), a thick, yellowish milk packed with antibodies (more on those later) and essential nutrients. Colostrum is sometimes referred to as 'liquid gold', and while it's typically small in quantity, it's pretty mighty by nature, acting as your baby's first shot or boost of shared immunity, to help protect them against infections. You may have even harvested some colostrum by hand-expressing just before your baby was born.

After those first few days, your breast milk evolves to what's known as transitional milk, usually at around days two to five. From then on, your milk gradually increases in volume and changes structurally, balancing proteins, fats and carbohydrates to match your baby's developing digestive system and nutritional needs.

By days 10–14 you will be producing 'mature milk' and at this stage your milk is rich in nutrients and antibodies.

From then on, breast milk continues to adjust based on the time of day at which you feed, and in line with your baby's feeding habits and health. There is a feedback loop (like a phone line) between a breastfeeding mother and baby, meaning a mother's body and the milk it makes is always on call for the baby's changing needs. For example, breast milk later in the day contains more sleep hormone (melatonin) to help ease your baby into slumber. If a parent or baby is ill, breast milk evolves to produce specific antibodies to help fight that illness within a matter of hours.

Macronutrients in breast milk

Macronutrient

Macro = big, aka needed in large amounts

+

Nutrient = something your body needs to provide energy and/or to support essential body functions and health

Breast milk contains all the 'big' nutrients that your baby needs, which are carbohydrates, protein and fat. These nutrients not only help maintain the energy content of breast milk, which is approximately 67–70 kcals per 100ml, to support your baby's growth, but they also play crucial roles in your baby's overall development.

Here are some key pieces of information about these macronutrients:

Nutrient	A bit more about it . . .	What does it do?
Carbohydrate	The main carbohydrate in breast milk is lactose, which is the naturally occurring sugar in milk. It makes up about 7 per cent of breast milk overall. Lactose is what makes breast milk taste sweet.	A key energy source for your baby to support growth and development. Supports calcium absorption. Helps brain development. Promotes the growth of friendly bacteria in the gut. Supports hydration.
	Human Milk Oligosaccharides, aka 'HMOs', are another type of carbohydrate in breast milk and are the third most 'solid' part of breast milk. (More on these later.)	Feeds the good bacteria in your baby's gut, to support a healthy gut microbiome. Supports healthy immune system development.

Protein	Protein makes up around 1 per cent of breast milk, and breast milk contains two main types of protein: whey and casein (think Little Miss Muffet – curds and whey!).	Essential for your baby's growth and development.
	Whey is liquid and easy to digest, while casein forms a curd in the stomach and is digested more slowly. When your baby is first born, the whey: casein ratio in colostrum is about 90:10. As breast milk matures, this ratio changes to about 60:40.	An energy source for your baby. Supports digestion and absorption of specific nutrients, such as calcium and iron.
	The protein content in breast milk drops when your baby is six months of age, as the requirements start to shift and solids are gradually introduced.	Specific proteins have immune-support benefits. Helps produce the hormones your baby needs to grow and develop.
	Breast milk also contains specific proteins that have immune benefits, like lactoferrin.	

Fat	Fat provides nearly half the energy in breast milk, making up around 4 per cent of breast milk.	A significant energy source for your baby.
		Essential for your baby's brain development, which is occurring rapidly.
	The main fats in breast milk are something known as triglycerides (fats with a specific shape/structure).	Supports development of baby's vision.
	Essential fatty acids called linoleic acid and alpha-linolenic acid are also found in breast milk. These are also the building blocks for other types of fatty acids the body needs but cannot make, including docosahex-aenoic acid (DHA).	Supports the development of your baby's immune system.
		Supports the absorption of fat-soluble vitamins (A, D, E and K).
	There are enzymes (mini scissors) in breast milk that help to digest fat found in breast milk.	**A note about fat in breast milk:** As the fat content of breast milk fluctuates, parents often worry about getting 'fatty' milk for growth, but please be reassured the *amount* of milk your baby consumes is more important than fat content. If you feed responsively, your body will adjust to provide the right balance.
	Certain fats in breast milk, found in large amounts, have a particular shape/structure that supports digestion, how easily nutri-ents are absorbed by the body, poo consistency and gut health.	

Developed from Kim, S. Y., & Yi, D. Y. (2020). Components of human breast milk: From macronutrient to microbiome and microRNA. Clinical and Experimental Pediatrics, 63(8), 301–9. https://doi.org/10.3345/cep.2020.00059

Fluid in breast milk

While not a nutrient as such, I think it's important to acknowledge that breast milk is around 87–88 per cent water, meaning it's also going to provide your baby with all the hydration they need. Babies have high fluid requirements compared to their body size.

Micronutrients in breast milk

> **Micronutrient**
>
> Micro = small – needed in smaller amounts
>
> +
>
> Nutrient = something your body needs to provide energy and/or to support essential body functions and health

Breast milk also contains all the micronutrients your baby needs in those first six months – vitamins, minerals and trace elements. Each micronutrient has an important job in the body, and many work together to provide health benefits. (See pages 431–5 for a list of all the essential vitamins, minerals and trace elements and descriptions of what they do for the body.)

What a mother eats and her body reserves can influence some of the micronutrient levels in breast milk. However, studies show breast milk is resilient and adapts well to meet a baby's needs. Be reassured, even if you have a more limited diet than normal, your baby can still get everything they need. Vitamins D and K are exceptions that typically require supplementation in exclusively breastfed babies. Vitamin K is particularly low in breast milk, so it is usually provided to babies after birth as an injection. In the UK, breastfeeding mums and exclusively breastfed babies are recommended to be supplemented with vitamin D daily.

Beyond nutrition – what else is in breast milk, and why it's important

Breast milk is more than just a source of nutrition for your baby, it's a living, dynamic fluid containing hundreds, if not thousands, of 'extras' that are often referred to as bioactive factors. These include antibodies, good bacteria, enzymes, hormones and more. Put simply, bioactive factors are natural substances that can have a positive effect on health, often supporting functions like the immune system or gut microbiome. It makes complete sense that breast milk is packed full of these! Your baby has a very immature immune system and gut at birth, which is why many of these bioactive factors play a crucial role in protecting your baby from illness, fighting infection and supporting the development of a healthy, happy gut microbiome. While not nutritional in the traditional sense (like calories or nutrients), bioactive factors are important because many work alongside nutrients to bolster your baby's growth and development. Many of your baby's body systems, like the immune system, are also primed and fine-tuned (like a radio) through the combination of nutrition, and these bioactive factors during early life, paving the way for future health.

I wanted to highlight a handful of bioactive factors in breast milk, as they are often not given much airtime but they relate closely to breastfeeding benefits that health professionals frequently do share, as I have below. There might be some pretty scientific-sounding terms, but I'll try to explain them as clearly as possible!

✧ **Human Milk Oligosaccharides or 'HMOs',** aka breast milk's food for good gut bacteria. HMOs are found in large amounts in breast milk and are a type of carbohydrate that your baby can't digest. But why does nature invest energy in including these in breast milk if babies can't digest them? Because they are rocket fuel for your baby's growing community of gut bacteria.

HMOs travel to a baby's gut, where they feed and encourage the growth of 'good' bacteria. I like to think of them as breast milk's prebiotic, akin to fibre in our diet. Hundreds of different HMOs exist in breast milk, varying from mother to mother. They help maintain a healthy gut microbiome, support the immune system and protect against harmful germs.

✧ **Breast milk biome,** aka breast milk's community of helpful bacteria or 'probiotics'. Breast milk contains a whole community of bacteria of its own. These aren't the 'bad' kind of bacteria you might think of; they are good bacteria that can help keep your baby healthy. This community of bacteria plays a vital role in building your baby's gut microbiome, which is like a friendly neighbourhood of tiny organisms living in the digestive system. A healthy gut microbiome is important for your baby's digestion, health, immune system and much more.

✧ **Nucleotides**, aka breast milk's construction crew. I know they sound like something from outer space, but these tiny components found in breast milk help to form the building blocks of DNA. They also play a role in building a healthy gut microbiome, supporting the development of the immune system by helping to create beneficial immune cells and helping tissue growth and repair (which is happening fast for your baby!).

✧ **Immunoglobulins,** aka breast milk's immune defenders. You could probably make a well-informed guess from the name that these have a role in your baby's immune-system development. Immunoglobulins are also known as antibodies, and one of their key roles is to be part of the immune system's defence system – identifying harmful substances like certain bacteria and protecting your baby from infection or illness. Immunoglobulins in breast milk can transfer immune support from mum to baby, bolstering their developing immune system.

This is known as passive immunity – baby borrows it from mum! One of the most common immunoglobulins in breast milk is Immunoglobulin A (IgA). Secretory IgA helps protect your baby by forming a physical mucus-type barrier in their gut and respiratory tract to help prevent harmful germs that cause infections from getting in.

✧ **Lactoferrin,** aka breast milk's iron-binding friend and immune protector. This particular protein in breast milk provides more than nutrition. It is very good at attaching itself to iron, making it easier for your baby's body to absorb. While harmful bacteria or viruses can use iron to grow, lactoferrin helps prevent this and supports your baby's immune system and gut health. It's almost like a 'natural disinfectant'.

I hope this section gives you a glimpse into breast milk's incredible benefits beyond nutrition and gives some context behind statements often made about breastfeeding, such as, 'it's good for baby's gut health' and 'it supports their immunity'.

Breast milk benefits for mum and baby

Building upon the discussion about bioactive factors in breast milk, it makes sense to highlight the broader advantages of breastfeeding, as many listed below for babies are associated with these beneficial 'extras' in breast milk.

Aside from the science, there are also practical benefits to breastfeeding for many parents, including:

✧ Convenience with feeding when out and about.

✧ There is no need to store or sterilise bottles and other feeding equipment (unless pumping or combination feeding).

✧ Feeding gets more manageable over time.

✧ Feeling like they have a 'magic power' for soothing during times of discomfort or upset (or more).

	Baby	Mum
Short term benefits	Reduced risk of infections, such as ear infections. Reduced risk of gastroenteritis ('tummy bugs') or more serious bowel problems in newborn or premature babies, such as necrotising enterocolitis (NEC). Reduced risk of sudden infant death syndrome (SIDS). Reduced risk of childhood leukaemia.	Reduced risk of post-natal depression.
Long term benefits	Reduced likelihood of being overweight or obese into childhood. Reduced risk of infections common in childhood. Positive links to higher performance scores in intelligence tests during childhood and adolescence. Reduced risk of asthma.	Reduced risk of • Breast cancer. • Ovarian cancer. • Type 2 diabetes.

Many of the benefits above are supported by studies focusing on exclusive breastfeeding for at least the first six months. However, these benefits are often dose-dependent, meaning that any amount of breast milk is beneficial, with greater health advantages tied to longer durations of breastfeeding. I also think it's important to note that while individual experiences vary, in that not *all* breastfed babies will avoid the above, the population-level impact of breast-feeding is clear.

Fun fact: Breastfeeding can be beneficial when starting solids!

Babies experience a variety of flavours through breast milk, influenced by a mother's diet. This early exposure can affect the acceptance of different foods during weaning and beyond. One study found that the longer babies were breastfed, the higher their fruit and vegetable intake was as children. Another showed that by age six, breastfed children were more willing to try new vegetables and eat more of them. Breastfeeding is also known to support jaw strength and oral development – both important for eating solids when the time comes.

Looking after yourself when breastfeeding

Eating a variety of foods and having balanced meals can help you get all the nutrients your body needs to stay healthy, and this is especially important while breastfeeding. Your body's working hard to produce milk, and research has shown that depending on the stage of lactation, women need an extra 400–700 kcals of energy per day for this. Producing breast milk consumes 25–30 per cent of the body's energy, while the brain uses 20 per cent!

Focusing on including a range of different foods in your diet can be tricky as a new parent, and I don't want to set unrealistic expectations. Yes, there will probably be days where beige foods are the only options you can grab, but below I've translated some ideal nutritional considerations into 'grab-and-go options' for when your hands are full.

Nutritional considerations	Grab-and-go options
Five portions of fruit and vegetables daily, ideally of differing types and colours, to provide a wide range of nutrients.	Smoothies – add frozen fruit and vegetables like spinach. Fresh fruit. Bags of dried fruit. Pre-prepared chopped vegetables. Batch-cook soups, stews or curries or pasta sauce with lots of vegetables.
Breastfeeding mums need more protein, especially in the first six months. Aim to include protein-rich foods like meat, fish, eggs, beans, dairy or nuts at least twice a day, ideally three times a day.	Nut butters or tahini spread on toast, crumpets, bagels. Boiled eggs (do a batch ahead). Tinned fish or precooked fish fillets for sandwiches or pate. Precooked meat. Baked beans on toast. Greek yoghurt or cottage cheese with fruit or nuts. Hummus with veggie sticks or crackers. Edamame beans or roasted chickpeas as a snack.
Include healthy fat sources such as nuts, seeds, avocado, oily fish (no more than twice per week) and plant-based oils, such as olive, rapeseed.	Mash avocado or sardines on toast or bagels. Snack on nuts or seeds. Add nut butters to cereals, porridge pots or toast. Add oil to salads and use in cooking.
For energy, include carbohydrates like oats, rice, pasta, potatoes and bread in meals and snacks throughout the day. Wholegrain options offer slower energy release and added fibre.	Cereals (with milk/dried fruit). Wholemeal toast/bagels. Oatcakes or wholegrain crackers with toppings. Precooked pasta or rice salads. Granola bars or energy bars. Pitta bread with hummus or dips. Microwaveable grains/rice.

Aim for 3–4 portions of dairy or well-fortified milk-free alternatives as a source of calcium, iodine and fat-soluble vitamins.	Individual cheese portions. Cream cheese on toast, crackers. Yoghurt with dried fruit, crushed cereal or granola or tinned fruit in juice. Milky drinks, such as tea, coffee. Milk or fortified alternatives on cereal.
Don't forget hydration!	Focus on water, but tea, coffee, unsweetened fruit juice and milk all contribute too! Be mindful of caffeine intake from tea, coffee and soft drinks. Try to always have a drink within reach (I used to leave bottles around the house) and drink until you don't feel thirsty.

Supplements for you and your breast-milk-fed baby

Vitamin D is one of the few nutrients that is not found in great quantities in breast milk and is one of the most common nutrient deficiencies we see in the UK in children and adults. In the UK it's recommended that breastfed babies are given a daily vitamin D supplement from birth, containing 8.5–10µg vitamin D, unless your baby is combination feeding (breast and formula) and having over 500ml per day of formula milk.

Most vitamin D preparations for babies are provided in a small-drop form, which can be given via a small spoon directly into their mouth (in some cases) or dropped onto your nipple before a feed. You can now also find spray versions that can be sprayed into your baby's cheek or under their tongue.

It's also recommended that breastfeeding mothers have a daily vitamin D supplement that provides 10µg per day. Many breast-feeding mothers may also choose to take a breastfeeding-specific multivitamin and mineral to help keep up with higher nutrient requirements during breastfeeding. For vegetarian or vegan mothers, additional supplementation is also encouraged, such as omega 3, and specifically vitamin B12 and iodine for vegan mothers. There is no set guidance on the specific amount of these supplements. I would encourage seeking advice from a health professional, such as a dietitian, about extra supplementation if you are excluding certain foods or food groups – for example, dairy while breastfeeding – and/or have conditions which can impact absorption of nutrients such as coeliac disease or inflammatory bowel conditions including Crohn's disease.

When choosing supplements for you and your baby:

✧ Check the supplement contains the correct amount of vitamin D. Many provide less than the recommended amount.

✧ If vegan, check the packaging to make sure you are choosing a suitable vegan option (lots of vitamin D is derived from animal sources, such as lanolin found in sheep's wool).

✧ If you're in receipt of certain benefits you and your baby will be eligible to receive free supplements via the UK's Healthy Start scheme. Check online or with your GP, midwife or health visitor on how to access this in your area. In Scotland, free vitamin D supplements are also available for mothers who breastfeed, in addition to infants and children under three years old (see page 442).

✧ Leave it somewhere you'll remember to give it every day – think toothbrush, changing table or kettle!

Breastfeeding basics: your quick guide to some essentials

While this isn't a breastfeeding book, I wanted to cover a few key breastfeeding basics alongside the nutrition side of things, but as I can't cover everything here, I have provided links to some in-depth support and resources at the back of this book.

Your baby's first breastfeed

After a baby is born, mothers are encouraged to experience what's known as the 'golden hour' with their newborn. This gives you time for plenty of skin-to-skin contact, initial bonding and your baby's first feed. Many babies will instinctively look for the breast after birth, known as the 'breast crawl'. This natural reflex helps them latch onto the breast and begin feeding, receiving some of that first breast milk, colostrum. This time is important for establishing breastfeeding, and in most cases is possible if you ask your midwife to delay steps such as weighing and cleaning your baby. For a small number of mothers, immediate skin-to-skin and initiation of breastfeeding may not be possible due to urgent medical interventions for baby or mother, or mum and baby being separated. If this is the case, do not worry; just have skin-to-skin and a first feed as soon as you can.

Whether you get this first hour or not, you should receive ongoing support from healthcare professionals, such as midwives and breast-feeding support staff, to initiate breastfeeding. In all honesty, at times I have seen and heard how difficult the reality of accessing this support can be, which can be a barrier for those who want to breastfeed. While you'll undoubtedly be in the headlights in your first hours or days of parenthood, I'd encourage you to have confidence in advocating for yourself and your baby by requesting support or asking others around you to do so. Don't hesitate to reach out, ask questions and insist on the help you need. This support can include assistance with latching your baby, ensuring a comfortable breastfeeding position and helping you to learn the signs that your baby is feeding well. After all,

breastfeeding is new for both you and your baby, and is a skill you will
need to learn together – and will be for weeks ahead.

Stomach size expectations

When I talk to parents about this topic, I always reassure
them that their baby doesn't need much milk in the early
days. The first breast milk, colostrum, is concentrated and
packed with everything your baby needs. Your baby is born
with a tiny stomach, which gradually increases in size.
Here's a rough guide to help you visualise and reassure you
that those small but powerful colostrum feeds are enough.
As long as your baby is latching and drinking effectively,
they do not need any additional milk, such as formula.

The average size of stomach:
✧ Days 1-2 – the size of a cherry (5-7ml)
✧ Days 3-5 – the size of a walnut (22-27ml)
✧ Day 7-10 – the size of an apricot (45-60ml)

It's easy to forget that in part our stomachs are a storage
organ and babies' stomachs are small with much less
capacity. This, alongside that high demand for energy
(calories), is one of the reasons they need feeding so much!

How often will your breastfed baby want to be fed?
Despite my background in baby nutrition and feeding, the early
days of breastfeeding still caught me by surprise. I was amazed at
how often and how long I spent feeding, and I know I'm not alone
with this realisation. While this isn't everyone's experience, I think
it's important to set realistic expectations about breastfeeding

frequency, especially to reassure mothers who worry about milk supply or lose confidence when their babies feed often.

Newborns and young babies need to feed a minimum of eight times a day, and it's quite normal for breastfed babies to feed 8–12 times a day, and sometimes more. This isn't necessarily just reserved for these early days and weeks. While many tend to find more of a rhythm with breastfeeds with time and experience, breastfeeding should come with the label 'subject to change'. More-frequent feeding can be common throughout your breastfeeding journey, for example during growth spurts, warm weather, or quite simply to help your baby meet other physiological needs, such as comfort.

In the early days of breastfeeding, cluster feeding is also normal. This is when your baby feeds on and off for many hours at a time, seemingly never satisfied, often in the evening or overnight. It can be intense, and I remember being up what felt like all night in the first few days after birth, with Aurelia latched on almost constantly.

Cluster feeding is a normal phase that helps to boost and establish your milk supply, stimulates hormones (chemical signals) such as prolactin and oxytocin involved in milk-making – it doesn't necessarily mean your baby isn't getting enough milk. My best advice is to be prepared for cluster feeding so you're not surprised or worried when it happens. Arm yourself with a TV series and have plenty of fluids and snacks to hand!

Regular feeding for a breastfed baby is also, in part, due to breast milk's composition. Breast milk is high in carbohydrates (lactose) but lower in protein – and the majority of protein is whey. This means it's quick and easy to digest, which means it's very normal for breastfed babies to need feeding frequently. In fact, in comparison with formula-fed babies, studies have shown that young breastfed babies reach a fasting state quicker, usually by around two hours, compared to three hours for formula-fed babies.

Throughout your ongoing breastfeeding journey, how often to feed should be led by your baby and their needs, not by a clock or schedule – unless this is medically advised. The caveat to this is that some newborn babies can be quite sleepy, so they may need waking to feed, including overnight, if they are not rousing regularly to feed or often fall asleep at the breast or between offering breasts. Babies will feed during the day and night, and I often remind parents that breastfeeding overnight is not only very normal but biologically helpful. One of the hormones that breastfeeding mothers make, prolactin (which stimulates milk production), peaks in the early hours of the morning, helping to establish and maintain milk supply.

Checking in with yourself and your baby during feeds

Your baby's general behaviours and demeanour, along-side a mother's experience during feeding, can tell us a lot about how breastfeeding is going. Here are some signs to check in on during feeds.

✧ *Frequency* – Is your baby feeding at least eight times in 24 hours?
✧ *Baby is transferring milk during feeds* – Watch and listen to your baby feeding; a typical start to breast-feeding begins with rapid fluttering sucks that trigger the milk ejection reflex ('let down') and the start of the milk flow. Once flowing, feeding changes to slower, deeper, rhythmic sucks. Your baby may pause some-times. Other signs to look for are that you can hear your baby swallowing and that their cheeks stay rounded (not dipped or hollow) when sucking. (These all apply from once your milk has come in.)

✧ *Mum* – Breastfeeding is meant to be a comfortable experience without pain in the breast or nipple. In the early stages, some initial discomfort or pressure (for up to 30 seconds) when the baby latches can be normal, but this should ease over time. If you experience ongoing pain or discomfort, it is recommended that you seek breastfeeding support. After feeding you may feel calm and relaxed (sometimes even sleepy), and your breasts may become softer; however, this may not be the case in the early days as your milk is coming in. Your nipples may look longer and wet after feeding, but there should be no trauma, evidence of flattening on either side, pinching or a distinct change to colour, such as turning white. If you are unsure, take some pictures or videos and share them with your midwife or health visitor.

How can you have a successful start to breastfeeding?

1. **Ask for support** – I cannot stress this point enough, as I honestly believe it's probably one of the most important variables for how a mother's breastfeeding journey starts and, ultimately, how and if it continues. I couldn't have breastfed without asking for help. Breastfeeding support should be provided by the hospital team after birth, then can be followed up by your midwife and health visitor. In the community, support can be variable. If once you're home you find support is challenging to find or access, I'd recommend checking online or with your health visitor for local or national breastfeeding support services (see page 440) and cafes. Levels of training and qualifications in breastfeeding vary both within professions and among professionals. Please be aware that not all breastfeeding support is equal. The highest-qualified breastfeeding professional is an IBCLC –International Board Certified Lactation Consultant. They may be part of the

breastfeeding support teams in your local hospital or community, but more commonly they offer various private services. If you can afford to invest in support this may be your best option.

2. **Plenty of skin-to-skin** – Accept this as permission to lie in bed and just cuddle your baby as much as you'd like in those early days, weeks and months! Skin-to-skin is when your baby is naked except for a nappy and the mother is topless (no bra). If you are worried about your baby being cold you can cover their back with a blanket. Skin-to-skin has lots of benefits, including:

   o Transferring friendly bacteria to your baby, which helps to support their immune system.

   o Regulating their breathing, heart rate and temperature – a great way for babies to get used to their new world outside the womb.

   o Helping your body to release hormones, such as oxytocin (the 'happy' hormone), which boosts milk supply.

   o Helping you get to know your baby, including spotting the early signs that they are hungry.

3. **Learning about latch** – Before you start breastfeeding, it's easy to think latching a baby to a breast for a feed will be like joining two jigsaw puzzle pieces – breast goes into mouth, and voilà! The reality is that latching can be more complicated than it looks, and will be something you need to practise, adjust and re-practise. A deep latch is important for effective milk removal from the breast. A poor latch can lead to sore nipples, difficulty with milk removal and associated consequences such as challenges with establishing milk supply, poor weight gain and increased risk of complications like blocked ducts or mastitis.

4. **Offer both breasts with every feed** – Offer your baby both breasts at every feed. This will help ensure your baby receives as much milk as while stimulating both breasts regularly to help establish milk supply. Let your baby show when they're done with the first breast before offering the other one, or if initially

falling asleep at the breast after one side, rouse them and then move to the other breast.

5. **Responsively feed (often called feeding on demand)** – Initially, your newborn may not show feeding cues reliably and might need to be woken for feeds (including overnight or mid-feeds) to reach eight or more feeds a day. Over time, they will become more attuned to hunger and fullness signals and will instinctively respond to these. It's important that you observe and react to these cues. Follow your baby's lead, not a clock or schedule. (For more on responsive feeding, see page 61.)

Providing support for a breastfeeding partner

One of the biggest, but often unspoken, factors surrounding a positive start and journey with breastfeeding is the support from those around you. In my experience this comes in different forms and may also come from different people. Here are some ways to support a breastfeeding partner, friend or family member:

Practical

✦ Providing food and drink.

✦ Doing household activities and chores.

✦ Looking after the baby while your breastfeeding partner rests.

✦ Changing nappies.

✦ Bathing baby.

Emotional and validation

✦ Recognising times when feeding may feel difficult, and doing so without dismissal or immediately suggesting alternative routes.

✧ Acknowledging and supporting a breastfeeding partner's wishes or goals around feeding.

✧ Supporting emotional changes and challenges associated with feeding (and being a new parent!).

✧ Simply being there to listen and empathise without judgement.

✧ Celebrating milestones, big or small.

✧ Providing encouragement and support.

Advocacy

✧ Being aware of a breastfeeding partner's wishes around feeding and supporting their choices.

✧ Turning away or managing the number of visitors.

✧ Supporting breastfeeding outside the house.

✧ Booking or arranging breastfeeding support.

✧ Recognising hard days and times when the balance may shift around feeding, meaning difficult conversations about moving away from breastfeeding may need to be had.

✧ Taking an active role in understanding breastfeeding.

✧ Going to medical or feeding appointments, for mum and baby.

✧ Supporting your breastfeeding partner to make time for self-care.

SOS – Frequently asked questions or worries about breastfeeding

I'd love to promise you all that you won't experience any feeding hurdles or questions in the first few months of your baby's life, however, there is a reason why the 3am google becomes a widely recognised phenomenon within weeks of becoming a parent, and undoubtedly many of these queries are feeding-related. For most concerns, your first port of call should be advice from health professionals, but I've covered a few common queries or worries below.

How do I know my baby is getting enough milk?

This is an exceptionally common worry when breastfeeding, as awareness of volumes or quantities of milk are an unknown unless you're pumping and feeding your baby. Concern about milk supply is also one of the reasons many women discontinue or 'wobble' during their breastfeeding journey. For this reason, I have covered this in detail on page 66 in this chapter.

When should I seek more breastfeeding support?

There are so many reasons why you and your baby may benefit from individualised breastfeeding support, some of which I have outlined below. However, I really want to emphasise that you can and should seek support whenever you feel like you need it.

Reasons to seek support with breastfeeding

1. For reassurance and confidence, at any time, about any aspect of breastfeeding.
2. If your baby is not gaining weight as expected (see page 69).
3. If your baby does not have wet and dirty nappies as expected (see page 67).
4. Medical reasons, such as blood in stools or prolonged jaundice, once you have seen your GP, Midwife or HV.

5. If your baby isn't latching frequently or seems frustrated during feeds.
6. If your baby exhibits unusual feeding patterns, such as very short or excessively long feeds.
7. Breast-related issues such as engorgement, blocked ducts, milk blebs (a dot on your nipple) irritation or deep pain or discomfort.
8. If you notice signs of a potential infection, such as redness (or darker, purple or grey tones on darker skin), swelling or flu-like symptoms (which could indicate mastitis).
9. If you're experiencing pain and/or nipple damage when feeding.
10. If you'd like support with expressing and pumping.
11. If a health professional suggests or is treating you/your baby for thrush but feeding symptoms continue.
12. If you're experiencing anxiety, stress or depression if specific to feeding, otherwise first-line advice should be from your GP.
13. If you suspect a feeding challenge, such as a tongue-tie (see page 72).
14. If you want to discuss your feelings around feeding choices and experiences.
15. If you plan to return to work or transition to bottle feeding and need guidance.
16. If you suspect any of the scenarios below might apply to you and/or your baby.

I'm worried my baby has a food allergy and is reacting through my breast milk.

Food allergies in breastfed babies are often debated, but they are something I come across in practice, the most common being Cow's Milk Protein Allergy (CMPA). CMPA is much rarer in exclusively breastfed babies than those that are formula-fed, affecting around 0.5–1 per cent of babies. For these babies their immune system mistakenly sees tiny fragments of cow's milk protein, transferred through breast milk, and considers these (wrongly) a threat. I always remind breastfeeding mothers that exposure via breast milk is different – since mum digests the milk protein first, only small, broken-down fragments reach the baby. Most reactions are mild or moderate and delayed type reactions. Research shows that protein fragments from cow's milk, egg, soy and wheat can appear in breast milk, though the amounts vary between women. *You can find common allergy symptoms outlined on pages 118–19.*

If your baby is experiencing symptoms that you suspect to be food-allergy-related I would encourage you to:

✧ Complete a food-and-symptom diary.

✧ Explore support from a lactation professional or GP, as many symptoms that are commonly interpreted as food allergy can overlap with both normal breastfeeding behaviours, breastfeeding challenges or illness, including but not limited to:
  o Maternal milk oversupply.
  o Fast let down.
  o Shallow latch.
  o Transient lactose intolerance or lactose 'overload'.
  o Tongue-tie.
  o Gastrointestinal infection.
  o Newborn baby rash (sometimes called baby acne).

To diagnose a food allergy in a breastfed baby, the recommended approach is to eliminate the suspected allergen – such as cow's milk – from the mother's diet for around two to four weeks. This allows time to see if removing the allergen improves a baby's symptoms. After this elimination period, the allergen should be reintroduced into the mother's diet to see if the symptoms return. Although this reintroduction can be challenging, especially if the baby's symptoms have improved, it is a crucial step. It confirms whether the allergen is the cause of the symptoms or if the changes were due to other factors, preventing unnecessary long-term dietary restrictions for both mother and baby.

It is exceptionally important that breastfeeding parents are aware that you do not have to stop breastfeeding a baby with suspected food allergies. You should be supported to continue breastfeeding if you want to.

If you suspect a food allergy in your breastfed baby, I would first advise seeking guidance from a healthcare professional, such as a GP, paediatric dietitian or allergy doctor. They can provide the necessary support to ensure both you and your baby receive adequate nutrition while avoiding unnecessary dietary restrictions.

While we're talking about breastfeeding and food allergies, you might also find the following information helpful/interesting:

✧ Breastfeeding may have a protective effect against children developing allergies.

✧ There is no current evidence that suggests excluding certain foods from your diet while breastfeeding (or indeed when you're pregnant), such as milk or peanuts, will help prevent food allergy. You only need to avoid allergens if you're allergic to them yourself.

✧ There are some small studies that suggest a link between CMPA and babies who are supplemented with formula milk in the early days or weeks of life, then go on to establish exclusive breastfeeding. While formula supplementation can be necessary for certain situations, especially when there are concerns about weight gain or inadequate breast-milk supply, I find many parents are keen to be aware of information like this.

Will certain foods or supplements boost my milk supply?

Many foods and supplements claim to boost breast-milk supply, but little scientific evidence supports these claims. The key to maintaining a healthy milk supply is regular and effective milk removal from the breast and developing a responsive feeding relationship that establishes and maintains the supply-and-demand cycle necessary for milk production. Ensuring you're eating well and managing stress levels support this too.

Will certain foods I eat cause my baby to be windy?

I am often asked this question, and while anecdotally parents still report a link between 'windy food' (think beans, broccoli, cabbage) consumption while breastfeeding and a subsequent gassy baby, this is a little more difficult to explain with science. This is because breast milk is primarily made up of components from a mother's bloodstream, which means the foods she eats are broken down, i.e. 'processed', by her body before they enter her milk. Gut bacteria typically produce the gas we experience from certain foods when they ferment specific fibres in those foods. However, this process occurs directly in the mother's digestive system.

Is my breastfed baby constipated?

I warn you, there will be a fair amount of poo chat in this book! In the case of breastfed babies, constipation isn't a common phenomenon. The frequency of bowel movements in breastfed babies can change as they grow. In the early days, your baby may have several poos a day, especially as colostrum acts as a natural laxative. However, as the weeks and months go by, you might notice that your baby poos less often. It's normal for a breastfed baby to have bowel movements anywhere from several times a day to once every few days – each baby will be different (see pages 67–8 for more detailed information on your baby's poo!).

That said, infrequent bowel movements can sometimes signal an issue. Here are some signs to watch out for that may indicate a problem:

✧ They are uncomfortable and showing signs of abdominal discomfort or pain, such as drawing up their knees, atypical amounts or frequency of gas, or distension of their stomach. Having a poo relieves these symptoms.

✧ Their feeding significantly drops the longer they go without having a poo, then they appear very hungry again after passing a stool.

✧ When they poo there is a very large volume of it and it may be hard or dry.

✧ Other symptoms are present alongside, such as increased regurgitation, vomiting or skin changes.

The first thing to be sure of if you're worried it could be constipation is that your baby is getting enough milk. Checking in on their wet nappies and growth can be a good starting point for this. If you have any concerns, I'd encourage seeking guidance and support from an IBCLC or breastfeeding counsellor, and if needed your GP or health visitor, who will help rule out or explore any other potential contributing factors.

Help! My breastfed baby won't take a bottle.
If you're breastfeeding and want to introduce a bottle, unfortunately it may not be as simple as popping some expressed breast

milk into a bottle and your baby drinking it up. A bottle means many of your baby's normal feeding cues and expectations will be different. While some babies adapt easily to this, for others it can take a bit longer. Be reassured, bottle refusal can be very normal in breastfed babies.

Generally, it's recommended that breastfeeding is well established before offering a bottle, although for some babies it may have to be offered early on, for instance for medical reasons. If you'd like some individualised support with this or are struggling despite using the first-line advice below, I'd recommend speaking to an IBCLC.

Here are some top tips recommended for establishing a bottle with breastfed babies:

1. Stick with a newborn or slow-flow teat. Many parents tell me they find using a round teat with a wider base more helpful, but different teats can work for different babies. Don't get sucked into marketing, generally I'd recommend choosing a bottle and sticking with it, as swapping through them if initially unsuccessful can make the learning process more difficult for your baby.
2. When first introducing a bottle, try to do it when your baby is happy, relaxed, awake and alert – ideally, you want a balance between them not being too hungry but also not being too full, such as immediately after a breastfeed.
3. If you can, offer some expressed breast milk in a bottle initially, as this taste and smell will be familiar to your baby. You may want to dip the teat in the milk before offering and you can warm it if preferred.
4. When offering the bottle, reassure your baby with plenty of eye contact and soothing reassurance and hold them in a familiar position. (*Note: if you are struggling with this, some parents find a small adjustment to feeding positions, such as being more upright,*

or positioning for a paced bottle-feeding method can be helpful, see page 51.)

5. While any caregiver can try offering a bottle, your baby may benefit from consistency initially. Many mothers assume it would be better for another caregiver to initiate bottle feeding, which in some cases works, however, for other babies they associate feeding times with mum. Remember, every baby is different, and it is important to try to follow their cues and do what works for you and them.

6. Try to keep calm. I know this is easier said than done if you're keen for your baby to take a bottle, but becoming stressed or frustrated (which your baby may well be too when first offered a bottle) can make the whole experience unpleasant for them or create some negative associations with the bottle.

7. Encourage your baby to open their mouth wide for the bottle by gently rubbing the teat on their top lip and waiting.

8. Remember, practise and consistency are key. Your baby may not take to a bottle immediately, and it's a whole new skill to learn bottle feeding, but be patient.

How long can I store expressed breast milk?
A huge amount of effort goes into expressing breast milk, so safe and efficient storage is key. On the next page is a quickfire guide to safe storage, and don't forget to keep breast milk in a sterilised container or a bag and label it with the date it was expressed.

How do you warm stored breast milk?
You can warm breast milk to body temperature by putting the bottle in a jug or flask of warm water or holding it under running warm water. Please don't use a microwave to heat up or defrost breast milk.

Expressed breast milk	How and how long
Room temperature after expressing.	Use within four hours.
Stored in the fridge (avoid keeping in the door).	Keep for up to eight days ensuring fridge temperature is 4°C or less. If higher than 4°C use within three days.
In a cool bag with icepacks after being stored in the fridge.	Use within 24 hours.
Stored in the freezer.	Keep for up to six months, ensuring freezer is -18°C or colder.
Defrosted.	Once fully defrosted (ideally in the fridge), breast milk can be kept for 24 hours in the fridge. **Top tip – be sure to keep your frozen breast milk on 'stock rotation', using 'older' milk first where you can.**

A final note

For many families I speak to, their breastfeeding journey did not go as expected or planned, or it was associated with significant stress or emotional challenges. It's important to recognise that these experiences are completely valid and not uncommon. The pressures to succeed, meet personal or societal expectations can often make an already difficult journey feel even harder. If you're feeling uncertain, unhappy, frustrated or disappointed, know that it's ok to seek support and talk through your experience. A debrief, whether with a lactation consultant, healthcare provider or support group, can be helpful for many families. It's also ok to redefine your goals around feeding in a way that aligns with your unique circumstances and wellbeing.

Formula-Milk and Bottle Feeding

A significant percentage of babies in the UK are formula fed. Some parents choose to feed this way from birth, or after a certain period of time they combine bottle with breastfeeding, whereas other families may be unable to breastfeed or have to discontinue breastfeeding. Regardless of reasoning, let me first reassure you that formula milk can provide all the nutrition your growing baby needs. Interestingly, despite the majority of babies in the UK being formula fed at some point in their first year of life, many parents over the years have shared with me that information about formula milk or feeding can at times feel less accessible or supported. This shouldn't be the case, and supporting parental feeding choices and understanding the practicalities around this can help ensure a positive start with feeding overall. Over these next few pages, I'm going to cover:

✧ **Formula-milk nutrition 101**

✧ **Understanding other ingredients in formula milk**

✧ **How to prepare formula milk safely**

✧ **Making sense of different types of or 'special' formula milk**

✧ **How to bottle feed your baby**

✧ **How much formula milk does your baby need?**

✧ **Supplementation for formula-fed babies**

✧ **SOS – common questions about formula or bottle feeding**

Formula-milk nutrition 101

Formula milk provides all the nutrition your baby needs to support healthy growth and development. Breast milk is used as a blueprint for formula milk, which aims to replicate all the nutrition it provides. Nonetheless, because formula is artificially produced it does differ from breast milk; for instance, the composition of formula milk remains constant, whereas that of breast milk varies with each feed and day to day.

Formula ingredients and nutrient levels are strictly regulated in the UK and Europe to ensure safety and to meet high nutritional standards. Health authorities like the European Food Safety Authority (EFSA) oversee these guidelines, covering everything from permitted ingredients to required nutrient levels. Regulations are regularly updated, based on scientific research, to support the best outcomes for formula-fed babies. For instance, in 2014 the EFSA recommended reducing protein content in the formula to better match breast milk, following studies that linked high protein intake in infancy to rapid weight gain and increased risk of obesity later in life.

For many parents, reading the list of ingredients in formula milk can be a little confusing, so over the following few pages I'm going to outline what's in it and how this benefits your baby nutritionally.

Choosing a formula milk for your baby

I am often asked what the 'best' formula milk is, and before I say anything else, please know that cost or aesthetically pleasing packaging shouldn't add weight to your choice! What's in formula milk is so heavily regulated that whatever first infant (baby) formula you choose you can be reassured that it will be nutritionally complete, safe and suitable for your baby – assuming they do not have a specific medical condition that requires a specialist milk option. These tight rules for formula milk mean that even though different

brands may have minor ingredient differences, they won't significantly affect the overall nutrition. The other thing worth knowing
about formula milk is that a first infant formula (or stage-one milk)
is appropriate to continue past six months of age and will still
provide all the nutrition your baby needs while you start introducing your baby to solids.

Macronutrients in formula milk

Formula milk contains all the macronutrients, 'big' nutrients, that
your baby needs – carbohydrates, protein and fat. Together these
make up the energy content of formula milk, which is around
66–67 kcals in 100ml, and each nutrient has other vital roles in
your baby's development. Here's a bit more on each:

Nutrient	A bit more about it . . .	What does it do?
Carbohydrate	Formula milks may use one or a number of different carbohydrate sources, including (but not limited to): Lactose – this is the most common carbohydrate source in most first formula milk (like breast milk), and is the naturally occurring sugar present in cow's milk and other animal milks used for formula milk, such as goat. Maltodextrin – this is sometimes found in formula (often follow-on or specialist formula milks) and is a type of carbohydrate made from starch, typically derived from corn, rice, potato or wheat. Glucose syrup – this type of carbohydrate (sugar) can be found in some types of formula milk.	Carbohydrates provide a key energy source for your baby to support their rapid growth and development. Lactose can support calcium absorption and feed friendly gut bacteria.

Protein	The protein source in formula milk will depend on the type of formula it is. The majority of formula milks available are derived from cow's milk, meaning that cow's milk proteins will be used – including whey and casein.	Essential for your baby's growth and development.
		An energy source for your baby.
	Different formula milks may use different amounts of whey and casein, typically they replicate mature breast milk with 60 per cent whey and 40 per cent casein, however, different formula types may have different ratios; for example, 'hungry baby' formula contains more casein, with a ratio of 80 per cent casein to 20 per cent whey.	Supports the immune system and hormone production.
	The proteins in other formula milk types may be from other sources, such as goat's milk.	
Fat	Fats in formula milk are typically a blend of various oils and milk fats. This mixture is balanced to resemble the types and amounts of fats found in breast milk. Fats that may be used in formula milks include: • Rapeseed oil • Coconut oil • Sunflower oil • Soy oil • Palm oil (less so now) • Milk fats Since 2022, UK regulations have mandated the inclusion of specific types of fat in infant formula, particularly omega 3 essential fatty acids like DHA (docosahexaenoic acid), which are essential for brain and vision development. DHA in formula milk is typically provided either through fish oil or algae oil.	Significant energy source for your baby. Essential for supporting your baby's rapid brain development. It supports the development of visual acuity (vision development). Supports the development of your baby's immune system. Helps with absorption of fat-soluble vitamins.

Micronutrients in formula milk

Formula milk contains all the essential micronutrients – vitamins, minerals and trace elements – that your baby needs. These can be confusing on the ingredients label, as they will be listed as the scientific name. For example:

✧ Calcium carbonate = Calcium

✧ Ferrous sulphate = Iron

✧ Choline chloride = Choline

Understanding other ingredients in formula milk

Breast milk is rich in unique bioactive factors that promote positive health outcomes for babies, including supporting gut and immune health. Although attempts to replicate these benefits in infant formulas have been made, the intricate variety, volume and extensive effects of breast milk's bioactive components are impossible to replicate fully. However, some formula milk manufacturers have started incorporating ingredients that may provide similar benefits to a limited number of these bioactive factors. Their inclusion is not mandated by law, so they might not be present in all formulas. Many of these ingredients have lengthy and complex names, which can understandably confuse parents, so let me demystify some of these for you.

✧ **Galacto-oligosaccharides and fructo-oligosaccharides,** also known as GOS/FOS, are types of carbohydrates that are not easily digested, similar to fibre. They serve as prebiotics that feed beneficial bacteria in your baby's gut. Some studies, which include many funded by the formula industry, indicate that formula milk containing GOS and FOS can positively influence the growth of certain bacteria in a baby's gut and help them poo more regularly.

✧ **Probiotics** are friendly or 'good' gut bacteria, and the aim is to introduce these bacteria directly to your baby's gut to support their health. Preparation advice for these formula milks is different, usually recommending cooled, boiled water. The challenge is that in the UK it's recommended that formula milk is made at home with water that is at least 70°C. This is necessary to remove all harmful bacteria, especially while the baby's immune system is developing. However, it is also likely to stop the probiotics from working or kill them completely, thus reducing any potential benefits. Research into the potential benefits of probiotics added to formula milk is ongoing, as different types of bacteria and amounts may be needed to offer specific benefits.

✧ **Nucleotides** are tiny substances naturally present in breast milk, and as such have been synthetically produced and added to formula milk for over 60 years. They usually have a role in forming the building blocks for DNA and helping with gut health and infection prevention. The current science is pretty inconclusive about whether these offer any positive benefits in formula, but they are considered safe. You might see these on the formula milk tin on the ingredients, listed as big scientific words like 'Guanosine 5'-monophosphate'.

✧ **Milk oligosaccharides (types of carbohydrate/sugar)** are synthetic milk oligosaccharides like 2–FL, designed to mimic the human milk oligosaccharides (HMOs) found in breast milk and their benefits. These ingredients are still being researched, so the advantages are still unclear. Some companies may even market formulas with these components as being specifically for 'C-section babies'. While this type of marketing may make you feel like these formulas are essential, there is not enough evidence to support this claim, so there's no need to feel pressured to buy them.

✧ **Specific types of fat** used (or not) in formulas will be mentioned by many brands on their packaging. Here's some information about these so you can understand why they may be mentioned:

o *Whole milk fats* – Some formula brands now use whole milk fats, in place of alternative fats like oils. These fats can have a milk fat globule membrane (MFGM). This special casing surrounds the fat droplets and includes proteins, types of fat and other important compounds. While research on MFGM is still in the early stages, some studies (mainly funded by formula companies) suggest it might help support brain development and immune function.

o *SN2-Palmitate* – Without worrying too much about this name, this fat structure has been used in formula milk for over 30 years. It copies a prominent fat structure found in breast milk and has been shown to help fat and calcium absorption and may help babies have softer poo.

o *No palm oil* – Many manufacturers no longer include palm oil in their formula milk in favour of alternative fats. This is in part due to sustainability concerns, but also because studies have shown that palm oil can attach to calcium, forming something called 'calcium soaps'. These calcium soaps have been shown to decrease calcium absorption, which could impact a baby's bone development. Calcium soaps can also cause firmer and more-difficult-to-pass poo in babies, contributing to constipation.

How to prepare formula milk safely

Careful preparation of formula milk helps reduce the risk of illnesses such as infections caused by harmful bacteria that can sometimes contaminate powdered formula. This is important while your baby's immune system is still developing. There are clear recommendations for steps to make up a bottle of formula milk for babies:

1. **Wash your hands** – Start by thoroughly washing your hands for at least 20 seconds with soap and warm water.

2. **Prepare your area** – Clean the surface where you're preparing the bottles with hot, soapy water.

3. **Prepare your equipment** – Wash your bottles and teats in warm, soapy water, checking there is no damage to either part, then rinse everything well in clean, cold water afterwards. You can clean bottles and teats in the dishwasher, but be aware this will not sterilise them.

4. **Sterilise** – Sterilise your bottles and teats using your preferred method (boiling water, microwave, steriliser) and following the manufacturer's instructions clearly.

5. **Boil water** – Boil some fresh tap water, ideally at least 1 litre, and let it cool to around 70°C (leave in the kettle for a maximum of 30 minutes).

6. **Measure water** – Pour the cooled, boiled water into the sterilised bottle, checking the level carefully so it matches the instructions on the formula-milk packaging.

7. **Add formula** – Use the scoop provided with the formula to add the correct amount of powder to the water, first levelling off the powder in the scoop with the edge of a clean knife or flat surface.

8. **Mix** – Put the lid on the bottle and swirl or shake it well to dissolve the powder completely.

9. **Cool down** – Let the bottle cool to a safe temperature (body temperature is best) – you can do this by running the bottom of the bottle under a cold tap.

10. **Check temperature** – Test the milk temperature by dropping a little onto your wrist to make sure it's not too hot before feeding your baby.

11. **Use quickly** – Feed your baby immediately and discard any leftover milk after a feed. Ideally, make up feeds as your baby needs them to help reduce risk of infection.

Words of warning

✧ Always follow the manufacturer's instructions for making up formula milk. Do not be tempted to add more powder (concentrating the formula milk) or less powder (diluting the formula milk).

✧ Preparation machines for formula milk can be hugely convenient for many families, however, it's worth being aware that neither the World Health Organization nor the NHS currently recommend them. This is because they make formula milk differently by adding a hot-water shot first and then cold water. While there are no extensive scientific studies about this yet, the concern stems from some reports that have questioned whether the water reaches a hot-enough temperature to kill potentially harmful bacteria. Concerns about mould and bacteria build-up around filters have also been raised. If you choose to use one of these machines, please follow the manufacturer's guidelines around cleaning and maintenance.

Formula-milk affordability

One often-overlooked conversation about formula milk is affordability. The reality is that formula milk can be a significant expense for many families. If you're having any financial changes or concerns that impact your ability to afford formula, here are some important considerations:

✧ Please remember that all first formula milks are safe and appropriate for your baby. Consider choosing supermarket 'own-brand' options, which can often be cheaper than branded options and contain all the essential nutrients your baby needs.

✧ Please do not be tempted to dilute your baby's formula milk and add more water to their usual powder. This can impact your baby's growth, health and development.

✧ If you live in England, Wales or Northern Ireland and receive certain benefits you may be able to access the Healthy Start scheme and benefit from vouchers towards the purchase of formula milk. If you live in Scotland, you may be able to get help from Best Start Foods, which is a prepaid card that can be used in a similar way to vouchers. Ask your GP or health visitor for more information, or see page 442 for more details on the Healthy Start and Best Start Foods websites.

Making sense of different types of or 'special' formula milk

Walking down the formula aisle can feel a touch overwhelming, with so many options on offer making it hard to know what to choose. This decision can be even more challenging when you start comparing prices, health claims or feel the lure of terms like 'comfort', which will speak to many parents' concerns. Here I'm going to cover the range of different formula milks available in the UK.

Organic formula milk

Organic formula will only use ingredients derived from sources that have strict standards for farming and organic certification. They will often be more expensive. However, be reassured that you do not need to choose organic products for your child to be healthy, because nutritionally there is no significant difference to formula without organic certification, but if an organic product is an important consideration for your family, they are available.

Ready-to-feed formula milk

This is formula milk that is ready to feed from the bottle or, as the name suggests, 'pre-prepared' rather than needing to be made up with powder and water by you. It can be a convenient option for many parents, especially when on the go or on holiday, but it is more expensive than powdered formula. Generally, there are no significant nutritional differences between ready-to-feed and powdered formulas, so ultimately, it often comes down to personal preference, time available, convenience and affordability.

Goat's milk formula

This formula milk is made using goat's milk instead of cow's milk. Some sources suggest that goat's milk is easier to digest than cow's milk due to differences in the types of protein, however, there is limited robust scientific evidence for this claim, so whether you choose to use it comes down to your preference.

Goat's milk formula is not suitable for babies with Cow's Milk Protein Allergy (CMPA). This is because the proteins in goat's milk are very similar to those in cow's milk, meaning the immune system struggles to tell the difference and will react to goat's milk proteins too. This is known as cross-reaction.

Infant formula milk with specific claims

✧ Hungry-baby formula
✧ Comfort formula
✧ Anti-reflux ('stay-down') formula

The following milks are specialised infant formulas developed to target common challenges like colic, constipation and reflux. They are marketed as suitable from birth. They meet the same regulations as mentioned earlier, so they will provide all the nutrition your baby needs. Although these types of formula are available off the shelf, it's advisable to consult a medical professional before using them to discuss any feeding or health concerns, as a thorough assessment of issues like colic or reflux is important. In my experience, many parents swap through formulas to soothe unsettled babies, but these products aren't a guaranteed solution. Currently, there's no solid scientific evidence suggesting their benefits, although some parents do find they provide their baby with symptom relief. Of course, if they work for your baby and their symptoms, that's wonderful!

Hungry-baby formula
Often marketed for 'hungry babies', these formulas claim to 'delay weaning/starting solids'. Many parents also explore this option in the hope that it will help their baby sleep for longer or be more settled. These milks contain more casein than whey protein, meaning they take longer to digest, staying in the stomach longer. It's important to point out that there is no difference in calories (energy) between these formulas and standard infant formula. There is also no evidence to suggest that they benefit babies, delay starting solids, help them sleep or settle better. In my experience, hungry-baby formulas can also be associated with side effects such as discomfort and constipation.

Comfort formula
Comfort formula is typically marketed for babies with 'tummy or digestion troubles' such as colic or constipation. The cow's milk proteins in these formulas have usually been chopped

into smaller pieces, which is known as 'partially hydrolysed'. Some comfort formulas will also have lower levels of lactose, which is replaced with a different carbohydrate. Some may also contain a thickener. Many manufacturers will state that this formula milk is 'easier to digest' because of these protein types and lower levels of lactose, However, no solid scientific evidence suggests they more easily settle babies or benefit their digestion.

Note: These shouldn't be confused with specialist formula milk, which is **extensively** *hydrolysed and prescribed for babies with Cow's Milk Protein Allergy.*

Anti-reflux formula

Anti-reflux formulas are typically marketed for babies with regurgitation or reflux symptoms. These formulas tend to contain a thickener such as different starches (potato, rice) or gums like carob or locust-bean gum. A health professional should advise giving your baby these – ideally after working through other reflux-management strategies first. These formula milks are often recommended to be made using water at lower temperatures to stop it from going lumpy, and it's essential to take extra care with this because of the risk that lower water temperatures will not kill harmful bacteria in powdered formula (see pages 42–3). If you're considering anti-reflux formulas, it is recommended you do not combine them with medications such as Gaviscon or feed thickeners. You may also have to increase the teat size on your baby's bottle.

Specialised medical formula milk

✧ Lactose-free formula milk
✧ Formula milk for babies with Cow's Milk Protein Allergy
✧ Other formulas for medical reasons

The following types of formula milk are those used for medical purposes and should be prescribed by a GP or health professional.

Lactose-free formula milk

This formula milk has the milk sugar – lactose – completely removed. It is used for babies with suspected or diagnosed lactose intolerance. Lactose intolerance occurs when there isn't enough of the enzyme lactase (which acts like a pair of mini scissors) in the gut to digest lactose properly.

The most common reason for lactose intolerance in babies is what's known as secondary lactose intolerance. This usually happens after a tummy bug, where a baby experiences diarrhoea and vomiting, leading to a temporary reduction or loss of the lactase enzyme from the gut. Symptoms can clearly indicate this enzyme is missing or in short supply, as lots of undigested lactose reaching the gut will cause frequent diarrhoea, flatulence and gripey tummy pain. Most babies will only need a lactose-free formula for a number of weeks while the lactase enzyme builds back up again. After this, babies can return to their regular formula milk. A health professional should be able to diagnose lactose intolerance and provide support management.

Lactose-free formula milk is unsuitable for babies with a Cow's Milk Protein Allergy because only the milk sugar has been removed, and an allergy to cow's milk is to the protein, not the sugar, found in milk.

Formula milk for babies with Cow's Milk Protein Allergy

Babies who have a suspected or confirmed diagnosis of Cow's Milk Protein Allergy (CMPA) need specialist formula milk where the cow's milk protein (which is what they are allergic to) has been broken down to a small-enough size that their immune system no longer recognises it and therefore they do not react to it. A doctor or dietitian may recommend or prescribe any of these three types of specialist formulas.

Extensively hydrolysed formula milk – Most babies with a diagnosed or suspected CMPA will be started on extensively hydrolysed (very well-broken-down) formula milk. This is where the milk proteins have been broken down from long, tangled-like structures to much smaller pieces, the size of which are set by specific guidelines. Some of these formulas may still contain lactose, but others will have it removed.

Hydrolysed rice-protein formula milk – This formula uses a broken-down rice protein and contains no cow's milk protein.

Amino-acid formula milk – A small number of babies with CMPA may require amino-acid formula milk. Typically, these babies continue to experience symptoms while on extensively hydrolysed formula or have a history of more severe allergic reactions to cow's milk. In these formulas, the protein is entirely broken down into amino acids – the building blocks of protein.

These types of formula milk tend to have a distinct bitter or sour taste, very different to the sweet taste of standard formula milk. In my experience, while young babies (under four months) usually tolerate this taste change without concern, older babies may take some time to adjust to the flavour. Short-term strategies, like titrating with their current formula milk or adding a small amount of high-quality vanilla extract, can make the milk more appealing for babies. Interestingly, some small studies have shown that having these broken-down formulas can support increased acceptance of bitter (such as green) vegetables later in childhood.

It should be noted that these milks can also be a little thinner, which may exacerbate regurgitation or reflux symptoms for some babies. If this is a concern for you, please discuss this with a medical professional.

Important: not all specialist formula milks for CMPA are Halal or Kosher, because animal enzymes can be used to help break down the proteins. Please discuss this with your prescribing doctor to ensure an appropriate formula is offered to your baby.

Other formulas for medical reasons

Certain babies may need prescribed formula milks for various health-related reasons. This includes specialised formulas for premature babies, containing extra energy, protein and essential vitamins and minerals. Additionally, there are higher-energy formulas for babies who are having difficulty gaining weight or have increased energy requirements due to medical issues. A medical professional will recommend and prescribe these options.

How to bottle feed your baby

This might seem a little obvious, but in my experience it's often a topic missed out when discussing bottle feeding. To support your baby to have some agency over their milk feeds (similar to if they were breastfed), including how much they drink and to help prevent overfeeding, a paced bottle-feeding approach is often recommended. This, as the name suggests, is a method that helps control the speed of milk intake. The positioning of the bottle and your baby, which I've described below, means the flow of milk is delivered steadily across a feed and creates opportunities for supportive pauses for your baby, should they need them.

1. **Both you and your baby need to get into a comfortable position** – Try to sit on a well-supported chair, and hold your baby securely during feeding. Hold your baby close, but rather than lying them flat or reclining them too much, aim to hold them in a semi-upright position.
2. **Encourage your baby to open their mouth for the bottle** – (think of it as like 'asking permission' for your baby to feed). You can do this by gently rubbing or brushing the teat on your baby's top lip and waiting for their mouth to open wide.

3. **Position the bottle** – Place the teat into your baby's mouth, aiming for it to be in a horizontal position with a slight tilt, rather than vertical and facing downwards. The teat will not be full. This positioning allows the milk to flow more steadily. Selecting a slow-flow or newborn teat will also prevent your baby feeding too much too quickly.

4. **Pay attention to your baby** – Their body and behaviour will give you signs that they need a break or are finished. These could include gulping, hand and/or toe splaying, turning away from the bottle, becoming upset, dribbling milk from the side of their mouth or simply stopping sucking. If or when they pause, it is because they need to. Avoid jiggling or tapping the teat to get them sucking again. Never make your baby finish the bottle.

How much formula milk does your baby need?

This is a common concern for parents, which understandably stems from the desire to ensure their baby is well fed and happy. One challenge with bottle feeding is that babies can easily consume more milk than they need. Factors such as bottle and teat design, milk flow, feeding positions and guidance from professionals, other parents or formula labels can lead parents to believe their baby 'should' drink a certain amount per bottle, making them intent on getting their baby to hit that target. For this reason, I often see parents spending considerable time getting their baby to finish the last ounce of milk – twisting or tapping the bottle, changing positions and so on.

I encourage parents to view recommendations on formula tins or the milk guide below as a *guide*, not a milk 'prescription'. Your baby is the best indicator of how often they need to feed and how much they want to drink. I've detailed how to follow your baby's lead with a responsive-feeding approach later in this chapter.

To emphasise this point, I want to highlight the variability in milk needs among babies of the same age. For instance, not all six-week- or six-month-olds require the same amount of milk, as each child's requirements are different – here's an example:

Age	Example formula tin recommendations	Estimated feed volumes for baby girl growing healthily along the 2nd centile	Estimated feed volumes for baby boy growing healthily along the 91st centile
6 weeks	5 x 150ml	5 x 105ml feeds/ 6 x 90ml feeds/ 8 x 65ml feeds	5 x 170ml feeds/ 6 x 140ml feeds /8 x 105ml feeds
6 months	5 x 210ml	5 x 135ml feeds	5 x 220ml feeds

Guideline amounts of milk for different ages

Age	How many feeds per day	Total
0–2 weeks	6–10	420–560ml
2–8 weeks	6–8	450–735ml
2–3 months	5–6	525–1080ml
3–5 months	5–6	900–1050ml
Around 6 months	5–6	840–960ml
7–9 months	4	Around 500ml
10–12 months	3–4	Around 400ml

Adapted from First Steps Nutrition

Remember, one of the best ways to be sure your baby is getting enough milk is to monitor their weight gain, along-side what's coming out the other end with the two 'Ps' – pee and poo (see page 67). These can be easy visual cues and reassurance that your baby is getting what they need.

Should I use a tracking app for feeds?

Nowadays there is lots of technology available to parents that allows you track and monitor everything from sleep to feeds. I'm often asked if these are beneficial, and my response is always 'it depends'. Some parents find tracking feeds, or feed volumes, initially helpful and reassuring. My word of warning, however, is that they can be time-consuming in their own right and cause some parents anxiety about feeding changes that are incredibly normal for babies, such as accepting less volume than the day before or at their last feed, or changes in usual feed times. If you use these, I would always urge you to remember your baby will have changeable needs and feeding routines. They are little humans, not little robots. If you find tracking apps move you away from helpful feeding practices like responsive feeding, or drive anxiety over timings and volumes, then perhaps approach them with caution.

Supplementation for formula-fed babies

Formula milk contains all the vitamins and minerals a baby needs. Therefore, if your baby is drinking more than 500ml per day, they will not usually need any extra supplementation. When drinking less than 500ml per day, a combined supplement of vitamins A, C and D is recommended.

Combination feeding (or mixed feeding)

This method of feeding, which involves a mix of breast-feeding or expressed breast milk and/or formula, has gained popularity among parents and caregivers in recent years. This is likely due to various factors, such as personal feeding preferences, the increased ability for parents and caregivers to share parental leave and caregiving duties, and work arrangements. Additionally, some parents may opt for combination feeding if they encounter difficulties with exclusive breastfeeding but still wish to provide their baby with some breast milk. In some instances, parents might need to combination feed for medical reasons.

SOS – common questions about formula or bottle feeding

Can I still bond with my baby if I'm bottle feeding?

Absolutely yes, you can! I hear from so many parents who worry that bottle feeding will interfere with connecting and bonding with their baby, but supporting a strong emotional bond is very possible when bottle feeding. Many of the suggestions below will come naturally to you as a new parent, but here are my suggestions:

✧ Skin to skin – hold your baby close and use skin-to-skin during feeding (either parent!). This has additional benefits for your baby, like helping to regulate breathing and transferring good bacteria from your skin to theirs.

✧ Give your baby plenty of eye contact during feeding.

✧ Use your body language and voice to reassure and connect with your baby, offering lots of smiles, gently talking to them or singing.

✧ Pay attention to your baby when feeding them, looking for signs they may need to pause or are full. This is called responsive feeding, which I discuss in more detail on page 61.

Can I use bottled water to make up formula?

Whilst it may feel like using bottled water can be a convenient way to make up formula milk, it is not recommended. Bottled water is not sterile, and it can contain high levels of sodium (salt) or certain minerals.

Can formula milk be reheated?

Formula milk that your baby has started to drink from should never be reheated. Do not warm formula milk in the microwave as this can cause hot spots which could burn your baby's mouth.

Is my baby's formula milk making them constipated?

Constipation can be more common in formula-fed babies than in breastfed babies. Constipation describes when your baby is pooing less often, and is passing harder or dry stools, which may be large or pellet-like, with possible straining and pain. You can read more about the symptoms of constipation on pages 382–3. Causes or contributors to constipation in formula-fed babies can include:

Possible cause	What you can do
Transitioning your baby from breast milk to formula milk, as breast milk is easier to digest.	Usually, the change to your baby's poo habits will settle down as their gut adapts to digestion of formula milk. In the meantime, try the general tips on the next page. If you're able to (it won't be the case for all families), gradually transition from breast to formula milk.
Incorrectly made formula milk, that is too concentrated (where more powder is added than recommended for the amount of water).	Check you are following the manufacturer's instructions for making up formula milk. Ensure scoops of powdered formula are levelled off, not heaped. Do not be tempted to dilute formula milk.
Dehydration, which can occur if your baby isn't having enough milk or during times when they may need additional fluids, such as warm weather or during illness.	Check that your baby is having regular wet nappies, and showing signs they are drinking enough milk. Offer additional milk feeds as needed or follow advice for offering water on page 129.
Formula milks that contain palm oil may cause calcium to bind with palmitic acid in the gut, forming calcium 'soaps' that can contribute to firmer stools.	Switch to a formula milk that doesn't contain palm oil. You will find the ingredients listed on the tin.
A possible allergy to cow's milk protein, which is much less common but can occur in up to 2–7 per cent of babies. Usually constipation will not be a 'stand-alone' allergy symptom, and occur alongside other symptoms (you can read more on page 382).	Seek medical advice from your GP if you suspect Cow's Milk Protein Allergy. You can read more about this on page 365.

General tips to manage constipation

✧ Bicycle legs – lay your baby down and gently move their legs, like they are riding a bike.

✧ Gentle tummy massage, or a baby massage sequence for their tummy can be helpful for some babies.

✧ A warm bath can get things moving for some babies.

If your baby's constipation is not improving, please seek support from your GP who may wish to rule out any underlying medical causes, or consider prescribing medication to help your baby poo.

Is there a formula milk suitable for vegan families?

Unfortunately, in the UK at present there are no suitable formula milks for vegan families. Some formula milks made from plant-based ingredients such as rice do exist, however, these may still contain animal-derived ingredients such as vitamin D from sheep's wool (lanolin) or ingredients cultured in milk-derived ingredients.

Can I make up my baby's formula feeds in advance?

It's recommended, wherever possible, that you make up your baby's feeds one at a time, as they need them. This helps reduce the risk of infection. Of course, there are times when you need to take feeds out of the house with you. If possible, bring pre-measured formula powder and a thermos of freshly boiled hot water, along with a sterilised empty bottle, to prepare formula when you're out and about. If you cannot follow this advice, you can make up a feed at home, cool it quickly under a running cold tap, or in a bowl/jug of cold water and place it in the fridge for at least one hour before you leave. When you are out it should be carried in a cool bag with an icepack. Use this milk within four hours, and within two hours if you cannot keep it cold.

As a general rule, made-up formula needs to be used within:

✧ 24 hours, when kept in a fridge.

✧ 4 hours, when kept in a cool bag with an icepack.

✧ 2 hours, when stored at room temperature.

My baby is refusing to feed, I'm worried my baby has a bottle aversion?

Aversion is a word that doesn't feel particularly pleasant to hear as a parent, isn't it? It's used in the milk and food world to describe a significant dislike of feeding, and in this case, with a bottle. Babies who have a bottle aversion may be letting us know by:

✧ Repeatedly refusing their usual bottle feeds.

✧ Clamping their mouth shut when offered the bottle.

✧ Rejecting or refusing the bottle after a very small amount of milk (despite being hungry).

✧ Showing distress around the bottle being offered or when getting into their usual feeding position.

Sometimes it can be a short-lived episode due to changes in routine, bottles, teats, milk or during illness, but if this occurs repeatedly and is not just a one-off 'phase', it can be hugely distressing for parents and babies alike. The anxiety of a small baby not feeding is understandably huge for parents and caregivers.

While bottle aversion can occur at any time in the first year of a baby's life, in my experience it commonly happens around four months of age onwards. This is because at around this time babies develop more volition (or 'control') around their acceptance of milk feeds, rather than feeding just being reflexive (something they innately 'do'). In practice, I find bottle aversion to be much more common in groups of babies who may have had a tricky start to their feeding journey, such as those with reflux, repeated vomiting, food allergies, being born prematurely, with a complex medical history or with a history of medical interventions around their mouth and face, such as tube feeding or ventilation.

If you are concerned that your baby has a bottle aversion, some initial suggestions would include:

1. Make sure you address any medical concerns that may be affecting feeding – anything from constipation to reflux, or developmental differences, can impact a baby's feeding experience.
2. Try to go into feeds as calmly as possible. This is definitely easier said than done (it's almost impossible to relax when someone tells you that you need to!), but your baby is well attuned to their parents, and can quickly pick up on your stress and anxiety. In turn this can exacerbate their distress and refusal. You may even wish to enlist the help of other familiar adults to support feeding if you need some time out.
3. Create a positive feeding environment. If your baby is getting upset as soon as you approach their usual feeding locations or position, try making a change, such as to where you usually sit, how you hold your baby, or the feeding environment. For example, play some relaxing music or have some flashcards or sensory toys out for your baby to look at.
4. If you've been cycling through milks, teats or bottles, try to offer consistency to allow you baby time to get used to these. It's easy to get buying-happy in the hope of a quick fix and in

desperation, but it can make feeding a challenge for your baby who has to keep adapting to these changes.

If your baby is repeatedly refusing a bottle and this is affecting their milk volumes to the extent that their growth or hydration levels are affected, seek support via your GP or a qualified health professional, such as a feeding and swallowing specialist speech therapist (SLT).

Getting to grips with breast and bottle feeding

Regardless of your method of milk feeding, there will be parts of the process that are relevant to all babies and parents. Across the next few pages, I'm going to cover:

✧ **Responsive feeding**

✧ **How can you tell when your baby is hungry and full?**

✧ **How do you know your baby is getting enough milk?**

✧ **SOS – frequently asked questions about milk feeding**

Responsive feeding

As a dietitian with years of experience supporting new parents, I clearly remember that feeling of 'how will I know when to feed her or what she needs?' The responsibility of nourishing a tiny human who cannot express their hunger verbally, combined with advice like 'just feed her on demand', can make new parents feel exceptionally vulnerable. You may also be overwhelmed by messages from various sources recommending the number of feeds or feed volumes for your baby at different ages and stages. This advice can also come from sources like formula packaging or health professionals who might 'prescribe' feeding schedules. These sources often imply that babies must adhere to specific feeding routines, which isn't the recommendation for how to feed healthy babies. Instead, regardless of whether you are breast- or bottle feeding, it's highly encouraged that parents and caregivers **responsively feed** their baby, which is sometimes called feeding on demand.

Before I explain more about responsive feeding, I want to set the scene for appetite regulation in babies and young children. Most healthy babies are born with an almost-perfect inbuilt appetite-control mechanism. They respond directly to their body's feelings of hunger and fullness (controlled by hormones), signalling for feeds when hungry and stopping when full. Appetite regulation begins at birth but becomes more effective as a baby learns to signal hunger and satiety (fullness). This is why initially sleepy newborns may need rousing for some feeds but within weeks have developed good regulation, responding to their internal body signals (cues). This continues throughout early life, with young children being led by their body and appetite signals, not external factors. Recognising this about healthy babies (and young children) lays the foundation for responsive feeding.

Put simply, responsive feeding is an attentive way of feeding your baby that focuses on feeding them when they show signs of hunger and stopping when they are full. It emphasises establishing trust in your baby to determine when, how often and how much they want to feed/eat, rather than using an app, the clock or advice from countless feeding forums about what your baby should be doing at this age.

Babies will also signal for comfort and connection; in the case of breastfed babies, this will also involve feeding. Responsive feeding works both ways for breastfed babies, as breastfeeding mothers are encouraged to listen to their own bodies' cues and desire to feed their babies, such as full breasts when mum needs to feed for her own comfort.

I find breaking responsive feeding down into roles and responsibilities helps with understanding this concept further. The example below is relevant to babies up to six months old, but responsive feeding is encouraged throughout childhood and is part of a broader parenting approach called responsive parenting.

Preparation – You're prepared to feed your baby when they express signs of hunger.

Baby signals – Look out for and respond to your baby's signals. They will use age-appropriate ways to communicate with you, such as facial expressions, movement and vocalisation to signal they are hungry (and when they are full).

Caregiver responsibility – To respond to your baby's signals, feeding when hungry and stopping when they show signs that they are full.

Your child's learning – Your baby will begin to understand that you will proactively respond and meet their needs, which builds felt safety and security.

Responsive feeding is an incredibly positive parenting skill in your arsenal, and one that is widely recognised to help promote healthy eating habits, positive feeding and mealtime relationships and support a child's physical, social and emotional development.

Now for a bit of honesty. As a new parent, it would be completely understandable if you feel slightly intimidated at the thought that you'll be at the mercy of your baby's metaphorical 'food, comfort and connection bell', which could go off as many times as it wants and at any time, day or night. Rest assured, over time you'll likely find a general rhythm with milk feeds, but leaning into and, as best as possible, embracing that the ideal feeding routine is one led by your baby will, I hope, help you feel empowered as a parent.

While in the throes of honesty, one of the biggest challenges with this approach to feeding is that it can clash with many of the strong opinions, messages and attitudes about feeding babies that have become prevalent over the years. These messages could come from grandparents, social media, apps, forums, other parents or even professionals. You will undoubtedly hear advice about rigid feeding schedules or how babies won't or shouldn't need feeds at night at a certain age, which can feel overwhelming and is often harmfully incorrect. Trust your instincts and your baby, and be wary of advice suggesting babies should follow specific rules and routines around feeding*.

For a small group of babies, a health professional may advise feeding plans and schedules, for example, if there is a concern about weight gain, or for certain medical conditions.

Benefits of responsive feeding

Baby's physical development
- Helps establish long-term positive feeding and eating behaviours.
- Supports healthy weight gain and growth.

Baby's emotional development
- Helps your child feel safe and secure in your care.
- Supports emotional regulation, promoting soothing and regulating behaviours and helps reduce stress.
- Encourages emotional resilience as your baby learns that their needs will be met consistently.

Parental benefits
- Promotes your confidence by encouraging responsive-ness and trust in your instincts.
- For breastfed infants – helps optimise mother's milk supply.
- Supports an understanding of your baby's cues and communication.
- Supporting bonding and emotional attachment, strengthening your parent–child relationship.

How can you tell when your baby is hungry and full?

This is the million-pound question, and parenting would undoubtedly feel much more straightforward if your baby could just tell you when they are hungry or full! Instead, I encourage you to focus on paying attention to your baby, as certain behaviours or cues ('signals') will communicate this to you instead. Grasping these cues may require some time, especially as they evolve with your baby's growth and development. However, understanding them enables you to quickly meet your baby's needs.

Remember, babies don't follow clocks or volume recommendations; they follow their bodies.

Signs your baby is hungry

Crying is often shared as the main 'sign' that a baby is hungry, and while crying indeed can be an indication that your baby wants to feed, it's one of the last communication signals they'll send us. At this stage, they have gone past being hungry and are getting towards being over-hungry, which can make feeding time more difficult – something we want to try to avoid as much as possible!

Here are the stages of signals/cues that tell you your baby is hungry.

Early signs, aka *I'm getting hungry, feed me, please*
✧ Stirring.
✧ Turning their head – seeking/rooting.
✧ Opening their mouth.

Progressing signs, aka *I'm starting to get really hungry, feed me, please*
✧ Bringing hand or fist to mouth, sucking on fist or hand.
✧ Sticking tongue out of mouth.
✧ Stretching.
✧ Increasing movements and restlessness, such as kicking and grunting.

65

Late signs, aka *I'm very hungry and need calming before you feed me*
✧ Crying.
✧ Scrunching facial expression.
✧ Tight fists.
✧ Agitated body movements, tensed body.

Signs your baby is full
✧ Slowed pace of feeding – sucking slows down and/or baby takes more regular pauses or stops feeding.
✧ Coming off and/or turning away the breast or bottle.
✧ Keeping their mouth closed, not opening or reopening to latch onto breast or bottle.
✧ Your baby is settled and relaxed – any body tension or clenched fists will have settled. Some babies will fall asleep.*
✧ Loss of interest in feeding.
✧ In older babies, pushing away the breast or bottle.

If your baby is a newborn, they may initially need waking to continue feeds. If your baby appears to be fatiguing regularly during feeds, and there are any concerns about milk supply if breastfeeding, growth or frequency of wet or dirty nappies, please seek feeding support.

How do you know your baby is getting enough milk?
Worries about whether your baby is getting the milk they need can be a common concern for new parents, regardless of whether they are breast and/or formula fed. For breastfeeding mothers, doubting breast-milk supply is one of the most common reasons for discontinuing breastfeeding, so I find that having the information to reassure that your baby is getting enough milk is hugely important.

Your baby's growth and what's coming out the other end are two of the best ways to get peace of mind around their milk volumes.

Your baby's wet and dirty nappies aka the two Ps: pee and poo
One of the best ways to check in on milk intake is by monitoring wet and dirty nappies. This is a useful way to monitor feeding progress, and your midwife or health visitor will routinely ask about it. Wet and dirty nappies will change in the early days and weeks, so here's what to expect with the two Ps, depending on your feeding method.

Breastfed babies

Your baby's age	Pee – Wet nappies in 24 hours	Poo – Dirty nappies in 24 hours
1–2 days old	1–2 or more.	One or more black or dark green 'tar-like' poo. This is known as meconium.
3–4 days old	3–4 or more – notably heavier nappies than first two days.	At least two or more which are changing in colour and texture, such as brown/green/yellow, looser consistency. Should be at least the size of a £2 coin.
5–6 days old	Five or more heavy nappies.	At least two or more, yellow stools may be loose/runny and larger than a £2 coin.
7+ days old	Six or more heavy nappies.	At least two or more yellow stools, may be loose/runny, at least £2 coin size.

Adapted from UNICEF Baby Friendly Initiative

I also want to pause a little more on poo here. Many parents are surprised or worried about breastfed baby poo. Here are some things you need to know for reassurance:

✧ It's very common and normal for breastfed baby poo to be quite loose or runny in consistency. Many parents worry this is diarrhoea, as for adults comparatively it might seem that way, but wet, loose poo is completely to be expected.

✧ It's common to see small grains or 'seeds' in breastfed baby poo. These are normal and are undigested milk fats.

✧ While poo is generally a mustard yellow colour, other colours can make an appearance such as green poo. The odd rogue colour can be normal, but if you want to understand more I talk more about poo at the back of this book.

✧ It's common for the frequency of poos in breastfed babies to change and reduce over time, and fewer poos after six weeks of age can be normal for some babies.

Formula-fed babies

Your baby's age	Pee – Wet nappies in 24 hours	Poo – Dirty nappies in 24 hours
1–2 days old	Your baby will have at least six wet nappies after the first day or so.	One or more black or dark green 'tar-like' poo. This is known as meconium.
After the first week	At least six wet nappies per day. These should be soaked through with clear or pale yellow wee.	After the first week your baby should pass pale yellow or yellow-brown stools. Ideally your baby is passing poo at least once per day.

Adapted from UNICEF: A guide to infant formula for parents who are bottle feeding

A note on poo for formula-fed babies:

It is common for babies who are formula fed to poo less than breastfed babies. Poos tend to be darker, firmer and smellier than breastfed baby poo. They can be a yellow, brown or even at times a dark green colour. How often they poo may change in the early weeks and months.

Weight gain and growth

Your baby's weight and growth give a good indication of how milk feeding is going, but I think it's important to share what to expect with growth in the first few weeks and months. Here are some key points:

✧ While your baby's weight will be monitored during their first two weeks of life, it's helpful to know that it is normal for babies to lose some weight in the first two weeks after birth, often due to fluid changes in their bodies and adaptation to the outside world, especially in breastfed babies. Hearing their baby has lost weight can send many parents into a pattern of worry and add pressure to feeding, but remember it is expected. You'll even notice a gap on most growth charts between zero and two weeks because weight loss is expected, and a baby's weight during this time doesn't reflect the centile (growth) line they'll continue to plot.

✧ Most babies will have regained their birth weight by three weeks of age. If your baby has lost over 10 per cent of their body weight or has not regained their birth weight by three weeks of age, you should be offered a feeding assessment and breastfeeding support. This will usually be from a midwife, health visitor or dedicated infant feeding team. A weight loss of 8 per cent or more by day five may also be an indication of a need for more support, if it can be accessed. It's easy to worry at this stage and feel like you're doing something wrong, but it doesn't mean you're a failure. I see this often.

✧ Support providers should help ensure your baby is feeding effectively, in particular if you are breastfeeding, in which case they should also consider your history, including anything that's impacted your milk production, such as birth history and/or medication. A feeding plan should be agreed upon with you and your support team, and depending on your individual circumstances, advice may also be given about expressing, cup feeds or temporary use of formula milk (which should always be accompanied with a plan for expressing if you want to continue to breastfeed). This will continue to be monitored.

✧ If your baby has lost more than 12.5 per cent of their body weight, a review by a paediatrician is recommended for your baby. Again, this can feel intimidating for many parents, but it's a safeguard to rule out any other medical reasons affecting your baby's feeding or growth.

✧ A baby typically gains weight steadily throughout the first few months, averaging around 150–200g weekly. Please remember this is just an average, and every baby is different. They should be weighed once per month until six months of age unless a health professional has recommended more frequent weighing. Their growth should be plotted along centile lines on a growth chart. You can understand more about growth in Chapter 5.

SOS – Frequently asked questions about milk feeding

Whether breastfeeding or bottle feeding, there are some questions that are relevant to both methods of milk feeding and that I hear often.

The weather is warm, does my baby (under six months) need extra fluids?

While we are never guaranteed hot summer months in the UK, we can all hope! You might also be heading away on holiday to warmer climates with your baby, and with either scenario, parents are always keen to know how to ensure their baby remains well hydrated. So, here's a quick reference guide, depending on how your baby is fed.

Exclusive breastfeeding	Continue to offer the breast regularly and responsively breastfeed. Your baby will likely feed more often and/or for longer during the day and night. Breast milk is 88 per cent water and will also adapt to the warmer weather with changes to water content. Breast milk remains the only source of hydration that your baby needs at this age (0–6 months) and water does not need to be given. Make sure you stay well hydrated yourself, and if you get sticky during feeding, put a muslin between you and your baby.
Exclusive pumping	Continue responsively feeding your baby breast milk, offering more frequently if available – you can supplement with stored milk if necessary. If you're concerned about your baby's hydration and breast milk is not available, you can offer small amounts of cooled, boiled water in a sterilised bottle after feeds. Again, make sure you stay well hydrated yourself. Ensure quick and proactive breast-milk storage in the fridge or freezer once pumped during warmer weather. We've all seen what happens to warm milk.
Combination feeding	Continue responsively feeding your baby, offering the breast more often than is typical for you, and continuing formula feeds as usual across the day and night. Water does not need to be given.
Exclusive formula feeding	Continue responsively feeding your baby formula milk. Cooled, boiled water can be offered in small amounts after feeds if necessary.

Help, I think my baby has a tongue-tie.

Tongue-tie diagnoses have surged in recent years, making it a hot topic in parenting discussions and forums. A tongue-tie is where the fold of skin (lingual frenulum) connecting the tongue to the bottom of the mouth is shorter or tighter than usual, which can make feeding more difficult.

Symptoms of tongue-tie can include those I've detailed below, but it's important to point out that many of these symptoms can happen for reasons other than tongue-tie too.

✧ Difficulty latching or maintaining a latch when breastfeeding.

✧ Difficulty maintaining a seal on the bottle teat – your baby may lose milk from the sides of their mouth.

✧ Clicking noise or lip-smacking during feeding.

✧ Challenges with feed times – short, frequent feeds may occur and/or prolonged feeding times (often accompanied by frustration or fatigue) if repeatedly re-latching to a breast or bottle.

✧ Poor weight gain due to challenges with breast and/or bottle feeding.

✧ Gassy and/or windy due to excess air being swallowed during feeding.

A tongue-tie can be assessed and diagnosed by several healthcare professionals, however, it's essential to be aware that specific training is required to assess and manage it.

A frenotomy may be recommended if your baby has a tongue-tie diagnosis. This is a short procedure where the lingual frenulum is released by scissors or laser (rarer), generally without a general anaesthetic, in babies under six months.

Tongue-tie diagnosis and decisions to treat it should be based on both the anatomy alongside a functional feeding assessment and mum's presentation. Before division, interventions should always include breastfeeding support, if feeding this way. If after support issues persist, a frenectomy can be considered. While this is generally considered a low-risk procedure, there are, of course, associated risks such as infection and reattachment.

How often and how should I wind or burp my baby?

Winding or burping is a common query for parents when first feeding their baby. As a society, we seem to love a discussion about wind (either end) with our babies! So here are some key points about winding or burping babies.

Firstly, why do it in the first place? Ultimately, this comes down to how babies feed. Some babies will swallow lots of air during feeding. Winding or burping can help a baby bring up some of that air, which may cause pain or discomfort if it stays trapped or builds up in the stomach. To begin with it's recommended that you wind your baby after every feed, especially if you're bottle feeding, and you may stop to wind during a feed too if your baby seems uncomfortable. From experience in clinic, I find that some babies go on to need winding during or after every feed, whereas others do not and repositioning after a feed can be enough to help expel any wind. Breastfed babies may not need winding at all – it's very individual.

It can be common that when the stomach valve opens to allow air to escape, some milk is brought up too. This is called posseting.

Secondly, what is the right way to wind? There isn't one perfect way, but you'll certainly get to know what works for your baby. Saying that, it's important that your baby's head and neck are always supported, and that their tummy and back are straight (not curled). You can then gently rub and pat their back. Some common positions for winding include:

✧ **Over the shoulder,** with your baby's chin resting on your shoulder. I also really love the 'Wonky winding' position that I've seen coined by Lyndsey Hookway. This is where you tilt your baby to their left and over your right shoulder, which can help trapped air bubbles escape more easily due to the natural shape and positioning of the stomach.

✧ **Sit your baby up** on your lap, facing out. Place the palm of your hand flat against their chest, supporting their chin and jaw gently in your hand (along the L shape of your thumb and forefinger) without pressing on their throat. Lean your baby slightly forward and use your free hand to gently rub or pat their back.

If your baby is struggling with tummy pain and excessive wind despite regular winding, I'd encourage you to seek a feeding review from your local infant feeding team. During feeding babies can swallow excessive air through gulping, spluttering and repeatedly latching on and off a breast or bottle. Reasons for this can include a shallow latch when breastfeeding, difficulty managing milk flow, or oral restriction issues, such as tongue-tie. There can also be other contributing factors to wind and abdominal discomfort in babies, such as food allergies or constipation, so individualised support can be beneficial.

*   *   *

As we wrap up these first crucial months of feeding, I hope you are feeling more confident and empowered with this first nutritional milestone. Before you know it, the next stage in their feeding journey will be here: starting solids, also known as weaning. This is an exciting and important step, and there's plenty of valuable information here to guide you as you prepare to explore the world of solid foods with your little one.

2

Solid Ground

First steps into the world of food, aka weaning: 6–12 months

Nutrition and feeding milestones between six and 12 months:

✧ Your baby is starting solids and over the next six months will transition from first tastes to family meals.
✧ Milk contributes significantly to your baby's nutritional needs, especially at the start of weaning. Gradually, as your baby gains the skills they need to eat a range of family foods, they will start to get more of their nutrition from solid foods, and their reliance on milk will decrease.
✧ Your baby is learning how to eat solid foods. These months allow your baby to start building these skills and experience for life.
✧ These six months offer key opportunities to support your baby's feeding and development, including helping them learn to feed themselves and accept a variety of tastes and textures, reduce the risk of food allergies, and introduce foods to support growth, as well as gut and brain development.
✧ By one year, your baby will be around triple their birth weight and will have grown (on average) 10 inches in length.

✧ Your baby's brain will reach 70 per cent of its adult size by 12 months.

✧ Your baby remains within the first 1,000-day golden window.

Congratulations on making your way through exclusively milk-feeding your baby! I hope you're at the stage where you feel confident and settled with your baby's feeds, and you're now reaching back to this book for a head start on the next feeding milestone – solid foods!

As your baby begins to explore solid foods, this stage can evoke a mix of excitement, anticipation and anxiety. I find parents frequently encounter an overwhelming amount of information at this time. To ease your worries, it's important to know that while the coming months are crucial for your baby's feeding development, there are many wonderful and effective ways to ensure a successful start to solids.

Before I walk you through the next few months, it's probably helpful to understand what 'complementary feeding', aka weaning or starting solids, means. The official definition from the World Health Organization is:

'When babies receive foods to complement breast milk or infant formula.' Or, 'The process of providing foods in addition to milk when breast-feeding milk or milk formula alone are no longer adequate to meet nutritional requirements.'

I don't have a strong preference for the terminology used, but I tend to favour the term 'starting solids', as it clearly describes the process and avoids confusion with weaning a baby off the breast in relation to breastfeeding. I might use the other terms interchangeably on these pages where it feels appropriate.

That said, there's a term not often used that I feel is an ideal description of the next few months: 'learning to eat'! Your baby's learning about food in the coming months is complex, far beyond just seeing and eating food; in fact, many experts recognise that eating is the most complicated skill your child has to grasp and one that will continue to develop for years ahead.

So, repeat after me . . .

Eating is one of the most complex skills my baby has to learn.
Weaning is not a race; let's follow my baby's pace.

Before You Get Started with Solids

✧ **At what age should you start offering solids?**

✧ **What skills does your baby learn and practise during weaning?**

✧ **Debunking common weaning myths**

✧ **Preparing yourself and your baby for weaning**

✧ **The best weaning method – spoon feeding or Baby-Led Weaning (BLW)?**

At what age should you start offering solids?

According to the World Health Organization and the UK Department of Health, most babies should begin solid foods at around six months of age and not before 17 weeks.

Like any developmental milestone, it's important to remember this is a guideline; every baby is different and there will be some variation in the exact time that each baby reaches the readiness signs below. I encourage parents to watch their baby, not just the calendar!

Four developmental signs indicate your baby is ready to start solids. Think of these as anchors that show your baby's body and brain are prepared to go! These signs are:

What	Why
1. Your baby can sit upright for a short time without support;	Babies must be able to maintain a stable upright posture and head control in order to eat and swallow safely.
and	
2. Hold their head upright.	(Imagine eating with your chin to your chest, leaning to one side, or flopping forwards – not easy!)
3. Your baby should be able to see an object, reach out, grab it and bring it to their mouth.	Babies need to have started to develop the motor skills (how we move and control our body) to feed themselves.
4. Your baby's tongue-thrust (extrusion) reflex should have started to reduce. As a guide, a baby should keep in and swallow more than 50 per cent of every mouthful.	Babies need to be ready to start swallowing some food, not just spitting it out. If solids are started too early, babies may seem to reject the spoon or food, when in fact they are rejecting the feeling of something unfamiliar in their mouth, not the food itself.

What skills does your baby learn and practise during weaning? (Hint: it's not just eating)

While your baby might meet the developmental milestones that indicate they are ready for eating solids, initially they won't possess all the skills required to eat a diverse range of foods. However, over the next six months they will develop and practise numerous skills in order to be able to eat a broad and varied diet.

The table below highlights skills your baby will learn and practise through weaning. I hope that raising your awareness of these helps you understand that 'success' with solids isn't solely defined by what or how much your baby eats at each mealtime. I hope sharing this also helps you shift the focus from 'getting' your baby to eat to supporting them as they develop the skills to eat. I often remind parents that learning to eat is part of your baby's development. As with any milestone, it can be helpful to remember that, as parents, we can support but not control development.

Skills and experience	Examples
Gross motor skills (Big movements we make with the large muscles in our body, like our arms, legs and core)	Postural stability (sitting up independently) Reaching and grasping Hand to mouth co-ordination Head and neck control Chewing and swallowing
Fine motor skills (Small movements made with hands, wrists and fingers)	Self-feeding with hands and fingers Early cutlery skills Hand–eye coordination Finger dexterity (using hands and fingers for tasks) Mouth control, such as lips and tongue movement
Oral motor skills (Mouth, jaw and tongue skills)	Clearing the spoon with their lips Early chewing skills, such as munching up and down Biting skills Tongue skills, such as moving tongue up and down and side to side Mouth mapping Diagonal chew (emerges from nine months) Rotary chew (emerges 12–24 months)
Sensory awareness Eating is one of the only things that is a multi-sensory experience!	Taste exploration Texture awareness Becoming aware and learning about different sensory experiences with food e.g. smell, taste, sound, temperature Oral awareness and sensitivity Coordinating multiple pieces of sensory information (when we eat our senses have to work together) Responding to internal feelings of hunger and fullness

While many of these skills develop innately, babies must have the opportunity and plenty of practice to develop and refine their eating and feeding skills. In simple terms, mastering eating involves gaining experience with a wide range of foods.

Each baby may reach the following developmental milestones at different ages. However, I generally advise parents to observe their baby's eating habits and the following skills for signs of progress.

Lips
✧ Closure of lips around a spoon; creating a seal around a cup or closing lips and clearing food from a spoon.
✧ A reduction in how much water is spilt from their mouth.

Tongue
✧ Reduced tongue thrust, with movement shifting to forward-and-backward and side-to-side motions.

Jaw
✧ Moving up and down (munching), diagonal movement, progress with rotary (round) chewing.

Gag
✧ Regression of the gag reflex as weaning progresses.

Hands
✧ Picking up food in the palm of their hand, picking up food with thumb and forefinger (pincer grip).
✧ Grasping and exploring cutlery, bringing cutlery towards mouth (may flip spoon initially), early scooping and spoon loading, improved self-feeding skills and independent eating.

Debunking common weaning myths

Numerous myths surround weaning, so I wanted to pause here to debunk a few of these for you before we get into the details about introducing your baby to solids.

Starting solids helps your baby sleep through the night
Honestly, I would have loved this one to be accurate. Although I know some of you will be hoping otherwise, two extensive studies have agreed that no evidence suggests that starting solids or early introduction of solids enhances a baby's sleep duration or reduces nighttime waking.

Your baby is ready for weaning when . . .
- ✧ They want more milk or start waking for additional feeds.
- ✧ They start drinking less milk.
- ✧ They reach a certain weight.
- ✧ They get teeth.
- ✧ They start bringing their hand or fist to their mouth.
- ✧ They are watching you eat with interest.

Despite what anyone suggests, none of the above are developmental signs indicating a baby is ready for solids or, in the case of teeth and weight goals, a necessity for weaning.

Is 'food before one just for fun'?
If you're about to start weaning or just getting started, I'd guess you've heard this phrase already. While I'm a huge advocate of finding the fun during weaning and keeping the pressure off, it's important to remember that starting solids has a bigger purpose. I tend to reframe 'fun' as:

Food before one is just for . . .

F – Fundamental skill development, for example, gross motor skills, fine motor skills, multi-sensory learning, oral motor skills.
U – Understanding mealtimes, for example, routines, socialisation, communication and language, feeding cues, skills needed to eat.
N – Nutritional needs, for example, the introduction of allergens

and inclusion of iron- and zinc-rich foods, as a baby's stores from being in utero start to deplete around this time.

The three-day rule – 'Offer one new food every three days'

A more gradual introduction to foods might be necessary for some babies with medical needs. However, for the majority, the 'one-food-for-three-days' approach drastically reduces dietary variety. Sticking to this method for three months limits your baby to approximately 30 different foods. On the other hand, offering a wider selection can help them experience double or triple that, or even more. Given the importance of variety during weaning – for fostering food acceptance and supporting gut health – I usually do not advocate this approach.

Preparing yourself and your baby for weaning

Parents often ask me how to prepare their baby for weaning. While waiting for developmental milestones, here are some suggestions:

✧ Bring your baby to the table during meals so they can observe and experience some social and sensory aspects of eating, such as how food looks and smells and what you're doing with it. You can also introduce them to empty cups and cutlery to help build familiarity.

✧ Continue plenty of tummy time, which supports the development of your baby's head control, neck and shoulder strength and core stability – all of which are needed for eating.

✧ Purposeful play can help babies develop weaning skills like reaching and grasping. You can start practising these through activities like reaching for toys.

✧ Weaning is a sensory experience, so introducing sensory play e.g. water play and textured toys, beforehand can be beneficial.

Before starting your baby on solids, you'll need some practical essentials. While there are many specialised weaning gadgets available, really only a few core items are necessary, which I've listed below.

✧ **A highchair** – The importance of secure and supported seating can be easily overlooked, but it's essential for ensuring your baby is stable, comfortable and in the ideal position to eat safely. There are a few things I recommend looking for in a highchair:

   o **An adjustable footrest** – we all need our feet to eat, and when describing to parents why a footrest is necessary, I encourage them to sit on a chair, lift their feet off the floor, and move their back away from the seat. Imagine using your hands and sitting to eat a whole meal like this. It's not easy! I'm sure if you've ever done this you felt your core muscles working hard to keep you upright and stable. It's like eating on a barstool. Not only is this pretty distracting, it also makes the eating process a whole lot more tiresome and less safe. Having feet grounded on a footrest (even if it's a makeshift one) will help support the optimum posture for eating and allow your baby (or child) to focus on the task in front of them while keeping them safe and stable.

   o **Safety features** – a highchair should have features that secure your baby safely and comfortably, such as a harness or clip-on baby seating attachment, a stable base and an upright position. Your baby should never be reclined when eating.

   o **Removable or adjustable tray** – this not only helps with cleaning up but also means you can bring the highchair to the family table when your little one is older.

✧ **Bibs** – Consider bibs as some of your damage control for the mess that weaning brings! There are many options available, from those with just a front cover to coveralls that can clip to the highchair and catch some of the food that inevitably drops into your baby's lap. Bibs that are easy to clean or wash are ideal.

✧ **Bowls and plates** – Choose options that are easy to clean. Ideally, they should stick to the tray and allow your baby to see and reach into them easily. Be aware that silicone crockery can quickly build up a soapy taste, which can transfer to food. So if your child suddenly refuses food when eating off these plates/bowls, have a quick taste test.

✧ **Cutlery** – Your baby will take months and years to become proficient with their cutlery skills, but introducing a spoon and, eventually, a fork early is great. When it comes to self-feeding, babies often do well with short, wider-handled cutlery (easier to grasp) and/or those with a double handle so you can pass it to them and they can take it from you easily.

✧ **Cups** – It can be tempting to buy every cup available, but each type requires your baby to learn a different way of drinking. I recommend prioritising a small open cup to support sipping. A weighted straw cup can also be an option to introduce. Avoid cups with a valve, where babies continue to suck, instead of learning to sip.

✧ **A blender** – If you plan on making purees or blending foods, you'll need some equipment to do this. You may already have a blender or food processor at home, which will work fine. If you don't, a cheap hand blender will do the job – don't buy anything expensive and fancy, as you won't use it for as long as you think!

The best weaning method – spoon feeding or Baby-Led Weaning (BLW)?

In recent years, discussions around weaning methods have become more heated, leaving some parents feeling confused about the 'best' choice or feeling guilty about the choice they've made, both in the moment and even years later. However, as with many aspects of feeding, there is no one 'right' way, and I would encourage you to be understanding and respectful towards all parents' feeding decisions.

The most important thing to remember is that no matter which approach you use, the end goal is the same: helping your baby to enjoy a wide variety of family foods and to develop the skills they need to eat. I remind all parents of the important similarities between approaches, such as the fact both methods can allow for responsive feeding, getting messy, and exposure to a wide variety of foods. You also don't have to choose one, you can combine both methods.

To help guide you on these different approaches, here's a quick rundown with some perceived pros and cons, but remember, the choice is ultimately down to you.

Spoon feeding

Spoon feeding, sometimes called 'traditional' weaning, typically starts with offering pureed, well-blended or mashed foods on a spoon to your baby. Over the following weeks and months, the texture is gradually adjusted to include mashed and lumpier foods alongside finger foods, eventually progressing to eating little portions of family meals.

Perceived benefits:
✧ **Controlled introduction and texture transition with foods:** Parents frequently tell me they enjoy being able to monitor and manage the texture of foods introduced. Some parents who are nervous about choking may prefer to use this approach, but it's worth being aware that the risk of choking exists with either

method of weaning. Texture progression is essential for skill development, allowing your baby to build the oral motor skills they need to eat a varied diet. If you're nervous about choking, read the SOS section beginning on page 143.

✧ **Less mess:** If you're mess averse, you're not alone. Many parents express a desire to use spoon-fed options during weaning for this reason, *but* babies benefit hugely from the learning associated with getting messy with their food. If you choose this approach, I highly encourage you to allow your baby to see their food, feel their food, self-feed and get messy! (See page 88.)

✧ **Nutrition:** Some parents opt for this method when they seek greater nutritional 'security'. This may be because it is easier to see how much their baby has eaten, incorporate additional nutrients (like fats or iron) into their baby's meals or support the early introduction of food allergens. Some babies may also consume more food more quickly.

Perceived negatives:

✧ **Parent–led feeding:** The primary criticism of spoon feeding is that it's parent-led rather than baby-led, which risks reducing a baby's independence around feeding. However, following a responsive spoon-feeding approach and introducing finger foods to support self-feeding skills can help negate this.

✧ **Time-consuming:** Preparing purees and separate meals can be more time-consuming than adapting a family meal.

Baby-Led Weaning (aka BLW)

Baby-Led Weaning is a term coined by Gill Rapley in the early 2000s, and it has become a more popular approach over recent years, although it has likely been used for much longer. It encourages babies to self-feed and explore a variety of family foods, including safely prepared finger foods, from the beginning of weaning. Generally, it is recommended that babies are at least six months of age and able to sit independently before introducing this method of weaning.

Perceived benefits:

✧ **Encourages independence:** Babies have a greater opportunity to learn to feed themselves and follow their bodies' hunger and fullness cues.

✧ **Develop fine motor skills:** Handling finger foods can support hand–eye coordination, hand and self-help skills.

✧ **Family mealtime inclusion:** Babies can join in family meals from the outset, making mealtimes more inclusive and allowing increased opportunities for role-modelling. Parents can also make just one meal.

✧ **Exploration of textures and flavours:** Babies are exposed to various textures and flavours early on, which may promote a more adventurous palate and allows babies to see foods in their 'real' form from the start. It is often cited that BLW will help prevent picky eating, and while parenting style and food exposures can support positive eating habits, no robust data proves it entirely prevents picky eating.

Perceived negatives:

✧ **Potential for choking:** There is a higher perceived risk of choking, although this risk can be minimised with proper supervision and age-appropriate food and texture choices. Research shows no increased choking risk in babies fed with a BLW approach compared to spoon feeding.

✧ **Messier mealtimes:** Self-feeding can often be messier than spoon feeding. However, as I've discussed above and below, while cleaning up the mess can be tiresome, getting messy is a positive for your baby's learning and sensory development around food.

✧ **Nutrient intake concerns:** Given the variety of textures offered at the outset of BLW, how much your baby eats will depend on the skills they have to manage that food, and initially, babies fed via BLW may consume less than those who are spoon fed. However, a very recent study (albeit relatively small) found no difference in total energy intake between babies fed purees and those who followed a baby-led approach during the early weaning stages. Some data shows babies following a BLW approach may also find it more challenging to consume enough iron initially and may be more likely to consume more salt, but with careful meal planning, these risks can be minimised.

The importance of mess

Yes, I've dedicated a whole box to embracing letting your baby get messy with food. While I can empathise with a sarcastic 'yay' under your breath as I'm setting the scene for extra cleaning, I promise the mess is worth the stress.

Getting messy greatly supports helping your baby learn about food and eating. Eating is an incredibly sensory experience; babies and young children innately learn about the world around them through their bodies and physical experiences. We call this sensorimotor learning. Exploring foods engages the senses of touch, sight, smell, taste, hearing and more. Babies explore food with all their senses, often all at once, which is also fantastic for their brain development. So allow your baby to explore their food, (even the smearing, wiping and smelling), as fostering this exploration helps to create an environment where they feel secure and unafraid of mess.

Here are a few tips to create a safe, exploratory environment for your child to engage with their food and support development:

✧ Avoid these practices when possible, as they can unintentionally limit sensory experiences or create negative ones:

  o Trying to keep your baby clean throughout the mealtimes by repeatedly wiping their hands and face - leave clean-up until the end of the meal.

  o Scraping a spoon across their mouth or lips between each mouthful - let them wear it.

  o Keeping the bowl of food to yourself in a bid to control the mess; instead, put some food on the highchair and the bowl/plate within their reach.

  o Not letting them reach and take the spoon - give them some autonomy with feeding.

  o Trying to keep food to their mouth only - let them see it, feel it and smear it across the tray or themselves.

✧ Invest in some good bibs and soft washcloths you can use (and wash and reuse) to gently clean your baby down at the end of the meal. Bring two - your baby can also learn how to wipe their hands.

✧ A non-slip floor mat or highchair catchy can be helpful, too.

Combination feeding

A combined approach involves offering your baby some pureed or mashed spoon-fed options alongside suitable finger foods, and I often advise this approach. For example, you may offer some pureed or mashed sweet potato alongside a finger of steamed or roasted sweet potato. You can easily adapt family meals to provide mashed or soft options alongside finger foods as weaning progresses. Combination feeding allows the benefits of both approaches to be harnessed, and parents can approach weaning with a flexible mindset.

Remember . . .

✧ Choose the approach that feels right for you and your baby. You can always change your mind once you've started solids.

✧ One approach may feel more financially appropriate for your family, which is a valid reason to choose that method.

✧ Both approaches to weaning can be 'baby-led'. I often reassure parents that, from my perspective, baby-led means letting your baby's cues and development guide the process. With either method, you can lean into and support your baby's independence and learning, practise responsive feeding (whether with finger foods or a spoon) and be attentive to your baby's cues.

✧ Both methods allow you to offer a wide variety of foods and expose your baby to a range of textures, albeit with slightly different timelines. This variety is key to developing healthy eating habits and preferences.

✧ Comparison is often the thief of joy. Everyone approaches aspects of parenting a bit differently, so try to avoid feeling disempowered if other parents' choices or the baby's progress do not mirror your expectations.

The Weaning Timeline

✧ **First foods – what's best to start with?**

✧ **Following on – what next, why and how?**

✧ **What about babies at high risk of food allergy?**

✧ **What foods should be avoided during weaning?**

First foods - what's best to start with?

One of the most common questions when starting solids is, 'What's the *best* food to start with?' Like many of the intricacies of weaning, this can be hotly debated! While having a clear plan for your baby's first foods can be fantastic, please know there are also *no rules* other than avoiding foods that shouldn't be offered during weaning. There are many ways to get off to a positive start.

In recent years, a popular approach to starting solids is 'vegetable-led' weaning or offering bitter foods first, such as green vegetables. Babies are accustomed to sweet tastes because breast milk and formula are sweet, making it easier for them to accept these flavours. As a result, introducing bitter flavours helps to expose them to a broader range of more challenging tastes. Research indicates that starting weaning with various vegetables and, importantly, *continuing* to offer them, can support young children to eat vegetables as part of the diet later in life. As with many topics to do with feeding, the key takeaway for me from this research was the importance of consistently offering these foods. This is a message I hope you will remember now, and in the years ahead, with your little one.

Introducing solids can begin this way, but please know you aren't limited to vegetable-led weaning. You can offer sweeter root vegetables, fruits, proteins and/or starchy foods like oats or a mixture of green or bitter vegetables and these options. When choosing initial foods and other choices for your baby, it's also essential to consider cost, preparation time, personal culture and food preferences. For instance, while fresh green vegetables are a great first option, they can be pricey or inaccessible for some families.

First-food ideas

Here we are, beginning the first days of solid foods! As a guideline, introduce one new food (taste) each day during your baby's initial five to seven days of weaning. Think of this as a runway to get going, and remember, it's very typical for your baby not to seem interested at all!

Big faces and grimacing communicate that 'it's new', not necessarily 'it's ewww'.

I've listed a few weaning options below that can be offered as a puree or finger foods, to guide and inspire you. Remember, there's no need for a one-size-fits-all approach, so feel free to adjust based on the foods you have or want to try!

	Vegetable-led weaning options	Budget-friendly first-food options	Cultural dietary considerations*
Day 1	Broccoli	Cooked frozen broccoli	Cauliflower
Day 2	Courgette	Cooked frozen peas (blended)	Yam
Day 3	Cauliflower	Tinned green beans in water (blended)	Pumpkin
Day 4	Spinach	Carrot	Rice porridge
Day 5	Carrot	Cooked frozen cauliflower	Spinach
Day 6	Green beans	Banana	Plantain
Day 7	Peas (pureed)	Potato	Peas (blended)

Day 8	Potato	Oats/porridge	Cabbage
Day 9	Parsnip	Swede	Soft-cooked and blended lentils – dal
Day 10	Avocado	Cooked beetroot	Sweet potato

While much weaning advice often highlights first foods commonly found in a typical Western diet, I encourage you to use the foods you cook with most often at home. Incorporating foods that are part of your family's usual diet makes mealtimes more enjoyable and helps your baby develop a taste for the flavours and ingredients they will grow up with. Those listed here are just examples.

For foods that need cooking to create a puree, you can boil, steam or even microwave until them they are very soft. If boiling and blending or mashing, I recommend using a splash of the cooking water to help loosen the puree or mash, as it replaces some of the water-soluble nutrients lost during cooking. You can also use a splash of your baby's usual milk if blending. If offering any of the above as finger foods, read on for more guidance about safely preparing these to age-appropriate sizes and textures.

When it comes to when to introduce foods, I encourage parents to free themselves from typical meal timings. Choose a time when your baby is alert and settled, and ideally, not too soon after a milk feed. Many parents choose to do the first 'meal' around mid-morning, but it depends on what works best for you – there is no 'right' or 'wrong' time.

Remember to make sure your baby is sitting securely, ideally facing you, and provide lots of reassuring facial expressions and gentle encouragement as you get going.

Following on – what next, why and how?
After what can feel like a very structured first few days or weeks of initial tastes and food exploration, you're probably now wondering, 'What next?' The good news is that there are few hard-and-fast

rules, aside from avoiding foods that pose a choking risk or are unsafe for babies during weaning (see pages 102–3). I also remind all parents that there doesn't need to be any distinction between 'baby food' or 'kids' food'– it's all just food!

In this weaning phase, I suggest parents mix different foods and flavours to ease their babies into family meals, emphasising variety. Begin with foods you regularly eat at home while focusing on the essential food groups or nutrients that I outline later in this chapter. Don't stress about whether certain foods traditionally complement each other – your baby is learning and should not be restricted by conventional meal expectations. It's perfectly acceptable to serve chicken with raspberries!

If you prefer a staged approach to weaning, I've summarised the key milestones and timelines below.

What foods?

Step 1 – First tastes: Single tastes of foods such as vegetables or fruits.

Step 2 – Food combinations: Start combining different foods and food groups – carbohydrates, fruit, vegetables, dairy (or suitable fortified alternatives), fats and importantly iron rich foods like meats, beans and pulses. Combining two to three foods at this stage is appropriate as you work towards building a balanced plate for your baby. You can also use herbs and spices to combine or add variety with flavours, but avoid salt. Offering a range of food types and combining different flavours will help your baby learn about food, support their acceptance of various tastes and textures and provide varied nutrition.

Step 3 – Balanced meals: Now your baby regularly has different flavours and food combinations, it's time to start their journey towards joining balanced family meals by building them 'mini meals'. To meet the unique nutritional needs of a growing baby, it's recommended that you combine certain food groups which likely align with the meals you're already preparing for yourself at home. I provide a guide on how to build balanced meals for your baby below.

What textures?

Puree progression – If you're using a spoon-led or combined approach, your baby can progress to more textured foods in the coming days and weeks. Most babies starting solids at six months don't need to stick with smooth purees for long and can transition with texture within a few weeks. You can add more texture to meals by:

✧ Blending foods for less time.

✧ Using very well-mashed foods.

✧ Incorporating grainier textures or small soft lumps within meals.

✧ Using foods from different food groups, as this naturally adds texture variety.

✧ Offering combinations of foods prepared at home, which often leads to more varied textures.

As your baby explores different textures, remember, there's more for them to grasp now and their mouths and tongues will be learning new skills, so expect some spitting out of lumps and some gagging. Don't be alarmed by this, but do stay near your baby to keep them safe (see page 145 for information about choking).

Finger foods – Introducing pieces of food that a baby can learn to feed themselves is encouraged for all babies. If you're following a BLW or combined approach, you'll offer these to your baby from around six months of age. If you've started with just spoon-fed options or puree, I'd encourage you to think about introducing finger foods by seven to eight months of age. There are a whole host of benefits to finger foods, including:

✧ Supporting your baby to learn how to self-feed.

✧ Autonomy around food.

✧ Development of fine motor skills (using hands and fingers).

✧ Development of oral motor skills (chewing, biting, moving the tongue).

✧ Sensory exploration of foods.

Some parents feel anxious about providing their baby with finger foods for fear of choking, so to support you in introducing your first finger foods to your baby, here is a quick guide:

F – Find the right size. To begin with, your baby will benefit from long strips or pieces of food that are roughly the size of one to two adult fingers. The food should be wide enough for your baby to close their hand around it easily (using their palm – called a palmer grasp) and tall enough so it pops out of their grasp. If the food is slippery, like avocado or banana, you may want to roll it in something like ground oats or breadcrumbs, or cut foods with a serrated knife or leave skin on the bottom. Your baby will be able to grasp this much more easily!

Once your baby develops their pincer grip and gains experience with eating, you can typically start offering smaller bite-sized food pieces from around nine months old.

I – In between your finger and thumb (and their gums). Initially, offer well-cooked or very soft foods that mash down or collapse if you apply gentle pressure between your finger and thumb (which mimics what happens in their gums). Think avocado, banana, cooked sweet potato. You can progress with textures of finger foods as your baby's eating skills develop and they gain more experience.

N – No choking hazards and not alone. Avoid any common choking hazards (see page 103), and always sit with your baby when they are eating – choking can be silent.

G – Gagging is to be expected! It is common for babies to gag on finger foods (in fact, all foods) during weaning. This happens because finger foods can easily reach different areas of the mouth and tongue, triggering the gag reflex. Babies have a highly sensitive gag reflex situated much closer to the front of the mouth than adults, ensuring their safety while they learn to eat. Over time and with repeated exposure to a variety of foods, including finger foods, this reflex gradually moves further back in the mouth and becomes less reactive.

E – Experience and exposure. Your baby will not have the skills to chew and swallow much finger food initially, but they may well lick or suck the food, hold, squash, throw it, munch and push it back out. These actions are typical and essential to their learning experience that will eventually help them eat these foods. Remember, experience and exposure to different foods build skills needed to eat.

R – Role-modelling. You can support your baby's skill development, and in this case with finger foods, by role-modelling and eating together. Your baby will be closely watching you, so try to eat the same foods and model what to do with them – exaggerating the skills like biting and chewing. This helps them to see and understand what to do with the food and encourages them to copy and practise these skills.

Here are some examples of great first finger foods by food group:

Fruits	Vegetables	Carbohydrates	Protein-rich options or dairy
Ripe mango

Steamed apple slices

Ripe peeled pear slices

Orange segment (no pips)

Banana fingers

Large whole strawberries

Watermelon fingers

Ripe peeled peach/nectarine | Steamed or roasted carrot batons/parsnip sticks

Ripe avocado slices

Steamed courgette batons

Large steamed broccoli or cauliflower florets

Roasted pumpkin or squash fingers | Steamed or roasted potato, sweet potato or yam batons/wedges

Very well-cooked fusilli pasta pieces

Toast with soft toppings, such as mashed avocado, cream cheese, hummus, fish pate

Pancake slices

Meltable maize 'puff' snacks*

*These can be great for skill-building but are not as nutritious as other starchy foods | Large flakes of fish or fish flaked into mashed potato tots/fish cakes

Long, flat strips of tender meat e.g. chicken

Lentil patties – sliced

Firm tofu fingers

Thin slices or sticks of cheese (use a vegetable peeler) |

From around nine months of age, most babies have started to develop their pincer grasp. This is where they begin to use their thumb and forefinger to pick up smaller pieces of food. At this stage, you can also start to offer foods prepared into smaller bite-size pieces so they can practise this new skill. For example, cubes of soft fruit, flattened blueberries or peas, small squares of toast or pancake instead of strips.

Hard munchables

Another helpful approach to introducing a type of finger food during early weaning – especially in those first few months – is to offer up large, sturdy options sometimes referred to as 'hard munchables' or 'food teethers'. The goal of these foods isn't eating, and they should be size-able enough that:

✧ Your baby can hold them independently.
✧ Most of the food remains outside your baby's mouth.
✧ They don't break apart and large pieces are unlikely to detach or be snapped off.

Examples are large whole peeled carrots, mango pits with most of the flesh removed, chunky ends of celery sticks and meat bones such as ribs.

These hard munchable options are the perfect tool for your baby to start exploring and mapping their mouths. They can practise mouth and tongue skills like gnawing/munching and moving their tongue side to side alongside exposure to different tastes and textures. Hard, munch-able foods can also help move the gag reflex.

What about babies at high risk of food allergy?

In recent years, growing scientific evidence supports proactively introducing specific food allergens, such as peanuts and eggs, early during weaning to help prevent food allergies. For babies at high risk, introduction before six months of age (between four and six months) may even be recommended under the advice of a health professional who will also consider factors like your baby's development and the safest way to introduce these foods.

To help understand your baby's risk of developing food allergies, take a look below.

Highest risk	Babies with severe eczema – such as those who may have had eczema from the early weeks or months of life, in whom it is widespread and/or needs regular use of steroid creams to help manage it.	May benefit from early introduction of food allergens such as well-cooked egg and peanut between four and six months of age. Discuss with a health professional such as such as a paediatric allergist or paediatric dietitian.
High risk	Babies with a food allergy already, such as Cow's Milk Protein Allergy.	May benefit from early introduction of food allergens above, around or before six months of age. Discuss with a health professional such as such as a paediatric allergist or paediatric dietitian.
Moderate risk	Babies with mild to moderate eczema.	Introduce food allergens from around six months of age after baby has commenced solids. Do not delay allergen introduction.
	Babies from a family (for instance, mum, dad, siblings) with a history of allergic disease including food allergy, asthma, eczema, hay fever.	
'Standard' risk	All babies who don't fit into the above categories.	

When I share the table above with parents, many want to understand why eczema is the most significant risk factor for developing food allergies. Here's an analogy I often use – imagine your skin is like a fortress wall that protects the city inside (your body). When the wall is intact, it keeps out unwanted invaders (in this case, allergens). However, invaders can slip through if the wall is damaged and has cracks (as with eczema). When food proteins found in the environment get through these cracks in the skin, they come into contact with the immune system in an unexpected way. Typically, food proteins are introduced into the body through the gut, where the immune system is trained to recognise them as safe. This is like inviting guests into the city through the main gate, where they are welcomed and recognised. However, when these proteins enter through the damaged skin, it's as if they are sneaking into the city through the cracks in the wall. The skin's immune cells, which are not used to seeing food proteins this way, mistakenly send alarm signals to the immune system, declaring these proteins dangerous. As a result, the immune system builds up a defensive response to these food proteins, wrongly treating them as threats. This explains why some children can have an allergic reaction even when they eat an allergen for the first time. Their immune system has already encountered these food proteins through the broken skin barrier, has become sensitised to them and is ready to respond.

If your baby has one or more risk factors for food allergy, I'd recommend the following:

✧ Ensure you have a clear, consistent (and working) plan to manage your baby's skin. Eczema is a skin condition associated with excessive moisture loss from the skin and inflammation, so good management starts with the skin. Consult a GP or derma-tologist for advice.

✧ Avoid using products on your baby's skin that contain food ingredients such as oats, coconut, tree nuts like almonds. Research is starting to show that this may increase the risk of children becoming allergic to these foods, as they've been exposed to the food proteins via their skin first instead of their gut. Given the regular food exposure to our hands, washing your hands regularly and using a scoop/spatula with pots of creams is recommended to reduce this exposure route.

✧ Speak with a qualified allergy specialist such as a paediatric allergist or paediatric dietitian to discuss weaning and provide some support.

✧ Don't delay the introduction of allergenic foods – the earlier the better once your baby has commenced solids.

What foods should be avoided during weaning?

The good news is that there are not that many foods that need to be avoided during weaning. Here's a quick rundown of what to steer clear of:

✧ Foods high in salt, such as processed meats, crisps, gravy granules.

✧ Foods high in sugar, such as cakes, biscuits, sweets, chocolate.

✧ Unpasteurised dairy products, due to risk of food poisoning.

✧ Lightly cooked or raw shellfish, due to risk of food poisoning.

✧ Fish, such as shark, swordfish or marlin due to mercury levels in them – tuna should generally be limited to two portions a week.

✧ Honey, until one year of age, due to a very small risk of a condition known as infant botulism, which can be caused by a bacteria found in honey.

✧ Rice milk alternative drinks as these contain high levels of inorganic arsenic.

✧ Cow's milk as a drink.

Foods that are a high choking risk to babies and young children should be avoided completely or modified to a shape and texture which is suitable for your baby, such as:

Food	Avoid or adapt?
Whole nuts and large seeds	Adapt by offering well-milled/ground or in smooth butter form (ideally loosened or stirred into other foods). Avoid offering tacky nut butter directly from a spoon
Mini chocolate eggs, boiled sweets, toffees or chewy sweets	Avoid until 5+ years of age
Jelly cubes and marshmallows	Avoid until 5+ years of age
Popcorn	Avoid until 5+ years of age
Stones from fruit	Avoid – remove from fruit
Chunks of raw, hard vegetables or fruit, e.g. carrot, apple	Adapt – cook, cut or grate to an appropriate size or texture
Grapes	Adapt – cut into quarters lengthwise
Blueberries	Adapt – squash flat or cut in half/quarters
Cherry tomatoes	Adapt – cut into quarters
Sausage cut into rounds/discs	Adapt – slice sausage lengthways

Baby nutrition 101

✧ **Macronutrients**

✧ **Micronutrients**

✧ **How many meals, and when?**

✧ **How much should my baby be eating?**

Feeding your baby can feel overwhelming for many parents, who frequently ask me if their child is 'getting enough'. While babies and young children share some nutritional needs with adults, they aren't simply 'little adults.' A key difference is that babies and young children require higher amounts of certain nutrients relative to their size. Additionally, we must pay special attention to specific nutrients like iron because stores which accumulate during pregnancy are running low by six months of age. Understanding these needs is important when choosing foods to incorporate into weaning.

Note: all foods mentioned below should be offered in a form appropriate for your baby's age, weaning stage or method.

Macronutrients

Energy

It will seem obvious, but babies need plenty of energy-rich foods to support their speedy growth and development. Please be reassured that as you begin weaning and throughout the first few months, your baby's milk (breast or formula) will still be their predominant energy source. Being aware of how to ensure their meals are energy-dense is helpful, as it allows you to gradually introduce a variety of nutritious foods that will complement their milk intake. Energy-rich foods include carbohydrate foods such as bread, rice, pasta, potatoes, couscous, noodles, millet, yams, quinoa, plantain and fat-rich foods, which I cover in more detail below. Babies and young children should not be offered low-calorie, low-fat or 'diet' versions of any food.

Fat

Babies and young children need plenty of fat to support their rapid growth and brain development. Ideally, up to 40 per cent of their daily energy should come from fat. With this in mind, babies should be offered fat sources in their meals throughout the day, such as full-fat dairy produce, eggs, oily fish, avocado, nuts and seeds, and oils like olive, rapeseed, sunflower, coconut or avocado. Including a variety of fats can be beneficial, and you can read more about types of fats on pages 186–7.

Micronutrients

Iron

The iron stores that your baby will have collected during pregnancy start to drop by six months of age, which means an eye on iron intake is important from weaning onwards. Iron will still be found in your baby's formula milk or breast milk (*note: while levels of iron are lower in breast milk, the iron is very bioavailable, meaning the body easily absorbs it*). However, your baby's iron requirement at 6–12 months is high compared to their size, so prioritising iron-rich foods is essential from now on.

Iron has an essential role in your baby's brain development and the transportation of oxygen around the body via red blood cells. (See page 296 for more about its importance in the first five years, and practical advice.)

What foods provide iron?

Iron is found in both animal foods (haem iron) and some plant-based foods (non-haem iron). Iron from animal sources can be easier for the body to absorb, but if your baby follows a plant-based diet, they can still get enough iron from a carefully planned diet.

Animal sources of iron (haem iron)	Plant sources of iron (non-haem iron)
Red meat – beef, goat, lamb, mutton	Lentils, beans, pulses
Poultry – chicken, turkey, the darker meat is higher in iron	Soya – tofu, tempeh, edamame beans
Eggs	Fortified cereals – these are cereals or oats where extra vitamins and minerals have been added
Oily fish, tuna	Dark green vegetables – kale, spinach, broccoli
Offal, such as liver – only offer in small amounts once a week to babies and young children	Nuts – almonds, hazelnuts and seeds such as sesame (offer very well ground or in 'butter' form)

How should you give these foods?

Once your baby has been offered first tastes of single foods, it is recommended that you regularly incorporate iron-rich foods into their diet – aim to include one portion in meals during weaning, such as:

Breakfast

✧ Scrambled egg with toast and fruit
✧ Fortified wheat cereal or oats with milk, nut butter and fruit

Lunch

✧ Lentil dal with rice
✧ Egg and spinach muffins
✧ Salmon fish cake
✧ Hummus with soft vegetables

Evening meal

✧ Red lentil or beef Bolognese with pasta
✧ Kidney bean or beef curry with rice and vegetables
✧ Spanish omelette fingers

Vitamin C significantly enhances the absorption of iron, which is especially helpful for plant-based sources. It can enhance iron absorption from food by up to four times. Foods high in vitamin C include fruits and vegetables such as kiwis, strawberries, oranges, new potatoes and peppers. A simple squeeze of lemon juice on a meal can also aid absorption.

Zinc

This mineral is essential in a baby's developing immune system, growth and protein production. Similar to iron, it is needed to support your baby's rapid physical and mental development.

What foods provide zinc?

Zinc can be found in various animal and plant-based foods, including:

✧ Shellfish

✧ Red meat

✧ Fortified cereals

✧ Nuts and seeds (well ground or in butter forms for babies)

✧ Beans and pulses

✧ Wholegrain foods, such as cereals, breads, grains

How often should you offer these foods?

Aim to include zinc-rich foods in one or two meals daily during weaning once your baby has regular meals and beyond. Many iron-rich foods are also good sources of zinc.

Omega 3 fats

Omega 3 fatty acids are essential fatty acids that the body cannot make. While they are found in your baby's breast or formula milk, it's ideal to introduce these to your baby in food. These fatty acids are vital to your baby's brain and eye development (see page 291 for more).

What foods provide omega 3 fatty acids?

There are three types of omega 3 fatty acids, which have very long names and are often shortened to DHA, ALA and EPA. DHA and EPA mainly support brain health and development in babies and children.

DHA and EPA are found in good amounts in oily fish such as salmon, sardines, pilchards and mackerel. You can also find some foods fortified with omega 3, like fish fingers, or with higher than usual levels, like eggs. Once your baby gets to grips with meals, aiming to include oily fish one or two times a week (no more than this), can help provide these essential fats.

ALA is primarily found in plant-based foods such as walnuts, chia seeds, hemp, flaxseed and their oils. If your baby doesn't eat fish, including these foods in their diet will be beneficial, as the body can make DHA from ALA. However, this process takes a long time and is not very efficient. Therefore, it may be worth considering a supplement with a plant-based DHA source for your baby, particularly once they are less reliant on milk.

See page 133 for advice on combining these foods in your baby's meals to create a balanced diet.

How many meals, and when?

Each baby will progress from one to three meals a day at their own pace, so I'd encourage you not to feel pressured by this or the advice of others. You may notice signs that your baby is ready for an additional meal, such as enjoying their current meals more, being content to spend a little longer at mealtimes, managing to swallow more and/or starting to grasp eating skills. As a general guideline, I recommend that babies aim to reach three meals a day by around nine months old. Babies who continue to feed frequently overnight may not be prepared for a third meal, typically breakfast, until they reach this age.

Here's a rough guide:

✧ Start of weaning around six months – one mealtime per day.

✧ 6.5–8 months – up to two mealtimes per day.

✧ 7–9 months – up to three mealtimes per day.

How much should my baby be eating?

This is one of the most common queries I receive as a paediatric dietitian. Many parents are surprised to learn that there are no set recommendations for portion sizes for babies under one year of age. While it's understandable to want a guideline, here are a few reasons why they don't exist:

✧ **Individual progress:** Each baby progresses with solids at their own pace; some grasp the skills quickly, others take their time. Recommended portions might add unnecessary pressure during this learning phase. I encourage parents to consider variety and experience over volumes.

✧ **Growth variability:** Babies' needs for growth are different. Those along lower centiles may need smaller portions than those on higher centiles. Growth depends on energy needs per kilogram of body weight, leading to natural variations in intake (a rule to remember now and looking forwards).

✧ **Food type matters:** The amount a baby eats can vary based on the food offered. Initially, they may eat more pureed or mashed foods, while finger foods might be consumed in smaller amounts until they develop the necessary skills.

✧ **Follow your baby's lead:** The best way to determine portion sizes is to follow your baby's cues. Babies are great at regulating their appetite, signalling when they want more or are full. Trusting their appetite fosters a responsive-feeding relationship and lays a strong foundation for healthy mealtimes throughout childhood.

Understanding weaning taste and texture opportunities

I've briefly touched on the different skills your baby develops while learning to eat, but I want to highlight two key windows of opportunity during weaning and why making the most of them is important – taste and texture.

Taste

If you haven't already seen a video of a baby sucking a lemon, I can guarantee you will. Why are they not just wincing and spitting it out? Babies are first exposed to a variety of tastes when in utero via the amniotic fluid, which is influenced by their mums' diets. This exposure to flavours continues if a baby is fed breast milk, as a mum's diet is reflected within her breast milk. Both of these may influence the acceptance of a wider variety of tastes and foods later in life. When a baby begins solids, there seems to be a sensitive period during the early months of life (approximately 6–12 months) when they are more open to diverse flavours. This presents a fantastic opportunity to introduce your baby to various tastes, and I strongly encourage you to take advantage of it! This early exposure can enhance your baby's acceptance of different foods now, and going forwards.

Top tips for taste exposure

✧ **Offer plenty of dietary variety** – You'll hear me use this phrase regularly throughout this book, and that's because dietary variety can be a highly beneficial way to support a child's experience with food, acceptance of foods, but also their health – from nutrients to feeding their gut bugs.

◇ **Focus on variety NOT volume** – Keep in mind that eating and liking are not the same, and acceptance differs across taste profiles. Babies usually find sweet flavours, such as those from fruits or root vegetables, easier to accept, while they may need more exposure to bitter, sour, spicy or savoury tastes. While it may feel natural to just offer more of the foods your baby enjoys, it's important to keep offering variety. Even when faced with grimaces or disinterest in certain foods, don't be discouraged – it's well established that babies and young children need multiple exposures to specific foods for long-term acceptance.

◇ **Don't be afraid to use herbs and spices** – These flavourings help to easily support variety or can alter dishes you may have offered before with minimal effort. For example, add mint to peas, cinnamon to apple, and various spices to dal or curry. The herbs and spices you use can be dried or fresh.

◇ **Adapt your family foods and meals** – Give your baby portions of family food where you can as there is likely to be much more variation in taste, especially compared to pre-prepared baby products. For example, a meat Bolognese dish, curry or stew is likely to vary slightly in taste each time you make it. Do separate out your baby's portion before adding salt to a family food.

Texture

Have you ever taken the time to slow down your eating and notice how your lips, jaw, tongue and mouth work together to handle the different textures on your plate? I suspect your answer might be, '*No, not really, Lucy.*' However, I encourage you to give it some thought during your next meal. While eating feels like second nature to most of us, it's a very complex skill your baby is grasping.

Encouraging texture progression during weaning is highlighted in UK guidelines, as there seems to be a sensitive window for introducing varied textures during weaning between six and 10 months of age. Babies are most receptive to different food textures in this period, and studies have found that later introduction of lumpier textures (after nine months) is associated with increased food refusal and feeding problems in toddlers. Managing textures is like any skill that needs plenty of practice and the right learning opportunities – babies need to experience textured foods to learn how to manage them effectively.

Top tips for texture progression

✦ Avoid sticking with super-smooth purees for too long. If starting with purees rather than finger food, aim to gradually introduce a variety of textures that can be graded, such as thicker purees and/or grainier textures, mashed foods, soft, chopped foods. Some babies can manage slightly textured foods right from the outset at six months of age.

✦ Offering a variety of foods is not just a tip for taste but for texture too. There's natural variation in texture across different food groups, and you can use this to your advantage. For example, add flaky fish to smooth mashed potatoes or cooked lentils to a vegetable puree or add different toppings to toast fingers.

✦ If you're not introducing finger foods from the start of weaning, aim to have started to introduce these by around seven to eight months of age.

✦ Be aware that pre-prepared baby foods will offer less variety with texture than adapting home-prepared foods.

✦ Remember, as your baby gets to grips with different textures, some gagging, spitting out food, or uncertainty can be normal!

Navigating pouches and pre-prepared baby foods

The baby food-and-drink market has significantly grown since the 1920s. As of 2022, it was estimated to be valued at around £706 million, so, unsurprisingly, I frequently receive questions about pouches and pre-prepared baby foods during weaning, such as whether they are advisable for weaning or if they are harmful to babies. Again, this seems to be another aspect of feeding where parents can be made to feel guilty or judged when it comes to feeding choices, with some pretty scary statements made about these foods. As always, there is a balance of being informed alongside a dose of pragmatism (like many aspects of parenting) when it comes to managing these foods.

Pre-prepared baby foods can offer immense convenience for busy parents and *can* have a place in a baby's diet when introducing solids. They can be particularly helpful for outings or when travelling abroad, making feeding your baby outside the home much more manageable. However, I *do* recommend using them thoughtfully, and with a degree of moderation. Ideally, pre-packaged options should be complemented with whole foods and homemade meals whenever possible, ensuring that they don't make up the majority of your baby's diet. This is important for several reasons, including:

✧ Giving your baby the best opportunity to have exposure to a wide variety of tastes and textures while learning to eat.

✧ Ensuring your baby's nutrient needs are met as they progress through weaning.

✧ Supporting your baby with a smooth transition to family foods.

So, considering all of this, here are my top tips to be aware of and to take into account when using jars, pouches and pre-prepared baby foods:

1. **Prioritise whole foods first** – This will ensure your baby sees and is exposed to a wide variety of different tastes and textures. You can use pouches combined with home-cooked foods, such as pasta with a vegetable pouch as the sauce and add some fish, or fruit stirred through yoghurt with a sprinkle of oats or ground seeds.

2. **Check the ingredients** – Many pouches promise certain flavours but often contain higher amounts of sweeter foods like apples or root vegetables. This makes them more appealing to babies already familiar with sweet tastes. Remember, ingredients are listed in descending order by weight, so the first items comprise most of the product. If you're unsure, taste it yourself! Many pouches also contain a low percentage of foods such as fish, meat or lentils, meaning the protein, fat and nutrient (such as iron) content is unlikely to mimic the equivalent homemade option. If you have a child with food allergies, please also be aware that common allergens slip into the most unlikely of baby foods, so always check the ingredients list on the packet. For example, I regularly see fruit and vegetable pouches containing milk or wheat.

3. **Be wary of halo marketing claims** – Please remember that you're being sold to! Many parents choose pouches or baby foods with claims such as 'natural sugars' and 'no added sugars', but the reality is that their free sugar content may still be high either due to the processing involved in producing the pouch (the cell walls of fruits are broken down when made into a puree) or 'natural sugars' such as fruit concentrates or dried fruits are used.

4. **Texture and taste differences (or not!)** – In this chapter I've already discussed how exposure to different textures is a key opportunity during weaning. However, the textures of

pre-prepared baby foods are limited, with each bite often being the same, unlike the different textures and texture changes you get with homemade food. Some textures may even feel somewhat artificial due to the high level of processing; for example, very smooth purees without lumps. Consistently offering such foods may not support your baby's feeding skills or their progress through mashed or soft-chopped family foods. There is also a lack of natural taste and colour variation between pre-prepared baby foods. For instance, when you cook the same spaghetti Bolognese at home, the taste will likely vary each time, even when using the same recipe. However, with pre-prepared baby foods, each batch will follow the same production process and have the same colour and flavour.

5. **Prioritise spoons over sucking** – I understand how convenient and mess-free feeding with pouches can be for babies and young children. However, it's becoming more widely recognised, especially by dentists, that when children suck directly from pouches (especially those with fruits and sugars), it can increase the risk of tooth decay. To reduce this risk, avoid giving your baby or young child the pouch to suck from.

6. **Minimal allergen exposure** – Many pre-prepared baby foods contain few or none of the common allergens in the UK, particularly eggs, peanuts, tree nuts and sesame. This can make introduction and ongoing exposure to allergens challenging.

7. **Cost** – Price is an important consideration – convenience items can be costly. For instance, banana puree pouches range from 70p–£1, while a whole banana costs about 10p. And remember, a higher price doesn't always indicate better quality!

Why and how to introduce common food allergens during weaning

Introducing common food allergens during weaning can make even the most laid-back parents uneasy. In the UK, around four to five per cent of children now have a food allergy, and media coverage on food allergies has notably increased in recent years. While it may be tempting to delay introducing these foods, UK research over the last 10 years has shown that one of the best ways to prevent food allergies is to introduce common allergens early, ideally before 12 months of age.

Note: Before you rush to the nearest A&E with a jar of peanut butter, rest assured that severe reactions like anaphylaxis are rare in babies and young children.

This might seem to contradict what you've heard, as over 20 years ago many parents were advised to postpone introducing foods such as peanuts to their children. This strategy, however, resulted in a rise in peanut allergies. Changes in recommendations followed research which was initiated after noting that cultures where babies were fed common allergenic foods, like peanuts, right from the outset of weaning had significantly lower allergy rates to these foods.

When I speak with parents, I often use this helpful analogy: delaying the introduction of allergenic foods is keeping the door open for allergies. To 'close the door', it's beneficial to introduce these foods to babies early on. In the next pages, I'll cover:

✧ What are the common food allergens?

✧ What is the difference between a food allergy and a food intolerance?

✧ What are the symptoms of food allergy?

✧ How to introduce common food allergens to your baby

What are the common food allergens?

While a child can be allergic to anything, there are nine food allergies that are most commonly seen in children in the UK. These are: cow's milk, egg, soy, peanut, wheat, fish, shellfish, tree nuts and sesame.

Across the world, the list of common allergens varies from country to country, as they tend to reflect the local diet. For example, legume allergy is more common in India, and bird's-nest allergy in Singapore. Interestingly, we are seeing an increasing number of children in the UK with allergies to foods such as peas, legumes, oats and coconut, which probably reflects that more of these foods have entered our food system and diet over the last 5–10 years.

What is the difference between a food allergy and a food intolerance?

Food allergy and intolerance are often confused, as symptoms can be similar, but they are very different conditions.

Food allergy – This is always a response from the body's immune system. The role of the body's immune system is to keep us safe from unwanted invaders like germs and harmful substances. With food allergy, the immune system (think of it like the bouncer at the door) gets it wrong and thinks a particular food protein, such as milk protein, is a threat. It generates an immune response when that food is eaten. The symptoms of a food allergy result from the immune system's response to that food allergen. Symptoms can be immediate (within two hours) or delayed (two to 72 hours) after eating a food – more on these two types of food allergy below.

Allergic symptoms can appear with the first exposure to a food. However, some children may become sensitised after initial exposures before showing an allergic reaction. This means the first exposure may not cause an allergic response, but later exposures could.

Food intolerance – This is usually when the body has difficulty digesting a particular food, which may be due to a lack of the necessary enzymes (mini scissors) to digest the food properly. Food intolerance doesn't trigger an immune response. Instead, it can lead to symptoms like tummy pain, bloating or diarrhoea after eating a particular food.

For babies, a common mix-up is between Cow's Milk Protein Allergy (CMPA) and lactose intolerance. CMPA is an immune-system response to milk protein, whereas lactose intolerance (rare in babies) occurs when the sugar (lactose) in cow's milk cannot be properly digested.

What are the symptoms of food allergy?

The symptoms of food allergies in children vary based on the type of allergic reaction. There are two categories: immediate (IgE mediated), where symptoms appear rapidly – within minutes or up to two hours after eating – or delayed (non-IgE mediated), where symptoms arise anywhere from two to 72 hours later.

Allergy symptoms usually affect multiple body systems and individuals react differently. Here are the most common symptoms of immediate and delayed food allergy.

Immediate-type food allergy (IgE mediated)

Skin: Hives (nettle rash, wheals), rash, itching, immediate eczema flare, redness and/or swelling.
Gut: Vomiting, diarrhoea, nausea.
Respiratory: Sneezing, runny nose, congestion, coughing, wheezing, shortness of breath, hoarse cry or cough.
Anaphylaxis: Immediate symptoms, which can include the above, affecting the airway, breathing and circulation. Requires immediate medical attention. See more information below.

Delayed-type food allergy (Non-IgE mediated)

Skin: Persistent eczema that does not improve with skin treatment (may be widespread), itching.

Gut: Reflux, vomiting, abdominal (tummy) pain, diarrhoea, constipation, excess mucus in poo, blood in poo. *Note: some children present with a rare type of delayed food allergy called Food Protein Enterocolitis Syndrome (FPIES). These children present with profuse, severe vomiting, one to four or more hours after consuming a food, often alongside other symptoms such as diarrhoea, dehydration and lethargy. It is often misdiagnosed as a tummy bug or even sepsis.*
Other: Refusing milk or food, slow growth.

If you suspect your child has symptoms of either type of food allergy, you should seek medical advice from your GP. In the case of any immediate reactions, especially anaphylaxis – a severe allergic reaction that can be life-threatening – seek immediate emergency support by phoning 999 and stating 'anaphylaxsis'. Anaphylaxis happens very quickly and includes symptoms such as swelling of the tongue or throat, difficulty breathing, feeling faint or becoming floppy or unresponsive, fast breathing and skin that feels cold to touch.

How to introduce common food allergens to your baby

After some initial first foods, you can start introducing allergenic foods, focusing on eggs and peanuts first based on the research we have and how common these allergies are. The order of introducing other allergens after these is up to you.

Before you start, make sure you and your baby are well prepared. Here are some of my tips:

✧ Only offer one new allergenic food at a time – if your baby does react, we want to know the culprit.

✧ Start with a small amount and build up gradually, for example, a quarter of a teaspoon, increasing slowly over the next few days. You may wish to leave two or three days between doses of some allergens, such as egg or wheat, to check for delayed reactions.

✧ Offer the food earlier in the day (and ideally on a day where you don't have too many plans) to allow you time to monitor for any signs of reaction.

✧ If your baby is unwell, avoid offering allergens for the first time. This way, you won't have to second-guess whether symptoms are illness-related or allergy.

✧ Ideally, if your baby has eczema, you want to ensure it's as well controlled as possible before offering allergens. The reality with eczema is that because it can flare for various reasons, there may never be a perfect time, but ensuring you have a good skin-management plan before weaning is ideal. Early, aggressive treatment of eczema may help prevent food allergies from forming.

✧ Don't worry if your baby won't eat it. The temptation can be to try to 'get it in', especially if you've emotionally worked up to introducing a specific allergen that day, but it's important to consider your baby's overall feeding experience. Force-feeding is never recommended.

✧ Consider the best way of supporting your baby's consumption of the allergenic food. Often, parents find that puree or mashed foods initially are easier to guarantee consumption of the allergen, compared to offering them as baby-led style finger food. This will depend on your baby's skills and progress with eating at the stage at which each allergen is introduced.

✧ Familiarise yourself with the common signs and symptoms of a food allergy before introducing these foods, which I've outlined above.

✧ You might find a planner, tracker or weaning diary helpful in remembering the allergens introduced and any concerns you have.

Should allergy tests be performed before introducing common allergens?

Most babies will not have allergy testing before introducing potential allergenic foods. The reality is that even children considered at higher risk of developing food allergies may have to wait weeks or months for testing. Food-allergy testing alone doesn't diagnose a food allergy but instead provides guidance on the likelihood of allergy. Therefore, introducing allergenic foods early and monitoring for any reactions is often recommended, unless advised otherwise by a healthcare professional.

While there are plenty of food-allergy or intolerance tests available online, <u>please don't be tempted to buy them</u>. They are not an accurate or effective way to diagnose allergy or intolerance, and I see so many children unnecessarily avoiding foods because of them.

Regardless of recommendations, you should also never rub food on your baby's skin. This method is not a valid 'test' for allergies before introducing new foods. It provides no insight into how your baby will react to a food, could irritate their skin and might lead you to delay introducing it unnecessarily. This practice could also increase the likelihood of sensitisation to the food for babies at higher risk, such as those with eczema. *Don't rub, just give them the grub!*

✧ If a food or allergen causes your baby to have an allergic reaction, or you suspect food allergy, avoid offering it again and seek support from a health professional – accurate diagnosis is important to make sure your child gets the right support, and isn't excluding any foods unnecessarily.

✧ Once an allergen has been successfully introduced (with no signs of reaction), keep it in their diet! I can't stress this enough. Maintaining that allergen within a child's diet is just as important as the introduction. To help, I've included some easy meal or food suggestions for maintenance for each allergen below, as well as how much to aim for (where we have evidence to support this).

Beyond what's mentioned above, when introducing allergens, the same principles also apply as for introducing other foods during weaning – the texture and type of food should be suitable for the child's developmental stage to minimise risks such as choking and keep them safe. So for each of the top nine food allergens, I've detailed some suggestions of how to initially offer this to your baby, alongside food options to help maintain each one within the diet.

Allergen	How to introduce	Ways to help maintain intake
Egg	Hard-boil an egg for 10 minutes, then blend the yolk and white together. Puree/mash – Mix the above with something your baby has had before, such as mashed vegetables. Finger foods – Omelette strips, or mix with mashed avocado and spread on toast.	Boiled egg fingers. Scrambled egg. Omelette. Frittata/quiche. Eggy bread. Egg muffins. Pancakes. Egg-fried rice. Add to fish pie or toast. *Note: The current recommended 'maintenance' dose for egg, particularly babies and children at higher risk of food allergy, is one whole egg a week – half an egg twice per week.*

Peanut	Choose a smooth peanut butter (100 per cent peanuts) or use well-ground/milled unsalted peanuts. Peanut butter can be tacky, so loosen with warm water or milk and never offer undiluted directly from a spoon. Puree/mash – You can stir nuts into porridge, yoghurt or fruit. Finger foods – Spread peanut butter onto fingers of sweet potato, pancake, toast or soft fruit slices.	Peanut butter spread on toast or pancakes, soft crackers or baby biscuits. Peanut butter or ground peanuts stirred into porridge, cereals or muffins. Peanut butter blended into curry, stir-fry sauce, such as satay, fruit purees or yoghurt. **The current recommended 'maintenance' dose for peanuts, particularly babies and children at higher risk of food allergy is 2g of peanut protein two or three times per week. One 2g dose looks like:** **1 heaped tsp smooth peanut butter, or** **20g (two-thirds) of a bag of Bamba™.**
Milk For babies who are formula or combination fed they are already having regular exposure to cow's milk protein	Puree/mashed – Plain natural or Greek yoghurt, cow's milk added to oats. Finger foods – Porridge fingers made with cow's milk, cream cheese spread on toast, white/cheese sauce on pasta pieces.	Milk in cereals or porridge. Yoghurt. Cream cheese, such as in pasta sauce, on toast, stirred through vegetables. Hard cheese.

Wheat	Puree/mashed – Wheat-based cereal mixed with milk (ensure cow's milk has been trialled already or use baby's normal milk), couscous or small pasta pieces mixed into a meal. Finger foods – Toast, pancake or muffin slices	Plain cereals, such as wheat biscuits. Bread and other products containing flour, such as pancakes, muffins, fritters, chapati. Pasta. Couscous. Bulgur wheat.
Soya	Puree/mashed – Plain soya yoghurt or soya milk mixed with your baby's normal cereal. Finger foods – Some babies also have their first exposure to soya in the form of soya flour, which can be found in many breads. Tofu fingers.	Soy flour – found within bread products. Tofu. Edamame beans (serve appropriately for your baby such as crushed/blended). Unsweetened soy yoghurt. Soy milk alternative. Soy-based mince.
Tree nuts, such as almonds, pecans, cashews , pistachios, Brazil nuts, hazelnuts, macadamia nuts, walnuts, hazelnuts. *Note: coconut and pine nuts are not tree nuts*	Choose a smooth nut butter (no added salt or sugar) or use well-ground/milled nuts, such as ground almonds (you can place whole nuts in a blender or food processor if you cannot buy them already milled). Nut butter can be tacky, so loosen it with warm water or milk and never offer undiluted directly from a spoon. Puree/mash – You can stir nuts into porridge, yoghurt or fruit that's been mashed or pureed. Finger foods – spread nut butter onto fingers of sweet potato, pancake slices, toast or fruit slices.	Nut butter on toast or pancakes. Nut butter or well-ground nuts added to yoghurt or fruit. Milled/ground nuts added to porridge, cereal or baking mix, such as pancake. Milled nuts stirred through stews and curries.

Sesame	Puree/mash – hummus, smooth tahini mixed into yoghurt or fruit/vegetables. Finger food – tahini or hummus spread onto toast, pancake or fruit/vegetable pieces. If using sesame seeds, make sure these are finely ground before offering (as babies need exposure to the protein inside the seed).	Hummus, such as on toast, in sandwiches, as a dip. Tahini – Spread on toast (great with fruit), stirred into yoghurt, drizzled over pancakes or porridge, included in baking, such as muffins, biscuits, in a dressing with oil and lemon juice, such as for potatoes, vegetables.
Fish	Softly cook or poach white or oily fish or choose a tinned fish (in spring water, not salty brine). Puree/mash – You can combine flaked fish with potato or a preferred vegetable. Finger food – flakes of fish, fish mixed into a fish cake or tot.	Fish pie. Fish cakes. Fish pieces – roasted or poached. Fish pasta such as tuna pasta bake. Fish fingers.
Shellfish (*Note: shellfish allergies are not common in children*)	Consider offering shellfish you commonly have at home. Ensure it is fresh and well cooked the whole way through. Puree/mash – Blend or mince and add to potato or a preferred vegetable. Finger food – mix into potato tot/cake, or add into any option to the right.	Prawn or crab cakes. Seafood pasta. Curry or stew. Crab or prawn as sandwich filling.

Note: When it comes to maintenance amounts, this is a guide. There will be times when this isn't feasible, and your baby will not take this amount and that is ok. The main message is to continue it in their diet regularly.

What if you don't eat certain allergens as a family?

In situations where a family avoids animal products, for example, you won't plan for common allergens like eggs or fish in your child's diet. In this case, I would generally recommend that if a food isn't going to be maintained in the diet in the long term, it isn't introduced as a one-off. If your child is at high risk for food allergies, consider discussing the risks and benefits of avoiding common food allergens with an allergy specialist, such as a dietitian or allergist, to help inform your decision-making.

What if there is a food allergy in the family?

This can make introducing that particular food tricky to your baby, but it can be done carefully, ensuring the allergic family member is safeguarded. Suggestions I often make to families include:

❖ Introducing or giving the food via a non-allergic caregiver or family member.

❖ Ensuring the food is stored carefully to prevent cross-contamination.

❖ Carefully cleaning the area where the food has been prepared and eaten following good hygiene practices, such as cleaning with warm water and soap.

❖ Ensure your baby's face, hands and body are cleaned up carefully after eating, and a change of clothes is provided, if necessary.

Should you introduce gluten to your baby if there
is a history of coeliac disease in your family?

Studies are exploring whether the timing of gluten introduction affects the risk of developing coeliac disease. However, there is currently no evidence to suggest that you should avoid introducing gluten to your baby. It's recommended to introduce gluten-containing foods gradually (as above) and continue to monitor your baby for symptoms going forwards. The age of coeliac disease onset can vary across childhood and adulthood.

Continuing fluids as part of weaning

As your baby starts solids, it's important to also introduce and start offering fluids as part of their diet. While breast or formula milk remains a key source of fluids during this time, as weaning progresses fluid from water and foods will become more important for your baby's hydration. Introducing water also helps your baby learn an important feeding skill – cup drinking! in the next pages I'm going to cover:

✧ **How to manage a baby's milk feeds during weaning**

✧ **Introducing water (and cups)**

How to manage a baby's milk feeds during weaning

As you start the juggle of offering your baby solids and milk feeds from six months of age, it's common for parents to wonder how milk feeds need to be managed. Here are some key considerations for managing milk feeds from the start of weaning and beyond.

✧ Remember that breast or formula milk feeds will still significantly contribute towards energy and nutrients to meet your baby's nutritional requirements during weaning.

✧ When you begin the weaning process, your baby will likely continue their usual milk feeds as they start exploring food and the skills associated with eating. It might be a good idea to provide a milk feed about 30–45 minutes before solids, then as needed afterwards, although this will vary from baby to baby.

✧ As weaning progresses, it's likely that your baby will naturally start to reduce the amounts of milk they accept. This may mean lowering the frequency of their feeds and/or the amount (volume) they want at each feed. Listen to your baby, as their ability to self-regulate means they are likely to accept as much as their body needs. In formula-fed babies, if you find milk volumes are not reducing several months into weaning and your baby has a lack of interest in food, it may be worth checking in on total milk intake.

✧ You may find milk feeds increase again at times when your baby is unwell or teething – and therefore temporarily finds eating more of a challenge. This is normal, so try not to worry. Your baby should pick back up with solids again once they are feeling better.

✧ It's likely as your baby progresses towards three meals a day that you may find yourself in more of a routine with milk feeds and solids; for example, milk feed in the morning, breakfast, milk feed mid-morning, lunch, milk feed mid-afternoon, evening meal, milk feed before bed. Feeding (milk or solids) may be every two to three hours.

✧ For breastfed babies, it's vital to remember they feed for other reasons, such as comfort, so routines around milk feeds often remain variable around food and may be less 'structured' than those of formula-fed babies.

✧ If you're worried that your baby isn't progressing with solids or is having too much milk, speak with your health visitor, who can advise on appropriate milk volumes and routine adjustments, or check back to page 53 for milk volumes by age.

Follow-on formula or 'Stage 2' milk

Follow-on formula milk is advertised as suitable from six months of age. Typically this contains slightly higher amounts of certain nutrients such as iron, vitamin D and zinc, and may have a different ratio of protein – such as more casein and less whey than first formula milks. It's important to know that you don't have to switch your baby from first-stage formula to follow-on formula at six months. In fact, follow-on formulas are generally considered unnecessary.

Introducing water (and cups)

Here's another exciting new thing to introduce – water! Naturally, it's yet another skill your baby needs to learn, so it will take some time.

When can you introduce water?

Water can be introduced to your baby alongside meals at around six months or when you begin weaning. Some babies benefit from having the water offered at the end of the meal initially to enable them to focus on one skill at a time.

Which water?

For babies under six months, offer cooled, boiled tap water if needed. From six months onward, tap water is safe to offer your baby, but avoid bottled and mineral water due to their high mineral content. If tap water is not an option when travelling abroad, choose bottled water that's low in sodium (ideally under 200mg per litre) and with less than 250mg per litre of sulphates.

How much should your baby be drinking?

As your baby progresses through weaning and gradually picks up the skills for cup drinking, they will begin to drink a little more, but there's no need to number crunch this or push specific water recommendations under 12 months of age. Remember, your baby also gets fluids from milk and food; most babies are good at regulating how much they need and want to drink. So just make sure you keep offering water with meals. Additionally, for breastfed babies, I often remind parents that breast milk is a rich source of hydration, so it can be common for babies still having lots of milk feeds not to drink much water.

One of the best ways to monitor your baby's hydration is their nappies! If they have regular wet nappies with light straw-coloured urine, they will likely get enough fluids throughout the day.

What about other drinks?

Babies only need water or their usual breast or formula milk. Cow's milk should not be offered as a drink to babies under 12 months of age. Avoid juices, 'baby' teas, or fizzy or flavoured drinks.

Which cup should you choose for your baby?

Cup choices can often feel overwhelming due to the wide variety available. I frequently hear from parents who have cupboards full of the things, usually because they've bought several types to encourage fluid intake. When selecting a cup, remember, the goal is to help your baby learn to sip from a cup with free-flowing liquid.

My top choices for weaning cups are:

✦ An open cup – You can find options designed for easy grip and small hands that hold only a small amount of liquid. These will help your baby get used to managing free-flowing liquids, and learn how to sip – and ultimately it's the type of cup most of us use day to day.

✧ A weighted straw cup – This is an excellent option for minimal spills, but it will take some time for your baby to master the lip closure and suck up a straw. I recommend introducing it around eight to nine months of age after you've begun with an open cup. Choose options with a short and firm straw.

✧ A free-flow sippy cup (without a valve) is also an option during weaning.

It's likely that it will take months for your baby to master drinking from a cup, and as they do so there will be water everywhere, along with some coughing, spluttering and plenty of mess. But please know that most babies can grasp cup drinking with plenty of practice; be consistent and stick with one or two cups, and be sure to model cup drinking yourself. Watching you drink from a cup will help your baby learn.

Building a balanced plate for your baby

The best way to support your baby to get the nutrients they need now and moving forward into the early years is to offer plenty of variety and a balance of foods across different food groups. I promise that being balanced and varied doesn't mean having eight foods on your baby's plate. Focusing on some key mealtime components is enough for most babies once they're on their way with weaning and you're building mini meals.

Here's a simple formula for meal planning for your baby:

Energy-rich food + iron-rich food + vitamin-C-rich food

My top tip is to start with your family meals and food as a baseline – what can you use or adjust from the meals you prepare for your family this week?

I'm very aware that for parents, thinking about baby and children's food in the context of nutrients can sometimes seem intimidating, and can risk making feeding too scientific. For these reasons, I wanted to break down the above formula into food and meal examples. I hope this reassures you that meals you have at home are likely to contain many of the key nutrients I've discussed already, so with a little bit of planning you can easily ensure you offer your baby all the nutrients they need.

In the next pages, I'm going to cover:

✧ **How to offer your baby a variety of foods**

✧ **Supplements for your baby at 6–12 months**

How to offer your baby a variety of foods

I will sound like a broken record in this book, but I will keep returning to the importance of dietary variety and diversity. In short, this means offering your baby and family different foods whenever possible. Research has shown, and continues to show, that providing variety in the foods we eat can:

✧ Improve nutrient intake.

✧ Support a healthy gut.

✧ Reduce the risk of food allergies.

✧ Enhance food acceptance and long-term eating habits.

Introducing a variety of foods early can make mealtimes more interesting for your baby and help foster a more adventurous palate as they grow. I also recognise that offering variety can increase the mental load of parenting and is influenced by your family's dietary habits and resources. With that in mind, here are some practical suggestions to introduce your baby to a diverse diet that I hope shouldn't overwhelm you or your routine.

Iron-rich food	Vitamin C-rich food	Energy-rich food
Meat, such as beef, lamb, mutton, goat Poultry, such as chicken, turkey Oily fish, such as sardines, salmon, mackerel Eggs Lentils, beans, pulses Soya, such as tofu Fortified cereals	Vegetables and/or fruit (These are also a great source of fibre)	Starchy carbohydrates, such as rice, potato, plantain, bread, chapati, rice, pasta, cereals, oats, noodles, buck-wheat, couscous, polenta, plantain, millet, yam Fat source, such as full-fat dairy, oils, avocado, coconut, nuts, seeds Full-fat dairy e.g. milk in food, plain yoghurt, cheese (or milk-free alternatives)
Meal examples (offer suitable texture/dependent on age)		
Lentil dal	Spinach and tomatoes in the dal	Chapati with butter or ghee and/or rice and full-fat yoghurt
Scrambled egg	Kiwi slices	Buttered toast
Roast chicken	Peas and broccoli	Mashed potato with butter and milk added
Stewed chicken	Okra	Millet and roasted yam
Wheat biscuit cereal	Grated pear	(Wheat biscuits) and full-fat milk and a sprin-kle of seeds
Stir-fried tofu	Mixed vegetables, e.g. peppers, onions	Noodles and oil for cooking

✧ Make a plan: Now might be a good time to get into meal planning and put more thought into what you're preparing across the week. We are all creatures of habit, and as parents we seek ease in many areas of our lives, so choosing the same foods during the weekly shop or meals is an understandable default. Planning ahead gives you time to think about easy swaps, new recipes or foods to introduce across the week.

✧ Don't dismiss the tinned or frozen aisles: You can get a range of foods such as fruits, berries, vegetables and pulses that are cost-effective and nutritious. For example, you could pick up a different type of tinned bean, fruit or bag of frozen vegetables each week.

✧ Make simple swaps to meals: If you usually have a cheese sauce with pasta, swap it for a vegetable-based sauce instead. Use different herbs or spices in a meal or pick a different vegetable that you wouldn't usually try at home.

✧ Easy add-ins: I love meals that are an easy vehicle to add variety easily. Using porridge as an example, you could:
   o Add different fruits – tinned, frozen or grated.
   o Stir in different extras like ground nuts, seeds or yoghurt.
   o Bake the oats or leave them to soak overnight instead of offering warm porridge.

Supplements for your baby at 6–12 months

The UK Department of Health has clear guidelines for vitamin supplements for all babies in the UK that are based on research and studies identifying the nutrients that children in specific age groups may lack. Below, I've summarised these recommendations based on your baby's feeding method.

Breastfed babies six+ months:

✧ Your baby should now move on to a combined vitamin A, C and D supplement*.

Combination and formula-fed babies:

✧ Your baby should move on to a combined vitamin A, C and D supplement* once they have <500ml of formula milk daily. This is because formula milk already contains these vitamins.

You should continue this supplementation until your child goes to school.

> ***Recommended amounts of each vitamin daily**
> A – 200 micrograms
> C – 20 milligrams
> D – 10 micrograms

Note: Of all the vitamins mentioned, vitamin D is arguably the most important for your baby. Since most vitamin D comes from sunlight, getting enough at certain times of the year can be challenging. There are few good dietary sources, so even a well-balanced diet may not provide sufficient daily intake.

While supplementation is still recommended for vitamins A and C, evidence suggests that babies and children with a balanced diet are likely get enough from food alone. Recent 2023 data indicates that the recommendation for vitamin C supplementation may be discontinued, although there are minimal risks if you continue to supplement. For reference, half a kiwi or a handful of strawberries meets your baby or toddler's daily vitamin C requirements.

Some babies may need additional vitamin and mineral supplementation under the advice of a health professional, including babies who:

❖ Are born prematurely.

❖ Are following a predominantly plant-based, vegetarian or vegan diet.

❖ Have one or multiple food allergies.

❖ Have delayed development and associated slower progression through weaning or difficulty achieving a varied age-appropriate diet.

Top tips for picking a suitable supplement

❖ The Healthy Start scheme allows England, Wales and Northern Ireland residents entitled to certain benefits to obtain free vitamin supplements for their babies and toddlers.

❖ All children under three years of age in Scotland are entitled to free vitamin D supplements via the Best Start Foods Programme.

❖ Check the following in your supplement:
　o Vitamin D is provided as vitamin D3 (Colecalciferol) whenever possible, as the body absorbs it more effectively than vitamin D2.
　o It contains the right amount of vitamin D, 10 ug/400 IU per day. Many multivitamins targeted at babies and young children simply don't contain enough.

❖ Put it in a place where you'll remember to do it! In the pits of sleep deprivation, I had to leave Aurelia's supplement somewhere I'd see it to remember to give it to her. I chose to leave it by my toothbrush, giving me two daily reminders!

❖ Ensure you give only reputable supplements that have been

sourced or purchased from a medical professional, pharmacy or trusted retailer (on the high street or online).

✧ Check the labels carefully if your baby has food allergies. Some preparations can contain common allergens such as milk, soya and peanuts.

Kickstarting a healthy food relationship: supporting your baby's feeding journey

✧ **Understanding responsive feeding once you start solids**

✧ **Understanding when your baby is hungry and full**

✧ **Responsive spoon feeding**

✧ **Creating the ideal mealtime for your baby**

Understanding responsive feeding once you start solids

It may be bold to say, but *how* you feed your baby may be nearly as important as *what* you feed them! Weaning is the ideal time to thoughtfully consider how to feed your baby in a way that fosters healthy eating habits and positive food relationships for life. The key to this goes back to developing a trusting and responsive relationship with your baby at mealtimes, which can significantly benefit your baby's eating habits and mealtime enjoyment.

The World Health Organization acknowledges the importance of responsive feeding through weaning and beyond. Like milk feeding (see page 61), responsive feeding with solids emphasises the two-way relationship between you and your baby. In a shift from rigid routines, schedules and monitoring volumes, responsive feeding with food emphasises nurturing and trusting your baby to recognise their hunger cues and interact with food as they choose.

Over the years I have found supporting parents' confidence with responsive feeding around food can benefit from shining a light on *common* feeding behaviours during weaning, which many parents worry about, such as:

✧ Babies engaging with and playing with food without consuming it.

✧ Mealtimes where little or no food is being eaten.

✧ Extended periods – days or weeks – with a declined appetite or less interest in food (such as when teething, during illness or when other developmental surges are occurring).

✧ Feeling like your baby isn't 'getting it'.

✧ Babies accepting a food one day and rejecting it the next time it's offered.

✧ Throwing food.

✧ Spitting food back out due to lack of skill development or still learning to accept the taste.

✧ Innate preference for certain foods and less so for others – it's normal for your baby to prefer sweet foods like fruit and easier textures like yoghurt.

I wanted to emphasise that these behaviours often trigger parents to think something's wrong with their baby's progress. This can lead to a 'fix-it' mindset, which may divert from responsive-feeding principles like trusting your baby's appetite. For parents, 'fixing' can look like dragging out meals, over-encouraging bites, ignoring cues or offering alternatives that their baby is more likely to accept – often sweeter or pureed foods.

Research shows that caregiver behaviour during meals can impact children's eating. For example, when caregivers are too focused on how much a baby is eating, the child is less likely to accept a variety of foods later. Emotions like anxiety can also increase food refusal, which makes sense biologically since anxiety is a 'contagious' emotion for survival reasons. Being aware of your own eating and mealtime experiences is also helpful. If you grew up and were expected to clear your plate at mealtimes, expecting your baby (or older child) to do the same is understandable and it might feel difficult to move away from this mindset.

When to seek help

There can be some behaviours that *would* signal your baby could benefit from a review or extra support with feeding. These include:

✧ Notable lack of progress across several months with over-all intake or volumes, texture acceptance or finger foods.
✧ No reduction in gagging frequency as weaning progresses.
✧ Behaviours that are not typical for weaning, such as:
  o Regular vomiting and retching.
  o Not swallowing foods at all (except at the first stage of weaning).
  o Holding foods in their mouth.
  o Excess salivation.
  o A panicked look when food is in their mouth.

Understanding when your baby is hungry and full

Once your baby begins weaning, the guide below will help you recognise typical hunger and fullness signals. Babies are great at listening to their bodies, eating when hungry and stopping when full. Watch for the cues outlined below during meals and follow your baby's lead, even if it means they are finishing the meal after just a couple of bites.

You can see some overlap between signs of hunger and fullness, such as crying. Some signals are also more common in older babies (from 8 to 12 months), so they might become more apparent as you progress through weaning.

Understanding baby's feeding cues during weaning

Hunger cues	Fullness cues
Fussing or crying	Closing mouth or clamping it shut
Leaning towards or opening mouth towards a spoon or food pieces	Pushing food, your hand or the spoon away
	Turning head and/or body away from food
Opening mouth	
	Crying or showing stress signals
Opening hands	
	Slowing pace of feeding or getting distracted more easily by surroundings
Gazing or looking at foods	
Exaggerated or expressive facial expressions, smiling, noise or cooing around food	Holding food in the mouth
	Fussing as you bring food towards them
Getting excited around food	Signalling a clear no – a head shake or signing (which can be great to teach babies, such as a sign for 'finished/all done')
Reaching for or pointing to food	
	Throwing food
Showing or expressing wish for certain food or 'more' with sounds , singing or words (older baby)	Vomiting

Responsive spoon feeding

As a parent, spoon feeding may feel like it allows greater control around food, and how much your baby is eating. However, it's important to allow your baby to explore and take the lead whenever possible. Here are some of my tips for being responsive when spoon feeding:

✧ Ensure some of the food you're feeding your baby is accessible to them, such as on the tray directly, or in a bowl/plate within reach. Your baby should still be able to experience the other sensory properties of that food, such as how it looks, smells and feels on their hands.

✧ Avoid the temptation to start whirring around like an aeroplane or choo-chooing like a train!

✧ Bring at least two spoons to the mealtime, and allow your baby to explore and practise with these, working towards feeding themselves. Two-handed spoons can also be great for enabling you to exchange the spoon easily between you and your baby.

✧ Load spoons and place them either directly in front of your baby on the tray or in the air, to allow them to reach and instigate feeding themselves.

✧ Don't forget to model yourself. If parents have a more hands-on role with feeding, it can mean it's harder to sit, eat and model for your baby. You can pause to eat in between supporting your baby's feeding.

✧ Follow your baby's feeding cues carefully, avoiding pressure or force-feeding.

Creating the ideal mealtime for your baby

It's important to consider your baby's mealtime and learning environment. There's nothing like trying to learn a complex set of skills and build confidence when various factors complicate this process! While there are straightforward steps you can take to create a calm and relaxed mealtime – such as turning off screens and ensuring your baby is comfortable in their highchair – the most important factor is you, along with any other caregivers participating in feeding.

Connection with your baby at mealtimes and a calm and supportive relationship will pay off in the long term. In the feeding world, we recognise that 'felt safety' is one of the most important aspects of positive and enjoyable mealtimes. Felt safety recognises that your child needs to feel secure and comfortable in their environment to enjoy and participate in mealtimes fully. Safety is something that children feel and cannot be told. As discussed above, this means creating a relaxed atmosphere, being patient, and responding to their cues and needs.

You can support this at mealtimes with your baby and well beyond into the early years by:

1. **Eating with them** – Try to sit and eat with them whenever possible (see pages 176–7 for more on this). Babies look to trusted adults for reassurance, and a primary way they learn anything is through modelling. Sharing meals fosters these skills and makes mealtimes enjoyable for both of you. I know you may not be thrilled about broccoli puree at 11am on a Monday, but rest assured, your baby won't be focused on how much you eat but rather on what you're eating and your reactions.
2. **Giving them some autonomy** – Babies need to be given time, space and patience to learn new skills, and this couldn't be more true than with feeding. While it's tempting to intervene when they keep flipping the spoon or missing their mouth, don't steal the struggle! Problem solving builds competence.

3. **Lending them your calm** – No one eats well when feeling anxious or tense. Your baby is naturally attuned to your body signals and uses them to gauge safety. If you're nervous or stressed at mealtimes, they'll sense it and may not feel comfortable eating, thinking something is wrong. I understand first-hand how stressful parenting can be, but if mealtimes are becoming tricky, try to calm your nervous system beforehand with a short walk, deep breathing (or 4–7–8 breathing), or by reading the feeding mantras at the back of this book.

4. **Remember your role in the feeding relationship** – Making your child eat something is not your job (read that again, because I know it feels counterintuitive). Yes, you can support the environment and the opportunity to explore and eat food, but ultimately, you can't make your child eat unless you start using tactics like force-feeding, distraction or pressure, none of which I would ever recommend. Many parents benefit from understanding a mealtime relationship coined by Ellyn Satter (registered dietitian, family therapist, and internationally recognised expert on eating and feeding) called the 'Division Of Responsibility'. This recognises that the role of the caregiver is to 'provide', for example, the mealtime routine and foods, and it's a child's job to 'decide' what they eat, how much they eat and in what order the foods are eaten.

SOS – Frequently asked questions or worries when starting solids

Here are the most common questions I get from parents about weaning.

My baby was born prematurely – when should I start solids?

Any baby born before 37 weeks is considered premature. However, there will be significant differences between babies born extremely prematurely – for example, before 28 weeks of age – and those born moderately to late preterm – after 32 weeks of age – regarding when they are developmentally in the right place to start solids.

Bliss, the UK's leading charity for babies born prematurely, recommends that five months <u>corrected age</u> is usually the youngest that a premature baby will show the readiness signs above and have the skills to start solids. (The corrected age is calculated by subtracting the number of weeks or months the baby was early from the time they were born. For example, if a baby was born 16 weeks ago and was 11 weeks early, their corrected age is five weeks.) Around six months corrected age, many premature babies are ready to start solids, although some may need a little longer. If your baby doesn't seem developmentally ready to go by around seven months corrected age, I suggest you seek support from your neonatal team or a dietitian.

From a practical point of view, premature babies often need adaptations to weaning equipment. For example, many will be smaller than their peers and seem lost in certain highchairs, requiring additional support or alternative seating options.

Should I start solids early if my baby has reflux or slow weight gain?

I regularly speak to parents who have been told to start solids early for one or both of these reasons. I've combined these questions here because for both circumstances no strong scientific evidence supports starting solids early (before six months of age) as a 'magic bullet' for managing either concern. I will briefly delve into a few points for each condition below.

Reflux – Early weaning is often recommended with the justification that solids may thicken stomach contents and, therefore, reduce reflux symptoms, but there isn't strong evidence to support this. Consider discussing other reflux-management options with your healthcare professional before early weaning.

Slow weight gain – If you have concerns about your baby's growth and haven't already done so, I want to urge you to discuss this with a health professional. While food seems a logical choice for weight gain, your baby's consumption in the first few weeks is likely minimal, and the calorie content of food may not be high. For example, your baby's milk is around 66–67 kcals/100ml, whereas vegetable puree may be more like 30–40 kcals/100g. I would always recommend optimised milk feeding first.

What is the difference between gagging and choking? How do I keep my baby safe?

Gagging and choking are often confused but they are very different events. Gagging is a common occurrence during the early days and weeks of solids. Signs of gagging in babies may include: facial redness, retching, tongue thrusting, watering eyes and coughing. It is a protective reflex designed to help protect the airway from foods entering it (choking/aspiration). Babies' gag reflexes are triggered further forward in the mouth as weaning starts and gradually move back to the adult position over a few months. Gagging also occurs more typically in babies as they are still mastering their oral motor skills, and it's not uncommon to struggle to control food in their mouths, causing gagging.

Choking occurs when a piece of food has entered the airway, causing a partial or complete blockage. It happens much less frequently (it is rare) but is a severe event, as it restricts or blocks airflow (breathing). Signs of choking include a silent or weak cough, inability to breathe or speak, loss of colour from the face or lips and a panicked expression. In darker-skinned babies, look for changes in skin colour, such as a grey or ashen tone.

If your baby is gagging, stay calm and let them handle it. Avoid putting your fingers in their mouth, as this can cause choking. Gagging helps push food forward to prevent choking.

If your baby is choking and can't breathe or cough, take immediate action to clear the airway and seek emergency support.

Learning baby CPR and first aid is very helpful, as it supports parents to respond confidently and effectively to choking. To reduce the risk, ensure your baby's food is prepared to the appropriate size, texture and consistency, and always sit with your baby when they are eating.

I've heard salt is bad for babies. How do I avoid them eating too much salt during weaning?

Babies shouldn't have more than 1g of salt per day (less than ¼ teaspoon) because their kidneys can't handle too much.

Salt can quickly add up! If you're doing baby-led weaning (BLW), your baby might encounter more salt than babies being weaned onto purees, as many family foods, such as bread items and cheese, contain natural or added salt.

As a guide, I suggest considering your baby's salt intake over a few days rather than daily number-crunching. It's ok if some days there is a little more salt used as long as there is minimal intake on other days. It can also be helpful to be mindful of or limit the following foods:

✧ Processed meats, like sausages or ham.

✧ Gravy powders and stock cubes – swap for low-salt salt or no-added-salt alternatives.

✧ Hard cheese, such as Cheddar or Parmesan – be mindful of portion size and incorporate lower-salt cheese such as ricotta or mascarpone.

✧ Pies, pasties, Scotch eggs, sausage rolls and other processed savoury foods.

✧ Condiments like ketchup – swap for lower salt (and sugar) options if using.

✧ Tinned foods with high salt content, like soups, baked beans or tinned spaghetti (you can choose tinned fish and vegetables in spring water instead of brine).

✧ Salted fish, such as saltfish or smoked salmon.

✧ Some breads – check the label carefully and aim for a bread that contains <0.3–0.4g salt per slice.

How can I help my baby use cutlery?

Learning to eat with cutlery takes time, and I always reassure parents that it's normal for babies and young children to use their hands to eat! Mastery of all cutlery can take until around seven years of age, and I wouldn't expect a baby to be very proficient with a spoon until one year or older (depending on how much practice they have had). You can support your child's cutlery skills in the following ways:

✧ Preload spoons and forks – let your baby pick them up and bring them to their mouth – they may miss or flip a spoon initially, but that's ok!

✧ Role-modelling – eat with your child so they can watch you using cutlery and start to mimic you.

✧ Choose ergonomic cutlery – those with wider, thicker handles are more manageable for your baby to hold, and those with shorter handles are easier for your baby to take to their mouth.

✧ Provide opportunities – the more they practise, the more efficient they will be. To help them, offer foods that are easy to stab with a fork or scoop with a spoon.

✧ Give them time – these skills take practice and patience.

My baby seems to have a sensitive gag reflex and I'm struggling to move past purees.

You can identify a sensitive gag reflex in your baby if they often gag right from the beginning of weaning and this does not seem to lessen as they gain more experience with food. Some groups of children are more likely to have an over-sensitive gag reflex, such as premature babies, those with reflux or developmental delay.

As a result of a sensitive gag reflex, you may find your baby can manage if a texture is very smooth or runny but struggles if it is thicker, lumpy or more mashed than pureed. If you're struggling to progress past purees due to a sensitive gag reflex, I suggest:

✧ Offering dissolvable/meltable finger foods (such as puffs, corn-based sticks), especially if you're nervous about introducing finger foods.

✧ Trying long, hard finger foods (sometimes called hard munchable – see page 99) that cannot break easily in a young baby's mouth, such as peeled whole carrot or celery stick, or a teether with a Y shape, that baby can use to explore further back in their mouth.

✧ Ensuring you're allowing your baby sensory experiences around food, such as touching, smelling and exploring, as well as the opportunity to take their hands to their mouth with foods on them.

✧ Check your baby is well supported in their seating position.

✧ Make small changes to your baby's food texture, such as moving from very smooth shop-bought purees to homemade purees, or homemade purees to very well-mashed or grainier food.

If gagging persists and you would like some additional support, discuss it with your GP or health visitor, who can refer you to a feeding and swallowing specialist speech-and-language therapist.

Does my baby have to avoid all wholegrain foods?

Making sense of fibre intake in babies can feel tricky. Much advice to date can recommend blanket avoidance of all wholegrain or very high-fibre foods, due to concerns about the impact of a baby having too much fibre on their overall energy and nutrient intake. There are no specific fibre recommendations for children under two, however, we do know that a variety of fibre in a child's diet, including during weaning, can support health and feed their growing community of good gut bacteria. With this in mind, wholegrains don't need complete avoidance, and you can include some wholegrain foods as part of a balanced weaning diet alongside fibre from foods like fruit, vegetables, beans, pulses, nuts and seeds. Many parents find using a variety of carbohydrate options helpful, so swapping or mixing between white and wholemeal bread, for example, or including a 50:50 version. The one option to give a wide birth to during weaning would be bran, as this is very high in fibre and may cause some digestive discomfort.

My baby has started throwing food, what do I do?

I can empathise fully with how annoying this phase is. I'm afraid to say it may not be limited to weaning, but I'm pleased to say it's a normal developmental phase. It too shall pass! Babies can throw food for many reasons, but in those aged between six and 12 months, they may throw food because:

✧ They are learning something called a trajectory schema – understanding how objects move through the air (in this case, downwards!).

✧ They are exploring cause and effect – seeing what happens when they throw food, how it sounds and looks, and how you react!

✧ They might be bored or not hungry anymore – signalling they're done with the meal.

✧ They are seeking attention – wanting to see your reaction.

To help manage this phase, I suggest to parents that they:

✧ Keep calm and a little nonchalant about the food throwing – avoid big reactions.

✧ Try offering smaller amounts of food on the plate or tray initially.

✧ End the mealtime if they think their baby has finished eating.

✧ Eat with their child, if they're not already, providing attention throughout the meal, rather than only when their baby demonstrates a certain behaviour like food throwing.

✧ Use clear and calm language instead of a 'no', and communicate clearly, such as 'Your food is down on the floor, but food stays up on the table'.

My baby seems to develop a red rash or blotches on their mouth and face after eating certain foods. Is this an allergy?
Some foods that babies consume during weaning can cause what is known as a contact reaction, irritation or contact dermatitis. This type of reaction presents as localised skin redness and blotchiness, usually where food has touched the skin on the face and hands. Redness in darker skin may be harder to see and appear dark brown, purple or grey. It is commonly caused by foods that

are acidic, salty or rich in natural chemicals such as histamine. Common culprits include (but are not limited to) tomato, kiwi, strawberry, acidic fruits (or products/jars that use acidic fruit juice in the ingredients), aubergine, spinach and more. This rash should not spread, should cause minimal irritation to your baby and will go down without treatment. While it's understandable to worry, this type of reaction is *not* a food allergy, and there is no need for your baby to avoid these foods. Babies have delicate skin, especially those with eczema, so if you find that your baby develops contact reactions like this, consider applying a barrier cream or emollient moisturiser around their mouth and face before eating.

Does my baby need snacks? When should these be introduced?

In the UK, the NHS advises that snacks do not need to be included in a baby's diet until they are around 12 months of age. For many babies you can continue to offer breast or formula milk in between planned meals as you progress through weaning. I cover more about balanced snacks and managing snacking on pages 160–2 and 191–2.

Can my baby have spices?

Spices (and herbs) can absolutely be included in your baby's diet from the start of weaning and are actually a wonderful way of supporting dietary variety and the development of a broad palate in children. Just be careful with hot chilli, it can cause upset for small mouths and stomachs.

My baby's poo has changed, is this normal?

Yes! Your baby's gut is adapting from a milk-only diet to eating a variety of new foods – so expect a variety of 'new' poo! Here are some poo changes which are common to see during weaning.

✧ **Changes in the frequency of bowel movements** – Many babies develop thicker and firmer stools and poo less frequently as weaning progresses. Some babies may poo more regularly, or you might experience fluctuation in stool frequency or type across the weeks.

✧ **Colour changes** – Often stools can become darker in colour, but it's also worth noting that they can be affected by the colours of food your baby is consuming too – lots of greens, expect a greener poo!

✧ **Smell** – Stools often become stronger or more distinct-smelling.

✧ **Undigested pieces of food** – Particularly fruit or vegetable skins, seeds, husks, grains or whole 'pieces' of food such as sweetcorn, which are difficult to digest, can often appear unchanged in baby's poo. Don't be alarmed when undigested food makes a surprise appearance – your baby doesn't yet have the teeth or skills to grind down these foods, which move more quickly through a baby's digestive tract.

Help, my baby's been constipated since I started weaning.
This is an issue many parents mention to me, with constipation frequently occurring when starting solids. It can make your baby grumpy, uncomfortable, windy and reduce their appetite.

Constipation describes when your baby poos less and passes hard stools (which may be large or droppings), and there can be associated straining and pain. The NHS describes symptoms as:

✧ Pooing fewer than three times a week.

✧ Poos that are often difficult to push out or larger than usual.

✧ Dry, hard or lumpy 'rabbit-dropping' poo.

I cover constipation in lots more detail on page 382 (tummy troubles), however, here are some first-step options you can try:

✧ Include fruits high in sorbitol, a natural fruit sugar that acts like a laxative by bringing water into the large intestine. Prunes, pears, plums and peaches are all excellent options.

✧ Try adding kiwi to your baby's weaning diet. It's not just a great source of vitamin C but has been found in some scientific studies to relieve constipation.

✧ Check in on your baby's fluids – are you offering water with meals, and are fluid-rich foods like yoghurts, fruit, etc. included in their diet?

✧ Try a fibre check – getting the balance right with a baby is important as too much fibre or too little could contribute to constipation symptoms. Avoid excess intake of high-fibre foods, such as brown or wholegrain versions of bread, pasta and rice. Foods high in soluble fibre, such as oats, beans and lentils, avocado, courgette and seeds can be increased gradually. Be careful with seeds such as chia or flaxseed, and start with small amounts, such as ¼ teaspoon or less, and make sure you include them within a fluid-rich meal or soak them beforehand.

✧ Try other practical options to ease constipation, such as gentle movements like cycling your baby's legs, putting them upright in a chair or sling or a warm bath with a gentle tummy massage.

Consider seeking advice or support from your GP if your baby has any of the below stool changes:

❖ Blood or evidence of bleeding in poo.

❖ Black stools.

❖ White or very pale stools.

❖ Persisting or worsening constipation.

My baby doesn't seem to be progressing with weaning or seems disinterested – am I doing something wrong?

First, you're not doing anything wrong. If your baby's progress feels 'slow', please let go of blame and take a breath. Just like other aspects of development, weaning can prompt parental comparisons with peers. Remember, each baby has a unique weaning journey influenced by growth needs, early feeding experiences, medical issues, family dynamics and much more.

Weaning progress should follow your baby's pace. For example, some may need small steps between texture changes, while others may adapt quickly. Research shows differences in appetite traits and food responsiveness in babies and children too, so temperament is also often involved. Feeding is a complex skill, and as this section has covered, your baby will be learning much more than just eating.

Here are some top tips I usually discuss with parents who are worried about slow weaning:

1. If you've only just started weaning, and are in the early days or weeks of it, check your baby's development signs for being ready for solids.
2. Check in on the mealtime environment and your behaviours. Are these supportive for happy and enjoyable mealtimes?
3. If you're not already, try eating with your baby. Even the task of eating takes your focus away from just watching and

feeding your baby, giving them some space to explore. It's also valuable modelling for your baby to see what you do with the foods, so they have the opportunity to copy.

4. If you've chosen one weaning approach, consider experimenting or exploring the other – for instance, try finger foods or loaded spoons.

5. Check in with your expectations; even three to four weeks in, your baby may have only had experience with a few foods, once or twice a day. Learning to eat takes months and, in reality, years! It can be ok if it seems they aren't eating much or doing much with food in the early weeks and months.

6. Check your baby is seated comfortably – can they easily reach the food on the tray? Are they upright or falling to the sides? Do they have somewhere to put their feet for some stability?

7. Focus on the responsive feeding principles and cues I talk about on page 137.

8. Give your baby some agency. Do they have some food to explore and hold and spoons to practise with?

9. Check your timings – is your baby happy, alert and not too hungry or full?

10. Remember, learning to eat is more than just eating food.

11. Sometimes, a cascade of teething, illness and developmental progression in other areas can mean that starting solids can have a steadier start or feel quite up and down. Please be reassured that this is normal, and keep going!

12. Finally, keep going and keep offering variety. It can be tempting to default to the foods they can more easily manage or seem to enjoy. Remember the importance of variety over volume!

If you have concerns, seek support from a health professional experienced in baby feeding and starting solids.

My baby is stuck on pureed sweet foods. How can I help them accept more variety?

I receive numerous messages from anxious parents who feel their baby is stuck on purees, especially the sweeter varieties. Babies naturally gravitate towards these traits – sweet flavours are familiar and enjoyable, while smooth textures are easier for them to handle skill-wise. Progress can stall due to issues such as gagging on textured foods or a complete refusal to try more challenging tastes. This often leads to a frustrating cycle where parents revert to familiar purees when their baby doesn't accept different flavours or textures. If this sounds familiar, consider these steps:

✦ Start making gradual changes, like moving from puree to a slightly grainier texture. If you're solely using jars or pouches, begin introducing some homemade options, or combining the two.

✦ Incorporate appropriate finger foods into every meal, and consider having at least one meal a day without purees, allowing your baby to explore a variety of suitable finger foods.

✦ Try to resist the urge to 'rescue' the meal with preferred purees. Instead, focus on offering diverse foods and the other skills your baby is developing.

If you continue to struggle with progress, seek support from a feeding specialist such as a paediatric dietitian or speech-and-language therapist.

My baby has started pushing the spoon away – help!

Several factors can contribute to this situation. Your baby might not be hungry, or they are teething and sensitive to the feel of the spoon on their gums, or they might simply want more participation in their feeding. If you're primarily spoon feeding, I recommend trying some of the responsive spoon-feeding techniques mentioned earlier, or consider introducing finger foods if you haven't yet. Additionally, if you're using silicone spoons, ensure they haven't acquired a strong, soapy taste.

My baby has been waking at night since we started weaning. Is it related?

Night waking is quite normal for babies, and it isn't always related to food. Babies wake up for several reasons: they might be too hot, too cold, hungry or simply want some comfort. Some babies may appear to wake in discomfort, which parents can often attribute to increased gas or trapped wind that can occur as a baby adjusts to solids. For some babies, as their digestive systems gets used to new foods they might experience temporary discomfort. Usually, this is just an adjustment period and things will settle down. However, if the night waking and discomfort persist, it's a good idea to seek support from a healthcare professional to ensure that there are no underlying issues.

*   *   *

Here marks the end of the first year in your child's first five years of feeding, and I know what you're thinking – there's more? While starting solids is a significant milestone in your child's feeding journey, and you're likely to be just about getting to grips with new feeding routines, things are about to change again. From one year of age, we look forward to the toddler years, a time I fondly refer to as 'the unpredictable eating era', but don't worry, I'm here to guide you through feeding for these years ahead too, as I know so many parents who feel like advice falls off a cliff after the weaning months are done!

3

Terrific Toddlers

Embracing the unpredictable eating era: 1–3 years

Nutrition and feeding milestones in the toddler years:

✧ Toddlers have high energy and nutrient requirements to fuel their rapid growth and development, *but* they grow more slowly than in their first year of life.

✧ Toddlers gain *on average* 12cm and 2.5kg between one and two years old, and 8cm and 2kg between two and three years old – but each child will vary.

✧ By age three your toddler's brain is around 80 per cent of its adult size.

✧ By age three your toddler will have established some of the main community of gut bacteria (gut microbiome) that they will carry for life.

✧ Nutrition remains very important during the toddler years and it is still recognised as a crucial time to optimise growth and development. Until two years of age, toddlers still sit within the 'first 1,000-day' window of opportunity.

✧ Your toddler will become increasingly skilled at self-feeding and using utensils.

✧ Big developmental changes will affect eating in a wide variety of ways, from wanting increased control and autonomy with food choices, to food neophobia (a fear of anything new or familiar) creating more caution around new foods.

✧ A toddler's eating pattern can be consistently inconsistent!

✧ Lifelong eating behaviours continue to form during the toddler years.

At the time of writing, I am in the throes of parenting a toddler myself and I can confirm that it's a turbulent ride! Toddlerhood signals a huge time of transition and change. On a daily basis I'm witnessing new words, skills and confidence and I often feel like I have a teenager, not a nearly-two-year-old. The desire for control, regular use of new favourite words like 'no', and making best use of her newfound language to dictate my every move can feel over-whelming on some days! But don't just take my word for it, I asked my social media audience to describe the toddler years in one word, and these were just some of their responses:

'Chaos', 'Exhausting', 'Fun', 'Rollercoaster', 'Enriching', 'Wild', 'Emotional', 'Whirlwind', 'Manic', 'Adventure', 'Entertaining', 'Carnage'

Toddlerhood is a time of rapid growth – and I don't just mean in size. As this list of words suggests, your child's thinking, move-ment, social and emotional skills are booming, with good nutrition fuelling this development too.

This section aims to guide you through the 101 of toddler nutri-tion, but also the transitions you are about to experience, expecta-tions for your toddler's eating habits, feeding development, and a few of the common worries, including picky (fussy) eating.

Toddler feeding transitions

✧ **Transitioning to a new mealtime routine and introducing snacks**

✧ **Milk transitions**

✧ **Transitioning off the bottle**

✧ **Transitioning to childcare**

✧ **Foods your toddler no longer needs to avoid, and those to limit**

✧ **Changes to expect with your toddler's appetite and eating behaviours**

By now, you've likely settled into a routine with feeding your baby and you might feel like you've found a rhythm with meals and milk feeds. However, things are about to change. I can hear your audible sigh as I write this, but please be reassured that these changes can be gradual over the weeks and months ahead.

Transitioning to a new mealtime routine and introducing snacks

From one year of age you can introduce snacks into your toddler's eating routine. Snacking can often be viewed negatively, however, for toddlers, snacks are a valuable opportunity for nutrition. Toddlers have high energy requirements and comparatively small stomachs, so regular opportunities to refuel are important. As a guide, it's recommended that toddlers are offered three meals and two snacks per day. Think of these as regular eating opportunities every two to three hours.

Mealtime routines and structure are fantastic for young children. They provide regular 'eating anchors' in their day. Since your toddler doesn't yet grasp the concept of time, these routines foster a sense of safety and predictability as they become more independent, while also supporting appetite regulation. Here's an example routine to use as a guide:

7am Breakfast
9:30am Snack
11:30–12pm Lunch*
2:30pm Snack
4:30–5pm Dinner*
*You may choose to offer a second course at these mealtimes, for example, alongside the main meal, or afterwards.

While the above is a guide, I am very aware from years of working with parents that snack habits can vary between children. If you find snacks significantly dampen appetite for main meals, you may wish to limit or reduce the number of these. For other children, for example, those who are picky, snacks can offer a valuable opportunity to offer nutrients. As always, pay attention to *your* child's habits and needs, and remember a routine can be applied with some flexibility!

As you begin introducing snacks, many parents find that replacing the mid-morning and afternoon milk feeds with food is a good starting point. I encourage parents to view snacks as another opportunity to offer key nutrients and variety – sometimes framing them as 'mini mealtimes' rather than snack times can be helpful. (There is more advice on building a balanced toddler snack on pages 191–2.)

While we're on the topic of snacking, let's talk about grazing. You won't be alone if you find your toddler suddenly starts requesting snacks or pointing at the cupboards throughout the day. Their developing communication and desire for control is in the driving seat, with their lack of impulse control riding in the passenger seat too – so when they see the snack cupboard, they want what's in it! I speak to many parents who suddenly find themselves at the mercy of multiple snack requests throughout the day, which can often be accompanied by food refusal or poor appetite at mealtimes. While occasional extra snacks are nothing to worry about, if you suddenly find your toddler grazing throughout the day, be aware that it may well impact their appetite for main meals, and as a result the range of nutrients they eat. Setting healthy boundaries and sticking to a routine like the above is beneficial, in my experience, for the majority of toddlers.

When considering your toddler's world, it's helpful to remember that they can also benefit from knowing when mealtimes or snack times begin and end. I've seen the benefits – both with my daughter and hundreds of families I've worked with or heard from – when a consistent cue (signal) at the start and end of mealtimes is used. There have been times when I've plucked my daughter away from an activity she's engrossed in to plonk her at the table and a full meltdown has ensued. It makes sense, as she's had no warning about what's happening next and I'm expecting her to follow *my* routines and agenda. Imagine someone knocking at your door in the middle of the day and demanding you drop everything to leave with them!

With this in mind, when it comes to mealtimes, I encourage parents to 'bookend' meals with clear communication or signals to support transitions. For example:

Pre-mealtime (a meal is coming)

✧ Give a clear verbal cue ('warning') that a mealtime is coming, such as 'lunch is in five minutes'. You might also use hand gestures to sign 'food'.

✧ Get your child involved in a routine action/task, such as taking them to wash their hands and/or bringing a placemat to the table.

✧ If your child struggles to leave play or toys to head to the table, options like a 'finished' box or tidy-up time before a mealtime can help, alongside reassurance that after the meal they can move back to play or their next activity.

To end the mealtime (the meal is finished)

✧ Give a clear verbal cue (signal) when the meal is finished, such as 'Lunch is finished. Time to tidy up.' You might also use hand gestures to sign 'finished'.

✧ Get your child involved in a routine action/task, such as placing any leftover foods in a tidy-up bowl/plate, passing the plate to a parent or taking it into the kitchen.

Milk transitions

From one year of age, your child can move on to cow's milk, or a fortified plant-based alternative, as a drink. Current advice in the UK is to offer whole (full-fat) or semi-skimmed cow's milk – you can choose either or both. Skimmed milk should not be given to children under five years of age. If using a plant-based milk alternative, choose an option that provides the key nutrients that your growing toddler needs (see pages 183–4).

You may be wondering how to make the transition over from your child's current milk or introduce their new milk. There are a few options for this:

1. Start offering milk in an open cup or cup with a straw instead of a bottle. Some children will accept a straightforward switch

or introduction without issue, others may need a little more time to adjust.

2. Gradually titrate with your baby's current milk. For example, if you normally offer a 150ml bottle of formula milk, drop out one ounce and add one ounce of cow's milk or milk alternative. This can help some children adjust to the taste difference between the two milks. You may do this in your baby's bottle initially, then once transitioned swap to a cup.

How much milk?

It can be easy for toddlers to over-consume cow's milk or milk alternatives, so I encourage parents to be aware of milk volumes. For context, 500ml of whole cow's milk provides around 40 per cent of a toddler's energy needs for the day, so this amount of milk or more is likely to reduce your toddler's appetite for food and intake of important nutrients. Studies show that drinking too much milk is also linked to iron deficiency and anaemia, with toddlers consuming more than 500ml of cow's milk daily at higher risk.

For this reason, I recommend aiming for a maximum of 350–400ml of milk per day, avoiding consistent intakes above 500ml. This includes milk you may add to foods like cereal. Please be reassured that toddlers can drink less milk than this, or in fact can drink no milk, and still get the nutrients they need. Aiming for two to three portions of dairy or fortified alternatives would be enough to meet their requirements for nutrients that come from this food group.

If you're breastfeeding your toddler, there's often a misconception that breast milk loses its value after one year, which is far from true. Breast milk continues to offer energy, essential fatty acids, vitamins, minerals and immune benefits to your toddler. Breast milk will continue to complement your toddler's diet well without the need to introduce cow's milk or fortified milk alternatives as a drink unless you choose to. You can use dairy or fortified alternatives (such as yoghurt, cheese) in your child's diet while breastfeeding too.

Does my toddler need a 'toddler' or 'growing-up' milk?

The short answer here is probably no! There is no need for most toddlers to continue with formula milk past the age of one or drink a 'toddler'-specific formula, despite what marketing may suggest. The exception to this guidance may be for children under medical and/or a dietitian's care who have a limited diet, specific nutritional needs or feeding differences.

Transitioning off the bottle

Most health organisations, including the NHS, recommend stopping bottle use from age one. While this can be challenging due to the comfort and routines it provides, it's advised because prolonged use is linked to tooth decay, excessive milk intake and iron deficiency. Transitioning to a cup also supports oral motor skills for speech and feeding development.

Please be reassured that you do not have to force this transition overnight, and that there is more than one right way to stop bottle feeds. Approaches I find that work well with many families include:

✧ Choosing a good time. Ideally, when your child is well and not going through any other 'big' transitions or routine changes.

✧ Stopping the morning bottle first. The volume of milk may be reduced gradually – dropping an ounce at a time over a few days, then bringing your child straight down for breakfast and a drink of water shortly after waking.

✧ Swapping out any mid-morning or afternoon bottles for a snack and a drink from a cup. Again, some parents choose to reduce volumes first, while others go 'cold turkey' and substitute milk for a snack directly.

✧ Being aware that the before-bed bottle can sometimes be the hardest one to stop. Again, some parents choose to go cold turkey and switch out the bottle for a cup of milk in one fell swoop, while others gradually reduce the amount of milk in the bottle first.

✧ Keeping the bottle out of sight and ensuring your child's cup or drinking bottle is accessible regularly during the day.

If you're breastfeeding or combination feeding and would like support on how to wean your baby from the breast, I have referenced some helpful sources of information on page 442, for when the time is right for you.

Transitioning to childcare

I wanted to sneak a section into this book about managing the transition for parents and children into regular childcare, because I find it's so often overlooked when it comes to food, nutrition and mealtimes. Here are a few things that come up a lot when I speak to parents:

✧ **New routines** – When your child starts nursery or with a childminder, their mealtime routine may shift, with lunch and dinner often being offered earlier than your child is used to. Many parents ask me if they need to offer dinner when their child returns home, and this depends on the child. If you eat early, you can offer a small portion or let them serve themselves. If not, some parents offer a lighter meal before bed. Children are great at regulating their appetite, so if they've eaten well at childcare, they might refuse dinner – and that's completely fine!

✧ **Feeding differences between home and childcare** – It can be common for children to take some time to settle into the foods and routines offered at their childcare setting, with many refusing foods or meals for days or weeks (my daughter did this!). Childcare settings are generally very good at communicating what children eat across the day, many using apps and feedback forms. Many parents also find that over time their child accepts a wide range of foods at their childcare setting but may not accept these same foods at home – a topic I cover more on page 242!

✧ **Discussing dietary requirements** – Before your child starts childcare, clearly communicate any dietary requirements or preferences to the staff, including food allergies, action plans and medications. Discuss alternative foods, how meals are served and seating arrangements. Many parents ask about nursery food standards, and in the UK there are government guidelines and example menus available for Early Years settings. The reality is that these are guidelines, so practices can vary, which can be frustrating. If you're unhappy with any nutrition or feeding practices, such as frequent sugary desserts or poor snack options, I recommend discussing it directly with your setting.

Foods your toddler no longer needs to avoid, and those to limit

Now that you have a toddler, there are some small changes to advice about foods to be avoided and nutrients that may need to be limited in their diet. Many remain as per the weaning section on page 102, but I have summarised some key changes below.

✧ **Honey** – You no longer need to avoid honey in your child's diet, however, it is still considered to be a free sugar and for this reason moderation is encouraged.

✧ **High-risk choking foods** – Continue to avoid or modify high-risk choking foods until your child is at least five. You can check the list on page 103. I always remind parents about these foods but you should also be careful about small items like button batteries and marbles, since toddlers become more mobile, curious and quick to put things in their mouths!

✧ **Slushed-ice drinks** – This one often surprises parents, but avoid giving slushy drinks to children under eight. These drinks contain glycerol, the additive that makes them sweet and gives the 'slush' effect. While safe in small amounts, the issue for young kids is the large amount they might consume in one go, compared to their body size. Too much glycerol can cause headaches, nausea, cramps or diarrhoea, and in higher amounts can lead to low blood sugar, unconsciousness or collapse, requiring urgent medical attention.

✧ **Fish** – In the UK, there's no strict guidance on how often to serve fish, but general advice suggests about twice a week, with at least one being oily fish like salmon, mackerel or sardines. Due to possible pollutants, it's recommended to limit oily fish to two portions per week. For young children, a portion is around 40g, or about 1 tablespoon of tinned fish, or a quarter to one small fillet of fish.

✧ **Salt** – The amount of salt your child can eat increases to 2g per day between one and three years of age. This is still a low amount, so it's important to watch the salt content in your toddler's food. You can find more tips on managing their salt intake on page 255, but to show how quickly it can add up in the diet, here's an example of how a toddler might reach the 2g of salt per day from everyday foods:

✧ Portion of multigrain loop cereal – 0.24g

✧ Cheddar cheese sandwich with 2 slices of white bread – 1.26g

✧ Two cream crackers and small portion of shop-bought hummus – 0.55g

Total   2.05g

Remember, it's ok if your toddler exceeds this recommendation on some days, as long as intake levels out across the week.

✧ **Sugar** – Another important nutrient to watch in your toddler's diet is sugar, especially added and free sugars. These can easily sneak into their diet from various sources. I explore this in more detail on page 256.

Changes to expect with your toddler's appetite and eating behaviours

I can't discuss changes in your toddler's eating routines and nutritional needs without addressing the common appetite and behavioural shifts that occur alongside. My goal is to explain the 'why are they doing this?' questions that often concern parents about their toddler's eating habits. Understanding these changes helps make sense of their unpredictability and I hope will help provide you with both the reassurance and patience that you need to get through this developmental stage!

Developmental feature or transition	What does this mean?	Behaviours you may see around food/mealtimes
Growth is slowing down – at both one year of age, then again at two years of age, the amount of energy your toddler needs per kilogram of their body weight drops.	Your toddler needs fewer calories to grow. Toddlers will continue to listen to their hunger and fullness cues.	Eating less at mealtimes. Skipping meals or snacks altogether. Fluctuating appetite from day to day or week to week.
Increasing drive for control and autonomy (the ability to make their own choices and act independently). Developing a sense of self.	Your toddler is now very aware they are a separate person from their caregivers, and can express their own preferences, make simple decisions and assert their independence. This stage is marked by a strong desire to explore their environment, imitate adult behaviours and take on tasks by themselves, such as feeding, dressing and playing independently. Supporting their drive for autonomy while providing appropriate boundaries and guidance is crucial during this developmental phase.	Wanting to do things themselves, and development of self-help skills, such as self-feeding. Wanting to choose things themselves/making wants known, such as for food. Using language to express preferences, such as 'no' to certain foods. Preference for choices, such as wanting to decide what they want to eat, choosing between two things. Tantrums when their autonomy around food or mealtimes is restricted – 'I want the blue bowl!' Exploratory behaviour – 'playing' with food but perhaps not eating it, or becoming distracted by other things in the room and wanting to leave to play.

Short attention span.	Your toddler has a much shorter attention span than adults and older children. Some sources suggest it is around two to five minutes per year of age. They are highly curious and shift quickly between activities.	Not wanting to sit at the table for very long – for instance, two to 10 minutes. Wanting to leave the table to engage in another activity or bring a toy to the table. May want to get up and down from the table. Curiosity about others' food and food on the table at mealtimes.
Ongoing development of cutlery skills.	Your toddler will still very much be developing their cutlery skills. Between one and three years of age you're likely to see increasingly proficient spoon feeding and development of fork use. Toddlers may be exploring use of an age-appropriate knife.	Frequent and ongoing use of hands to self-feed. Wanting independence with feeding self with cutlery. Holding cutlery in one hand and feeding with hand on the other side. Feeding self with preloaded spoon. Scooping or dipping spoon and becoming more proficient at getting it to their mouth (ongoing spilling is normal in younger toddlers). Attempting to stab food with a fork and bring to mouth.

Food neophobia, aka fear or reluctance to try new or unfamiliar foods.	Food neophobia is thought to be a developmental trait that harks back to a time when it was crucial for increasingly independent and curious toddlers to avoid potentially dangerous foods, like poisoned berries or rotten carcasses, outside of our ancestral caves. This instinct, which originally served to keep toddlers safe, is still present today, although our food environment has significantly changed. Food neophobia is commonly observed in children between 14 and 24 months of age.	Preference for certain food groups. For many toddlers this can be predictable foods like carbohydrates. Reduced range of accepted foods overall. Rejection of foods they are less familiar with and some they have eaten before. Rejection of foods from specific food or texture groups, such as vegetables, meat, fish, wet or mixed textures. Apparent 'fear' of certain foods.
Social learning and imitation.	Toddlers become increasingly social creatures, learning through watching and imitating others. This social learning helps them develop new skills and preferences.	Toddlers may show interest in your food when eating, even if they have the same food themselves. Eating with others – such as at a family meal or a childcare setting – may support imitation of eating and feeding behaviours, including food acceptance.

Ongoing emotional development.	Emotional regulation in toddlers involves learning to manage their emotions and reactions, a process that heavily relies on the support of primary caregivers and other trusted adults. Big emotions, fluctuating emotions and emotional outbursts such as tantrums are common.	Your toddler's emotions and regulation states may impact their eating, for instance, if they are upset, cross, tired or dysregulated, appetite may be poor. Toddlers will co-regulate from caregivers around food; for example, if you're anxious, they are likely to imitate this and in turn appetite or behaviour around food can change. Equally, if you're calm and relaxed they are more likely to be too!

I hope this helps set expectations for common feeding and eating behaviours in toddlers. Understanding that these behaviours are normal can relieve some of the pressure around feeding. It's also important to remember that your toddler isn't an adult; they may seem more mature, but their brains aren't developed enough for the adult expectations that we can inadvertently place on them. Here are a few key differences to keep in mind.

Adult	Toddler and young child
Has relatively consistent energy (calorie) requirements.	Will be going through periods of rapid growth and slowed growth.
Can override or ignore hunger or fullness cues relatively easily.	The majority of toddlers will follow appetite cues – eating when hungry, stopping or refusing food when full.
Has had many years of experience with food and eating. Can apply learned experience with food to new or less-familiar foods.	Has much less experience with food and eating and is still learning.

Decides on daily food choices, can serve a portion of food they feel able to manage.	Toddler may have no or limited choice around food on offer, and may have foods and portion size determined by their caregiver.
Developmentally 'stable' – may be learning some new skills but has already achieved the key stages of development – they are no longer a child.	Toddler's undergoing rapid development in motor, social, emotional and cognitive areas.
Has the skills to eat without creating mess, is able to use different types of cutlery with ease and aware of social norms and expectations around mealtimes.	Toddler is continuing to develop self-help and feeding skills, may seek sensory learning with food, such as handling, and will learn about food in a way that developmentally aligns, such as play. Cognitively, a toddler won't understand or interpret all social norms at mealtimes, such as table manners.

Now that I've helped you put yourself into your toddler's shoes when it comes to behaviours around food and mealtimes, here are some strategies I encourage all toddler parents to grasp with both hands, as they move through the next few months or years of feeding:

1. **Lean into trusting your toddler's appetite** – Letting go of the idea that you're able to control how much or exactly what your child eats at every meal or snack time will give you, and your toddler, much more breathing space. Accepting that appetite fluctuations are normal and that your child is simply riding the wave of what their body wants and needs often helps ease mealtimes worries and reduce added stress at mealtimes. Not only that, huge health bodies like the World Health Organization strongly advocate for continuing responsive feeding during the toddler years, highlighting the importance of children eating autonomously in response to their body's signals.

I won't pretend this is always easy. As humans we struggle with 'neurological surprises' – when our expectations aren't met – and when it comes to our kids' health these can feel even more pronounced. So, when your toddler, who's been eating you out of house and home, suddenly declares they've had enough after one bite, your brain may well interpret this 'surprise' as a threat, heightening anxiety. Be kind to these feelings (they are there because you care), then return to these pages to remind yourself this is normal.

Many parents relate well to a concept I've already mentioned in this book, called the Division of Responsibility, by Ellyn Satter, which divides the responsibility of caregivers and children up into the following mealtime 'responsibilities':

Parent/caregiver provides	Child decides
A balanced meal.	What to eat.
When meal is offered.	How much to eat.
Where meal is offered.	What order to eat food in.

I'd also encourage you to be aware that external pressures have the potential to undermine your toddler's trust in their own appetite. For instance, if you urge them to take one more bite to ease your own concerns, it can send the message that they shouldn't trust their own fullness. Imagine feeling full and your partner or friend insisting you had to keep eating. That one last bite is also unlikely to offer much more nutritionally! Pressure around eating is a huge topic and if you want to understand more, head to pages 205–8 where I cover it in more detail.

Of course, if you have any previous or current concerns about your child's growth or appetite, these changes can be a worry. In this situation, I would highly encourage you to discuss any worries with a health professional like a paediatric dietitian.

2. **Hand your toddler some control and choice around food and mealtimes** – Working *with* your toddler's desire for decision-making and control can not only ease stress and power struggles, but also help them develop confidence and curiosity around food. Ways in which you can offer control at mealtimes or around food include:

   o Offering meals family-style.
   o Offering simple choices such as 'would you like the blue or red plate?' or 'you can have cereal or toast for breakfast.'
   o Let them help you prepare food or set the table, choosing their preferred seating space, cutlery or crockery.
   o Support and encourage your child to feed themselves.

Top tip: Avoid too many open-ended questions such as 'What would you like for . . . ?' Far-reaching questions like this can be a big ask for your toddler's brain. You'll find they often pick what's very familiar, what they've eaten recently or they know is near by!

3. **Keep a routine** – A routine around meals and snack times can work with your toddler's development to create predictability around food and mealtimes in their day. Remember, mealtimes and snack times are an *opportunity* for your child to eat, not an expectation that they will!

4. **Eat together** – Toddlers love to learn from others, and the same goes for food. Eating with your toddler isn't just about exposure to different foods and supporting their intake. Your toddler has high levels of attention needs, and sitting together at meals is a great way to connect with their favourite people! Rather than striving for picture-perfect mealtimes, prioritise talking and having fun and making mealtimes enjoyable.

Top tip: I'm a big advocate of eating together, but I understand not every caregiver wants to eat at 5pm. In which case, look for regular opportunities to share meals each week that fit your family's schedule – like weekend breakfasts or lunches – or serve yourself a small portion of your child's evening meal for a chance to eat together at night.

5. **Be aware of your own goalposts and expectations (without blame)** – As parents our 'wants' and perceived 'needs' for our children can often play out, inadvertently, as setting expectations. I talk to many families where we discuss realigning those expectations or goalposts with their toddler's development and eating habits. For example:

   o *Exploring and exposure to foods vs. Eating* – When it comes to new foods, or foods your child has eaten before, try moving the goalposts from expecting them to eat the food to accepting that learning or re-learning about that food will look like exploration or 'play' with that food – looking at it, watching you or a peer eat it, holding it, squashing it, smelling it.

   o *Quality of time at the table vs. Quantity* – Your toddler almost certainly won't 'sit nicely' at the table for half an hour. Based on attention span, it's acceptable to expect a mealtime may only be five to 10 minutes or less. Instead of focusing on time, shift to thinking about how to support and engage your toddler at the table for the time they are there. Avoid strategies to try to keep them there longer, like using screens or toys.

   o *Emotions vs. Managing our own reactions* – It's easy to feel frustrated or anxious when mealtimes don't go as expected, and these are all valid emotions. Mealtime battles can escalate quickly when we let our stress or disappointment take over. Recognising that your toddler's eating patterns are a normal part of their development can help you to stay calm and patient, even during challenging moments, and help create a more positive experience for both you and your child. Full disclosure, though, you're human and some days your bandwidth for controlling your emotions will be harder – and that's ok.

Toddler nutrition 101

✧ **Food groups to include in your toddler's diet**

✧ **Building balanced meals and snacks**

✧ **Portion sizes for toddlers**

✧ **Managing second courses or sweet foods**

✧ **Common nutritional deficiencies in toddlers**

✧ **Supplements for toddlers**

✧ **Drinks and fluids for toddlers**

It won't surprise you to hear that nutrition for toddlers is not just 'little adult' nutrition. While food groups and some nutrition principles are similar, the explosion of your toddler's development needs the right fuel. Toddler nutrition continues to build on the foundations of baby nutrition principles, outlined in the earlier chapters of this book.

Food groups to include in your toddler's diet

Before discussing food groups, it's important to note that while your toddler's growth rate slows after the first year, their need for energy and nutrients remains high for their size; one- to three-year-olds need nearly twice the energy per kilogram of body weight as a young adult! For this reason, the aim for toddler nutrition is plenty of nutrient-dense foods, making the most of every bite.

The foods your toddler needs as part of a balanced diet to support their growth and development can be split into the following:

1. Carbohydrate ('starchy') foods – These foods are one of your toddler's main energy providers, but they also contain nutrients such as fibre, B-vitamins, folate, magnesium and zinc.

Carbohydrates should make up a big portion of your toddler's diet, with around **five portions offered per day.** UK dietary guidelines recommend that from the age of two, total carbohydrate intake should provide around 50 per cent of a toddler's daily energy requirements. There's a reason your toddler loves carbohydrates!

Example carbohydrate/starchy foods include rice, pasta, potato, noodles, bread and bread products, chapati, roti, quinoa, teff, buckwheat, barley, oats, cereals, polenta, sago, taro, spelt, millet, sorghum, plantain, cassava, mochi and couscous.

2. Fruits and vegetables – It's recommended that toddlers and young children consume **five portions of fruit and vegetables a day,** which means you could include one or two portions at each mealtime – or simply offer one option at each meal and snack time across the day. Fruits and vegetables provide fibre, fluid and a wealth of nutrients like vitamins C, A, E and folate. Fruits and vegetables are rich in beneficial compounds like phytonutrients and antioxidants that can help prevent long-term diseases. The vibrant colours of these foods indicate the presence of these helpful components and the phrase 'eat the rainbow' is very much supported by science. Here's a quick breakdown of these terms:

Phytonutrients: Natural chemicals in plants that promote health, such as flavonoids, carotenoids and polyphenols.
Antioxidants: Substances in food that protect our bodies from damage, like ascorbic acid and lycopene.

Don't worry too much about understanding or remembering these words. Often the reason I share them is to illustrate there can be some big and pretty scientific-sounding words present in nature. Not every scientific-sounding word when it comes to food means 'bad'!

Toddler portions of fruit or vegetables aren't necessarily the same as for an adult. It's easy to assume the whole apple or banana is a portion, but for young children a portion of fruit or vegetables may look like:

✧ ¼–½ large apple

✧ 1 small fun-sized banana

✧ ½–1 satsuma

✧ ½–1 kiwi/plum/apricot

✧ 1 slice of melon

✧ 1–4 small florets of broccoli

✧ ½–2 tablespoons of peas/sweetcorn/mixed vegetables/green beans

✧ 2–6 carrot sticks

In addition, all different types of fruit and vegetables count, including frozen, fresh, dried and tinned. There are also lots of foods that contribute to your child's fruit and vegetable intake that often surprise parents, such as tomato-based pasta sauces, soups, and beans and lentils (including things like hummus and falafel).

Finally, I find parents worry about their toddler having a preference for fruits over vegetables. Let me reassure you that this is exceptionally common. Please be reassured that the nutrients you find in vegetables, you find in fruits too. There's a common misconception that vegetables are superior to fruits, which I think unfairly downplays the widely known benefits of fruit for health!

Fruit and vegetables for toddlers can include:

Fruit – Apples, pears, bananas, kiwis, melons, pineapples, oranges, mangoes, passionfruit, tomatoes, dragon fruits, blueberries, raspberries, strawberries, cherries, plums, blackberries, blackcurrants, papaya, grapes, peaches, nectarines, lychees, avocados, apricots, grapefruits, jackfruits, durians, ackees, plantains, soursops, guavas, pomegranates, figs, Sharon fruit.

Vegetables – Carrots, parsnips, cabbage, onions, bell peppers, cucumbers, celery, spinach, broccoli, cauliflowers, sweet potatoes, squash, pumpkin, courgettes, lettuce, green beans, aubergines, okra, pak choi, cho cho, yams, taro, greens, bitter melon, sweetcorn, mushrooms, turnips, swedes, radishes, beetroot, leeks, peas, mangetout, fennel, asparagus, Brussels sprouts.

3. Protein- (and importantly iron-) rich foods

Protein has an important role to play in your toddler's diet, supporting their growth, development, immune health and repair of tissues. Protein sources are often also home to a variety of vitamins and minerals like iron, zinc, vitamin A and omega 3 fats.

Aim for **two to three portions of protein-rich foods daily**. If you're following a plant-based, vegetarian or vegan diet, aim for three. This can look like including protein at two meals and possibly a snack. Protein can be found in a wide variety of sources, and mixing these up can help to offer a range of nutrients.

✧ **Red meat** (such as beef, lamb, pork) provides iron, zinc and B12. Limit highly processed meats where you can due to health risks, and opt for fresh meats.

✧ **Poultry** (such as chicken, turkey) offers iron, zinc and B12. As with red meat, limit processed options.

✧ **Oily fish** (such as salmon, mackerel) are rich in omega 3 fats. Include one to two portions weekly.

✧ **White fish** (such as cod, haddock) is a great source of iodine and B12, essential for brain development and metabolism.

✧ **Eggs** are nutrient-packed, providing iron, zinc and choline. Parents often ask me how many eggs is too many, and while there's no one-size-fits-all answer, it's generally considered safe for most people, including children, to eat multiple eggs per day.

✧ **Soya-based foods** (such as tofu, edamame) are rich in plant-based protein. Many parents are wary about including soya in their children's diets, due to worries about the phytoestrogens naturally present in soya, which often still get linked with concerns about fertility. Please be reassured that including soya in a toddler's diet is considered safe. Plant-based phytoestrogens do not act in the body in the same way as the female hormone oestrogen. We also have more and more evidence linking soya to positive health benefits, from cancer prevention, to heart, bone and gut health.

✧ **Beans and pulses** offer iron, zinc and fibre, and ideally should be included multiple times weekly.

✧ **Nuts and seeds** are great for healthy fats and protein and can be served in safe forms for young children, like ground or in smooth butters. Given their health benefits, in some dietary guidelines across the world it's now recommended that a portion is included daily.

✧ Protein is also found in dairy and wholegrains.

Many parents worry their toddler doesn't eat enough protein. Reassuringly, UK data shows that most toddlers exceed their daily protein requirements, sometimes by up to three to four times. In fact, excessive amounts of protein during the younger years has been linked to an increased risk of overweight and obesity later in life. You can read more about how easy it is to meet protein requirements on page 240.

4. Dairy and dairy alternatives

Dairy provides valuable nutrients to rapidly growing toddlers, including protein and fat, but also micronutrients like calcium to support bone and teeth health, iodine for brain development and vitamin B12 for a healthy nervous system. It's recommended that toddlers aim for **around two to three portions of dairy (or suitable dairy alternatives) per day,** which you may split across any meal or snack times. For example:

1. 120ml milk in cereal in the morning.
2. 20g cheese with lunch, such as in a sandwich or with crackers.
3. 100g plain yoghurt with fruit as a snack.

If your toddler cannot have dairy products, it's important to select suitable milk-free alternatives. The goal is to provide nutrition similar to what dairy offers, but it can be overwhelming with so many options available. Here are some guidelines I encourage parents to follow:

✧ Choose a plant-based alternative, such as soya, oat, pea or coconut. Rice-milk alternatives should not be given to children under five years of age due to the naturally occurring arsenic content, and nut-based milk alternatives are typically too low in calories.

✧ Choose an option that is >45–50 kcals/100ml, ideally as close as possible to the energy content of semi-skimmed or full-fat milk (50–66 kcal/100ml).

✧ Ideally, use a higher-protein option such as soy- or pea-milk alternative, but if these are not suitable, protein can be easily provided in your toddler's diet elsewhere.

✧ Select an option that is fortified (has added) vitamins and minerals ideally; and also has calcium and iodine as a minimum – vitamins B12, B2 and D are also helpful.

✧ Ideally, ensure there are no added sugars, being mindful that some manufacturers will add these as juice concentrates.

When selecting milk-alternative yoghurts, as for milks, choose plain options without added sugars and those fortified with calcium and iodine. Unfortunately, cheese alternatives don't provide the same nutrition as dairy cheese; they often come from coconut or coconut oil, with added salt and flavourings. I recommend using these sparingly due to their high salt content and choosing options with added vitamins and minerals whenever possible.

Examples:

Dairy foods: milk, cheese, cottage cheese, soft cheese (ricotta/mascarpone/cream cheese), yoghurt*, fromage frais, crème fraîche, custard.

Where possible, try to choose plain yoghurt varieties for toddlers, without added sugars, such as 'natural', 'Greek', 'Greek-style' and 'Icelandic' varieties.

Dairy-alternative foods: soya/oat/pea/coconut/nut-based milk alternatives, yoghurt alternatives and cheese alternatives (hard and soft), custard made with milk-free custard powder and milk alternatives.

5. Fats

While this isn't a specific food group as such, I wanted to recognise the importance of fat for toddlers and young children. To support your toddler's rapid growth and brain development they need plenty of fats included within their diet, especially when they are under two years of age. It's recommended that one- to three-year-olds get around 35–40 per cent of their energy intake from fat. Fat provides the highest amount of calories (energy) per gram compared to the other macronutrients, like protein and carbohydrates. Fats can also help with absorption of important fat-soluble vitamins A, D, E and K, alongside providing specific fatty acids that the body cannot make, such as omega 3 fatty acids.

Day to day, including fats in your toddler's diet can look like:

✧ Prioritising full-fat dairy, including full-fat or semi-skimmed milk, full-fat cheeses and yoghurts (or dairy-free equivalents).

✧ Using oils for cooking or adding to foods, such as olive oil.

✧ Using full-fat spreads, such as butter or olive-oil-based spread on toast, crackers or sandwiches.

✧ Including higher-fat foods regularly into meals, such as oily fish, avocado, eggs, dairy, nuts and seeds.

✧ If following a vegetarian or vegan diet, aim to include a good fat source at each meal, such as oil, coconut, nuts/seeds, or higher-fat milk alternatives with the meal.

One tricky aspect of fats is that they aren't all created equal. Fats are made up of different fatty acids, and their structure and shape determine which category they fall into, so here's a quick rundown.

Type of fat	Examples	Advice
Saturated fat	Mainly found in animal-based foods and is hard/semi-solid at room temperature, such as animal fats, butter, ghee, hard cheese, lard, pastry, cakes, biscuits and crisps. Also found in some tropical plant-based fats like coconut and palm oils.	Moderate intake – while saturated fat will be included in a toddler's diet, to support both energy intake but also due to consumption of foods which provide other nutritional benefits, like dairy, eating too much can increase 'bad' cholesterol levels. I recommend moderating intake of saturated fat from foods like processed meats, cakes, pastries and crisps.
Unsaturated fat aka 'good fat' Polyunsaturated fat Monounsaturated fat	Are often found in plants and generally liquid at room temperature. Found in sunflower, corn and rapeseed oils, oily fish, some nuts and seeds – like walnuts and sesame seeds. Found in avocados, olives, olive and rapeseed oils, peanuts, almonds, pistachios and cashews.	Prioritise as main fat sources in the diet. Both types of unsaturated fats that are found from plant-based sources can provide your toddler with essential fatty acids, support energy intake and are known to have longer-term positive effects on health. Unfortunately, some types of these fats, like seed oils (e.g. rapeseed oil), have got a lot of negative attention in recent years, with claims that they can be 'inflammatory'. I want to reassure you that high-quality scientific evidence does not back up these claims, and in fact shows the opposite!

Trans fats	These are created when heating vegetable oils in a process called hydrogenation, which helps keep them more shelf-stable or able to be reheated. They are found in foods like margarine, cakes and pastries.	Avoid as much as possible – the good news is that there are not many trans fats left floating around the UK food system, but you may still find hydrogenated or partially hydrogenated vegetable oils in foods such as pastries, cakes and ready meals. They are known to be associated with health concerns such as high cholesterol and increased risk of heart disease.

✧ Omega 3 fatty acids are also a type of fat to prioritise in your toddler's diet, which can be found in foods such as oily fish, eggs and some plant-based foods such as walnuts or flaxseed. They have a super important role in your toddler's brain and eye development, so I've covered more about them on page 291.

Building balanced meals and snacks

With an understanding of food groups, I also want to share how you can build balanced meals and snacks. As a general guide, try to include the following at meals and snack times:

Carbohydrate food + fruit/vegetables + protein-rich and/or dairy food

There will of course be some nuance with this – some meals or snacks will have all groups, some will have two. To help demonstrate this idea I've included some meal examples below.

Balanced breakfast ideas:

✧ Fortified cereal with full-fat milk and a portion of fruit, such as chopped berries or grated apple.

✧ A slice of toast with spread, scrambled eggs and diced cherry tomatoes.

✧ Pancakes with yoghurt and banana.

✧ Porridge made with milk, added fruit or grated carrot, and ground nuts or nut butter.

✧ Muffin, bagel or toast with smooth peanut butter and sliced banana or mashed raspberries.

✧ Dosa with lentil soup.

✧ Egg muffins or frittata, such as eggs baked with vegetables and diced or sliced potatoes.

✧ Fried plantains and boiled or scrambled eggs, with an orange on the side.

✧ Cornmeal porridge made with milk and added fruit.

✧ Eggy bread with fruit and yoghurt.

✧ Paratha with yoghurt and mango.

✧ A small wrap or sandwich, such as an egg and avocado sandwich, or salmon and cream cheese with cucumber.

Balanced lunch ideas:

✧ Beans on toast with cheese, served with a portion of fruit.

✧ Sandwich or wrap, such as hummus and vegetables, cheese and tomato, cucumber or grated apple, eggs with mayonnaise or yoghurt, tuna and sweetcorn, tinned salmon and cream cheese, mashed chickpeas with tomato puree and cheese, mashed beans and avocado.

✧ Stuffed pittas – with any of the above, or some shredded chicken and vegetables with yoghurt.

✧ Mini pizzas – try using pitta bread, wraps or muffin halves topped with tomato sauce, cheese and veggies like bell peppers or mushrooms and/or ham, tuna or shredded chicken.

✧ Rice and peas – with some fish, meat or beans.

✧ Chicken or vegetable curry (could be leftovers), served with rice and a small piece of naan bread or roti.

✧ Cheese and bean quesadilla with a side of guacamole or mild salsa for dipping.

✧ Mashed sweet potatoes topped with a small amount of shredded chicken or beans and chopped cucumber.

✧ Mini sushi rolls, made with cucumber, avocado and cooked prawns or tofu, cut into toddler-friendly pieces.

✧ Quiche or homemade 'quiches' made using a tortilla wrap as a base.

✧ Vegetable and cheese omelette, served with a slice of wholegrain bread.

✧ Lentil soup with a small slice of crusty bread for dipping.

✧ Mild vegetable stir-fry with tofu or small chicken pieces, served with plain noodles or rice.

Balanced evening meal ideas:

✧ Any of the lunch options!

✧ Spaghetti with lentil or meat Bolognese and cheese.

✧ Gnocchi with peas, chicken or chickpeas and cream cheese.

✧ Pasta with pesto, peas and shredded chicken.

✧ Meat, lentil or vegetable curry with rice, chapati or naan.

✧ Salmon, noodles and stir-fry vegetables.

✧ Egg or grated tofu fried rice with mixed vegetables.

✧ Chicken breast or nuggets with potato wedges and peas.

✧ Fish fingers with mashed potato and sweetcorn.

✧ Roast dinner – meat or chicken served with roast or mashed potatoes and a range of vegetables.

✧ Beef, chicken, prawn or tofu tacos with tortilla wraps, cheese, avocado and sliced vegetables.

✧ Falafel with hummus, pitta bread and salad – perhaps quartered tomatoes, shredded lettuce, cucumber and/or peppers.

✧ Sushi bowls, such as deconstructed sushi with rice, cucumber, avocado, cooked fish or tofu and a sprinkle of sesame seeds.

✧ Chickpea curry served with basmati rice or naan bread.

✧ Noodle soup with rice noodles, shredded chicken or tofu, vegetables and fresh herbs.

✧ Pierogi with sour cream – soft dumplings filled with potato and cheese or spinach, served with a dollop of sour cream.

✧ Shepherd's pie with a side of vegetables.

✧ Meat keema – spiced meat, rice and vegetables.

✧ Cabbage rolls filled with a mix of minced meat and rice, served with a mild tomato sauce.

✧ Seasoned chicken with coconut rice and vegetables.

✧ Stuffed paratha – spinach, chickpeas and potato.

Balanced snacks:
Before I delve into snack ideas, I want to mention that in the real world sometimes snacks for kids will just be grab and go – a banana, a pack of breadsticks and cheese, an oat bar. This is absolutely fine, but where you have more time, use snack times as an opportunity to offer variety. Combining two or three food groups can be helpful for your nutrient-needy toddler – a carbohydrate + fruit/vegetable + protein-rich food. The inclusion of nutrients like protein and fat can also help keep them full for a little longer, delaying the next inevitable snack request!

Here are some balanced snack suggestions:

✧ Oatcakes or crackers with cream cheese or dairy-free cream cheese, smooth nut butter or tahini and fruit or grated vegetables, such as carrot.

✧ Small sandwich or wrap – one slice of bread or half a wrap with hummus and grated apple or carrot, peanut butter and banana, cheese and tomato or cream cheese and cucumber.

✧ Toast with nut butter and mashed fruit, mashed avocado, melted cheese and grated apple or carrot, tomato puree and cheese or hummus.

✧ Egg muffins or frittata.

✧ Vegetable pakoras.

✧ Pitta bread and cucumber sticks with hummus or tzatziki.

✧ Avocado and black bean dip with flatbread or breadsticks.

✧ Baked oats or oat bars.

✧ Rice balls and vegetable dumplings.

✧ Plain yoghurt with berries and oats.

✧ Apple or pear 'nachos' – thinly sliced fruit drizzled with peanut butter, sunflower butter or yoghurt and sprinkled with desiccated coconut or ground seeds.

✧ Chicken roll ups – thinly sliced cooked chicken topped with grated vegetables and cheese in a wrap, rolled up and cut into pinwheels.

✧ Toddler trail mix – dry cereal pieces or crushed rice cakes, berries and cubes of cheese.

Portion sizes for toddlers

I'm often asked, 'How much should my toddler be eating?' The truth is there isn't a fixed portion size that will suit all children. Factors like age, body size, appetite that day and temperament will mean toddlers eat varying amounts. As mentioned earlier, it's important to trust your toddler's ability to eat to appetite rather than having rigid expectations for portion sizes.

That said, some general guidance can help, especially since studies show that many parents struggle with portions, or unintentionally over-serve toddlers. Here are some tips:

✧ Start with smaller portions and offer more if needed. Large portions can overwhelm toddlers and lead to parental confusion about how much they've eaten. Plus, it helps reduce food waste.

✧ Use smaller, age-appropriate plates and bowls.

✧ If you're comfortable with the idea, consider family-style serving, where your child can serve themselves.

For a rough guide, this suggestion is often used as a starting point only:

✧ Protein: About the size of your toddler's palm.

✧ Carbohydrates: About the size of their fist.

✧ Fruits and veggies: About what fits into their cupped hands.

Managing second courses or sweet foods

To support a varied diet, many parents choose to offer a second course after lunch or dinner, which (especially in the UK) is often sweeter foods like fruit, yoghurt or plain biscuits. These foods can provide valuable nutrients and be part of a balanced toddler diet. However, some parents worry if their child becomes fixated on asking for their second course, particularly sweeter foods. If you're in this situation, here are some tips:

✧ Avoid making second courses something to be 'earned'. Offer them regardless of what your toddler eats at the main meal.

✧ Consider serving the second course with the main meal. It takes the 'shine' off sweet foods, keeping the focus on foods neutral. Many parents give me a side eye when I suggest this option and follow it with 'but they'll eat the fruit/yoghurt/cake first?' To this my answer is always the same – 'It doesn't matter, especially if it was being offered anyway.'

✧ Remember, it's normal for children to enjoy sweet foods. They're naturally drawn to them, and they can provide valuable nutrients. You control how much and how often they're served alongside other foods.

✧ Consider mixing up your second course. It doesn't have to be sweet – options like oat cakes and cheese or extra vegetables and hummus can work too. Just be mindful you're not creeping into offering an alternative meal.

Common nutritional deficiencies in the toddler years

Nutrient deficiencies can be common in young children, often because their dietary intake doesn't meet their high nutritional needs. The science shows deficiencies of nutrients like iron, vitamin D and fibre are all common in the toddler years. For more information about these see the section beginning on page 397.

Supplements for toddlers

I always begin discussions with parents about nutritional supplements by emphasising their purpose: they should be **supplementary** to, not a replacement for, a well-balanced diet. The supplement industry is vast, and with so much information out there, it can be overwhelming to determine what your toddler actually needs, so I've outlined some key considerations for choosing supplements for your toddler.

Recommended supplements for all toddlers

In the UK it's currently recommended that toddlers, up to the age of around five years, have the following vitamin supplementation daily, often as a combined supplement.

✧ Vitamin D – 10ug (micrograms)

✧ Vitamin A – 200ug (micrograms)

✧ Vitamin C – 20mg (milligrams)

New UK guidance suggests there is less need for vitamin C supplementation, as children generally get enough through their diet. A well-balanced diet can also provide sufficient vitamin A, however vitamin D supplementation is a necessity for most young children.

You may be eligible for free supplements through the Healthy Start scheme if you receive certain benefits, and free vitamin D for children under three in Scotland.

You can find age-appropriate supplements containing the above in drop, liquid, spray and chewable forms, although be mindful that many gummy or chewable options are not suitable under three years of age.

Which toddlers might need extra supplements?
Some toddlers may benefit from additional vitamin and mineral supplementation if they find it harder to get all the nutrients they need from their diet alone. These include children who:

1. **Follow a vegetarian or vegan diet** – Some nutrients, such as B12, iodine and DHA, can be more challenging to get on a predominantly plant-based diet. (See pages 420–2.)
2. **Are picky eaters** – Children who are picky/fussy may benefit from extra supplementation of nutrients if they struggle to eat enough of them, such as iron. A healthcare professional should ideally guide you as to the type and amount of supplementation, however, some parents opt for an age-appropriate broad-spectrum/A–Z multivitamin and mineral supplement.
3. **Have food allergies, intolerances or coeliac disease** – Children who have to exclude one or multiple food groups are known to be at higher risk of nutritional deficiencies. For this group of children, individualised support from a paediatric dietitian is recommended, as advice will depend on what foods they can or can't eat.

Common supplement queries: does your child need them or not?
It can be easy to think more is better when it comes to supplements, but lots of research suggests additional supplementation of nutrients isn't a necessity for most children. Here are a few supplements I'm asked about regularly:

Magnesium – Supplementation of this mineral has gained popularity, often promising every parent's dream: 'better sleep'. Changing dietary trends mean it's reasonable to consider magnesium may become a nutrient 'at risk' in children's diets, and while some adult studies suggest magnesium can improve sleep, there's currently no robust evidence to support the need for supplementation in children.

Magnesium is found in foods that kids often enjoy, like bananas, cereals, wholemeal bread, oats, nuts, seeds, carrots and apples. For children with restricted diets who are showing symptoms of low magnesium, like sleep issues, anxiety or mood changes, consult a health professional to explore further. Please be mindful that side effects of magnesium supplementation can include digestive troubles like diarrhoea, and while magnesium can be effectively absorbed via the skin (you'll see it in sprays and bath salts), correctly dosing this can be tricky!

Bilberry or elderberry extract – There's limited evidence to support using these extracts for children's health. While small studies (mostly in adults) suggest they may reduce the duration and severity of cold and flu symptoms, the science isn't conclusive. Bilberry and elderberry are dark coloured and so contain antioxidants like anthocyanins, which children can get from other dark-skinned berries and other blue, red or purple fruits, vegetables and beans instead!

For more about 'immune-boosting' supplements and probiotics, see Chapter 5.

How to pick a reputable and helpful supplement

Not all supplements are the same, and with so many being flogged online now, I wanted to share some green and red flags when buying them.

Green flags
✦ Third-party tested.
✦ Supported by scientific studies.
✦ From a reputable supplement brand.

✧ Contains the amounts ('dose') of specific nutrients likely to be beneficial.

✧ Transparent ingredient list, free from unnecessary additives or fillers.

✧ Clear labelling with dosage instructions and potential side effects.

Red flags

✧ Non-legal health or nutrition claims (such as 'no junk', 'immune-boosting').

✧ Lack of transparency about ingredients or manufacturing processes.

✧ No third-party testing or certification.

✧ Exaggerated claims or promises of quick fixes.

✧ 'Blends' that don't specify individual ingredient amounts or that contain excessively high doses.

✧ Over-reliance on testimonials without scientific backing.

Drinks and fluids for toddlers

Young children need plenty of fluids to maintain their hydration levels as, like babies, they can be at higher risk of dehydration. Good hydration is important for supporting concentration, regular bowel habits and your toddler's overall wellbeing.

What should toddlers drink?

Toddlers' drinks should consist predominantly of water and some milk. It's recommended that fruit juice and smoothies should be limited, and if offered they should be diluted (1 part juice/smoothie to 10 parts water) and ideally given at a mealtimes to help protect your child's teeth.

Toddlers and young children should avoid sugar-sweetened

drinks such as milkshakes, squash or juice drinks or fizzy drinks, to protect their teeth.

How much should toddlers drink?

Each child's fluid requirements will be slightly different, but as a general guide it's recommended that toddlers consume 800–1,000ml or 6–8 cups of 120–150ml per day. A toddler's fluid requirements don't just have to be met from drinks, fluids from food (such as fruit, vegetables and yoghurts) or added to food, such as milk in cereal, all count. In fact, foods can contribute around 20–30 per cent of a child's fluid requirements each day.

There will be times when your toddler will need more to drink. This includes during warm weather, after active play or sports/activities and during illness.

Remember, the amounts suggested above are a guide. If you are unsure about how hydrated your child is, one of the best ways to check is to pay attention to the following, as these are all markers of fluid status:

1. Their nappies – are they having regular wet nappies, is their urine dark, straw-coloured or light/clear? Is their urine strong smelling?
2. Their behaviour – irritability or drowsiness can be signs of dehydration.
3. Their body – look for signs such as an increased heart rate, dry mouth and even cold hands and feet.

How to encourage your toddler with their fluids

Young children can have a lower sensitivity to thirst, so they may need regular prompts or cues to drink. Like eating, avoid adding too much pressure to your toddler and instead:

✧ Offer drinks regularly, for instance, with every meal and snack time, during and after active play and before bed.

✧ Model drinking yourself, and role-model with toys or teddies too.

✧ Engage your toddler in the process, choose their preferred cup or bottle or get them to fill their cup themselves.

✧ Make small changes or add novelty, such as adding fruit to water, add adding ice during warmer weather.

Picky eating (aka fussy/ choosy/reluctant eating)

✧ **What's happened to your child's eating?**

✧ **Why is it happening?**

✧ **The trap of trying to 'fix' picky eating**

✧ **Debunking some myths on picky eating and rules around children's eating**

✧ **Practical strategies to support your picky eater**

✧ **When is it more than just picky eating?**

There is a reason why a good chunk of this toddler section is taken up with the topic of picky eating, and that's because it's pretty common during the toddler years. I've lost count of the number of families I've supported with picky eating, and I know from every conversation I've had that it can cause prolonged stress and anxiety for many parents and caregivers, alongside children. Many parents, especially mothers, tell me they feel dismissed when raising concerns about picky eating or their child's eating habits, because many behaviours are considered to be developmentally 'normal'. I want you to know that your concerns are valid and deserve to be heard.

Before understanding more, the most important thing you need to hear is that your child's picky eating isn't your fault. Read that again, because for parents, when you are struggling to understand what's going on for your child it is very easy to turn on yourself and look for something that you've done wrong. Let me tell you now, there is nothing.

What's happened to your child's eating?

Picky eating can feel like a conundrum for many parents. In clinic, parents share that their baby ate anything during weaning but now, defying all adult logic, their toddler is turning their nose up at endless foods, and mealtimes have started to feel like a negotiation station or 'battleground'. Undoubtedly parents also find themselves comparing their child's eating with one of their peer's who eats anything in sight, which can also be natural!

You're not alone. Statistics from across the world show that 25–45 per cent of children will experience a phase of picky eating during some stage in their childhood. The peak age for this is generally recognised to be between 18 and 24 months, however, research varies with some children seemingly hitting this closer to six to nine years of age. While I've included this discussion in the toddler years section, it can certainly be relevant to your child at any later age.

There isn't a specific definition for picky eating. It can fall under the banner of many other names including fussy, faddy, choosy or selective eating. What the science does agree on, though, is that 'picky eating' has some common features, as I've shared in the table on the following page.

Why is it happening?

There is no doubt that these eating changes are hugely worrying and frustrating for parents. Understanding why this is happening can often be the first step to taking the pressure off mealtimes. Many parents I encounter in clinic presume it's either something they are doing wrong or that something needs 'fixing' with their child, when, typically, it's neither of these things.

The science suggests	It might look like this at home
A child's range of foods may reduce to between 20 and 30 (occasionally fewer).	It feels like mealtimes are Groundhog Day at home. Your child might have the same meal every one to two days, or accept only one specific choice per mealtime. You feel worried about how many foods they now refuse.
Children may have stronger preferences for certain tastes or textures of food, or how it is offered.	They want the dry, crunchy crackers but not the broken ones, and they must be square, not circles. They want them from the purple plate. The beige phase is in full swing.
Children avoid or reject new and/or familiar foods.	Looking at a piece of broccoli (which they have eaten hundreds of times already) like it's just landed from Mars.
Children appear to be or are fearful of new foods. (Called food 'neophobia'.)	Rejection of what seems like a vast number of foods, especially those that could appear more 'threatening' due to their taste, texture, colour – such as vegetables, meats, fish.
Children may eat different foods in different contexts.	Fish pie is not a problem at nursery, but at home all hell breaks loose.
Children are more likely to be served specific meals, which may be different to what the family are eating.	In the kitchen making three different meals, even though you always promised yourself you'd just be making one family meal.

While children can experience picky-eating behaviours at any age, there is one key factor closely linked with why it's seemingly so common, and that's a child's developmental stage. Here are some common developmental milestones for this age group (toddlers) and how they might translate to what you see or hear from your child around the table, although many apply to other age groups too.

◇ **A huge drive for autonomy** – Toddlers face the daily conflict of wanting to make decisions themselves, but having adults around them who make the majority of these for them. Food can be something that is easier to try to exert control over. It can look like 'I don't like it, I want ice cream', refusal of foods previously eaten, requests for specific foods ('All they want is snacks'), tantrums and big emotions at the dinner table, defiance and boundary pushing.

◇ **Using language to express their wants/needs** – Alongside a want for control are more ways to communicate it. It can look like 'no', asking for 'more' of preferred foods, labelling foods as 'yucky' or 'disgusting', throwing foods off a plate or the table.

◇ **Engrossed in learning new skills and play** – During the toddler years, eating can be much less of a priority and much more a functional 'thing to do'. Children's cognitive development is flying right now, with a focus on big skills like language, motor, social and emotional development which they want to practise. It can look like wanting to leave the table to play or do something different, asking for toys or bringing them to the table.

◇ **Growth changes** – From around 12 months of age, and again at two years of age, a child's rate of growth slows down. Slowed growth means less energy is needed per unit of body weight, and changes in appetite reflect this. It can feel hugely counterintuitive that your 10-month-old ate more than your two-year-old, but in fact it's completely normal. It can look like 'They just pick at food', 'I don't know where their energy comes from', 'My child is surviving like a plant from photosynthesis!'

Alongside a child's development, there are several other reasons why children may be more predisposed to picky eating in childhood.

✧ **Genetics** – Like many aspects of a child's health and development, genetic factors can shape eating behaviours. A twin study released as I was writing this book found genetics to be a primary factor in influencing picky eating in children – a nugget of information I hope also reduces any feelings of blame you're still holding on to! Please be reassured that there's still plenty you *can* do to support your child. Helpfully, this same research, along with lots of other science, shows that interventions for fussy eating are usually most effective when commenced during the early years. Another great reason to get going now!

✧ **Personality and feeding temperament** – Some children may be naturally more adventurous around foods (and life), while others have a more cautious or anxious disposition. Science has also shown that children vary in terms of food 'responsiveness' and appetite traits, meaning that they differ in how they respond to food and how their appetite is regulated. Some may be more sensitive to external cues like the sight and smell of food, making them more likely to eat in response to these stimuli, even when they are not physically hungry. Others might have a stronger internal sense of satiety, meaning they can better regulate their food intake based on their bodies' needs. These variations are influenced by a combination of genetic, environmental and psychological factors.

✧ **Learned experiences with food or feeding** – I see many children in clinic with picky or more significant feeding differences who have a background where something has happened to impact their experience of feeding or eating in a negative way. This is something well documented in scientific studies too. For example, children with a history of prematurity, reflux, constipation, food allergies, tube feeding, complex medical conditions, delayed weaning or where feeding has previously been very medicalised, or a history of strict targets on volumes or calories imposed. Understandably, these often shape how a child experiences or interacts with food. Sometimes this predisposes children to being more than fussy eaters, and many of these are known risk factors for more significant feeding difficulties.

✧ **Sensory differences** – Eating is a huge sensory experience (the biggest our body has to do). For some children, their bodies can receive more or less information from certain senses, such as smell, touch and taste, and with this comes an influence on a child's preferences around food or experience of eating. A child's sensory 'profile' and needs have also been found to help predict persisting pickiness with food, such as food refusal or eating behaviours that persist past two to three years.

✧ **Parental influences** – How we parent children around food and deal with food refusal can impact mealtimes too. In fact, one study showed that among mothers who considered their child 'choosy' at 15 months old and were worried about this, 50 per cent of those children went on to be a picky eater, compared to 17 per cent in the group where parents were not worried about choosiness. While I want to reinforce the message that there is no blame or judgement being assigned here, what is evident from science and the discussions I have with parents is that our perception as parents of our child's eating can impact *how* we approach feeding them.

The trap of trying to 'fix' picky eating

Before diving into strategies for supporting your fussy eater, I want to address (which is very much without judgement, or blame) the tendency to try to 'fix' the issue. Now I empathise with this hugely. As parents, we instinctively want to solve problems affecting our children. When picky-eating habits arise, it can often be considered a serious issue, with research showing that parents' main drivers for anxiety are rooted in nutritional concerns, weight or growth worries or even worry that a child will have the 'label' of an avoidant or picky eater. Helping and supporting our children to eat well can feel deeply ingrained in parental instincts, and in our eagerness to fix things, or fuelled by concern, we may inadvertently adopt approaches that can be controlling, persuasive or perceived as pressure by our children. Despite these being well intentioned, they don't tend to lead to the best long-term outcomes when it comes to picky eating.

Here are some common strategies I see and hear parents trying to use:

✧ Offering one or more alternatives or 'rescue' meals (or milk) after a meal or snack has been refused.

✧ Over-encouragement with food or persuasive tactics, such as 'Just take one bite', 'You used to love avocado', 'Look, it's Mummy's favourite'.

✧ Negotiation or rules such as 'we have five more bites before the meal ends'.

✧ Force-feeding. This can look like feeding a child when they are showing cues that they do not want the food/meal, such as head-turning, pursing lips shut, crying or being generally upset.

✧ Stopping a child self-feeding and taking over.

✧ Spending long periods at the table (sometimes hours) to make sure a certain amount or type of food is eaten.

✧ Offering lots of extra snacks between meals (often fuelled by a concern about 'getting enough' nutrition).

✧ Introducing food-based rewards or punishments, such as, 'If you eat that green bean, we can have ice cream for dessert', or 'If you don't try the pasta, you can't have strawberries'. (I call this using food as currency.)

✧ Getting upset or frustrated with their child at a mealtime.

✧ Begging – 'Please, please, just one bite for Daddy'.

✧ Distraction techniques, such as introducing a screen to mealtimes.

You're certainly *not alone* if you've found yourself using one or all of the above – I can empathise fully with how parents reach this point. Feeding children is hard, however, such approaches, especially those recognised by your child as pressure, will often increase food refusal or avoidant eating. There is an alternative route, which I'll walk you through over the next few pages.

At this stage I want to give you permission to stop trying so hard to 'get' your child to eat, and if you take nothing else from the rest of this chapter, let it be this: the best thing you can start doing if you're in the throes of picky eating is to step back and explore what forms of persuasion or pressure may be around food and at mealtimes with your child, and think how you can start moving away from these. Put simply – try to take your child out of the spotlight at mealtimes.

Now the chances are that you know this already! So if you find this particularly difficult, stopping to explore what concerns are driving any of these behaviours can be a good start. I find this varies between parents and caregivers, from worries about nutrition, growth or sleep to medical pressures, your experiences growing up around food, comparisons with others or the highlight reel of social media*.

If you think insight and support with this are needed, consider reaching out to a health professional to discuss further. You're not expected to have all the answers.

Pressure, and its relationship with avoidant eating

While it has long been recognised that pressure around food and mealtimes was linked to food refusal and avoidant eating, for many years the chicken-and-egg debate stood strong. Does pressure around food make food refusal 'worse' or does food refusal increase pressure around eating? A large study has put this debate to bed, finding that, unsurprisingly, the relationship goes both ways, which is why for so many families it may feel things spiral, getting worse and worse.

Pressure around eating and mealtimes has been found to impact children and families in a variety of ways, including:

✧ How the child feels – their ability to feel safe, happy and well regulated around food or at the table. You can read more about the impact of stress on appetite and the nervous system later in this section – I know it feels scientific, but it's worth understanding.

✧ A child's enjoyment of eating – studies have shown that pressure at a mealtimes can reduce eating enjoyment, and in my experience this can often be the case for stressed-out parents too! (A quick reminder here that food is not just for nutrition, enjoyment is a reason to eat too!)

✧ Mealtime (and beyond) conflict – it's not uncommon for me to hear parents call mealtimes a battleground. Research has shown that pressure can increase conflict, as children often push back against expectations to attempts to 'get' them to eat.

Debunking some myths about picky eating and rules around children's eating

Before delving into what you *can do* to support your picky eater, I want to pause and dispel some of the (annoyingly) persistent myths circulating on the internet, and perhaps even from some professionals.

1. **'Just let them go hungry and they'll eat eventually/If they are hungry they will eat'** – This is completely unhelpful advice that doesn't work in the long term! Refusing to offer your child food that they will eat can create stress and anxiety around meals, often worsening picky eating. For many kids, hunger alone won't push them to eat foods they don't feel safe or familiar with.

2. **'Use a reward chart to help them try new foods'** – While reward charts can seem a good idea, and may have some benefits in specific scenarios, the problem with stars and stickers for trying new foods is that you're rewarding children with an extrinsic (external) motivator rather than allowing them to tune into their intrinsic (internal) motivation. Put simply, your child may be trying the vegetable because they want a sticker, not because they *actually want to eat the food*. I find this approach rarely stands the test of time. It can also be a public display of what your child isn't achieving (as much as what they are).

3. **'Your child is a fussy eater because you didn't do baby-led weaning'** – I've had parents come to me in tears, blaming themselves for using a specific weaning approach, assuming that's why they now have a picky eater. There's no robust evidence that using a BLW approach simply prevents picky eating. From my experience of working with children weaned by either method, it's clear that this alone cannot prevent the developmental shifts or other factors that contribute to picky eating.

4. **'It's going to take 8/10/15 exposures before your child tries a new food'** – While research shows that repeated exposure

helps kids accept new foods, and that 10–15 exposures may be enough for some foods, it isn't a magic number for *all* foods. Some foods will take many more child-led interactions – even hundreds – before being eaten (if at all).

5. **'Children shouldn't play with their food'** – Young children learn through play! If we are expecting them to learn about different foods with a view that one day they might eat them, it's important to recognise that learning about these may involve 'play' too.

Practical strategies to support your picky eater

I want to start by saying that I wish I could hand you a magic wand to solve picky eating, but the reality is it's a process that can take months or even years for some children. I encourage all parents to think of this as a long game, as there aren't really any quick wins. While it might be disheartening to hear that there isn't a simple fix, the steps you take now at mealtimes can greatly benefit your child's future relationship with food and mealtimes for years to come.

When it comes to picky eating, I tend to break down tactics into two steps:

1. **Creating the ideal eating and mealtime environment.**
2. **Choosing what foods to offer.**

The strategies I'm about to share require consistency and time, so I'd encourage you to trust the process. I'm extremely aware this isn't always easy, so I've included some mantras at the back of this book for days when mealtimes and your child's eating feel tough (see page 429). I would also encourage you to approach any changes gradually, and avoid trying to implement too much at once, thus overburdening yourself.

Step 1: Creating the ideal eating and mealtime environment
You might wonder why I'm not just diving headfirst into how to get your child to eat their vegetables. The truth is that foundations for supporting picky eaters are as much about *how* food is provided, not just *what* foods are offered. I tend to break this down into:

1. The eating environment (including routines, managing distractions, seating and language).

2. Encouraging autonomy around food.

3. Eating with others and family-style meals.

4. Expectations and emotions.

The eating environment
It might feel like I'm going into a world of intricacies around mealtimes here. But I want you to imagine that you've been served a plate of foods you don't recognise or enjoy, you're not hungry, you're on an uncomfortable chair, there is noise and frequent distractions around you, and someone's repeatedly prompting you to eat or take another bite. Quite frankly, you weren't even feeling ready for dinner. It doesn't sound pleasant, does it? Yet this can easily be the reality for young children. Here are a few pillars for creating an ideal eating experience.

Eating routines
Children typically benefit from routines, which support predictability in their day and ultimately help them to feel safe. Consistent routines increase the likelihood of children being happy to come to the table (or eating space) and engage with the offered foods, so I'd recommend checking back in with your child's usual meal and snack routine.

✧ Are they having regular eating opportunities – three mealtimes, two snack times?

✧ Are gaps between eating opportunities spaced relatively evenly – every two to three or three to four hours?

✧ Do they have any signs or signals as to when the next eating opportunity is going to happen, or are they expected to transition to the table without warning?

You may have noticed the power of routines and 'cues' when your child's regular mealtime routine is disrupted. For example, many children refuse foods or eat less initially when they start childcare or go on holiday.

Beware stealthy snacking – A pattern of excessive snacking or grazing can, of course, disrupt appetite regulation for young children. In my experience, parents of picky eaters often agree to multiple snack requests fuelled by the worry that their child isn't eating enough. While topping up can feel instinctive, it tends to come back to bite a child's appetite on the bum! If you think this could be relevant to you, spend a day checking how often your child eats or snacks, then return to the routines suggested on pages 161–3 for your child's age.

Other 'extras' to add onto the mealtime routine for a picky eater include:

✧ **Tips for transitions** – Prompts or cues to help your child transition to and from the table (see page 162).

✧ **Sensory awareness and preparation** – To help some children be in the right frame of mind and ideal body state to eat, it can be helpful for them to do some sensory preparation activities or empty their 'sensory cup' before mealtimes. Food is a big ask from a sensory perspective, as it ignites all our senses into action. Sensory preparation activities can help children become more comfortable and ready to eat. Examples could include deep pressure or 'heavy work' activities like pushing palms together for a slow count to 10, squeezing a stress ball or having squashes and squeezes with a parent or carer (child-led).

Top tip: View mealtimes and snack times as an *opportunity* for children to eat foods, not a guarantee about what or how much they will eat. Remember, if your child refuses a meal, they will always be able to eat again in a few hours.

Keep it calm (always easier said than done!)
A stressful or pressured environment doesn't prepare the body for eating; quite the opposite. We need to be in a 'calm and alert' state

A note on offering alternatives

A familiar trap that parents of picky eaters fall into is offering alternatives or 'rescue meals'. I empathise with why, because as a parent, it's natural to be concerned when meals are left untouched, especially before bed. However, offering alternatives comes with its own set of challenges.

✧ Your child may become less likely to try new foods or eat what's initially offered if you consistently provide a preferred alternative. This can reinforce fussy eating habits and limit dietary variety.

✧ The focus shifts from you providing a meal to your child taking control of the situation. When children learn that rejecting a meal leads to getting something more desirable, they gain control over the menu.

✧ It can create a pattern of power struggles at mealtimes where your child expects a specific routine, such as being offered particular foods. They may use food refusal to assert independence or gain attention, making mealtimes more stressful.

While an alternative may be needed on occasion, try to avoid it where you can.

for eating, avoiding situations that increase stress or trigger our fight-or-flight response. Do you recall being hungry or dreaming about a buffet lunch before a job interview or important meeting? Stress reduces our appetite and makes it difficult for the brain to be 'online' ready to absorb new information – neither of which is ideal for mealtimes. In your child's world, stress or pressure at mealtimes can lead to food refusal or hypervigilance about the food on offer.

With this in mind, here are a few pointers:

✧ Try to keep mealtimes a calm, relaxed environment. Talk to your child, smile, make eye contact and remember to try to **focus on feeding connection.**

✧ Focus on 'felt safety' around food and mealtimes. Felt safety can be described an unconscious state of feeling secure. You might be thinking, 'A dinner table is hardly a lion's den, Lucy', but if mealtimes have been stressful, fractious, painful (for example, because of gut symptoms or reflux), or even unpredictable, it can take some time for a child to feel settled and safe at the table. Remember, a child's body and brain (psychological) safety are felt, not told. Factors like routines, predictability at mealtimes (such as having accepted foods on offer) and dialling back any pressure will support this.

✧ If your child is in the midst of a tantrum or the 'hangover' phase afterwards, push back a mealtime until they are more settled and better regulated.

✧ Avoid too much background noise, distractions or toys.

✧ Check in on your emotions (there is more about this on page 227).

Limit distractions, including screens
In my fussy-eating consultations, parents often share that they've introduced a screen to help improve the amount of food eaten, time at the table or just out of sheer desperation.

What on earth does regulated mean, and why does it matter?

Throughout this book, you might notice me using the term 'regulated'. While it may sound like it's related to rules or legal contexts, I'm using it in reference to your child's body and brain.

As adults, we recognise that our brain and body don't always feel the same from day to day, or even throughout the day. Some mornings you might wake up feeling energised and focused, while other times you may feel fatigued or stressed. Your physical and emotional state shifts depending on things like sleep, stress, life demands, nutrition and even the weather. These fluctuations are natural and impact how we interact with the world around us, including our food.

This idea of regulation is closely tied to the nervous system and the rest of the body. The autonomic nervous system, which controls many of the body's involuntary functions, plays a key role in how we feel and react. It has two main branches: the sympathetic nervous system (often referred to as the 'fight-or-flight,' or 'stress,' system) and the parasympathetic nervous system (often referred to as the 'rest-and-digest' system). When a child is in a stressed or anxious state, their sympathetic (stress) nervous system may be activated, making them more likely to feel on edge, restless, freeze and refuse food. In contrast, when they are calm and regulated their parasympathetic nervous system is more active, allowing them to feel more relaxed and open to eating, digesting, learning and engaging with the world around them. An occupational therapist I work with loves the term 'you have to regulate to educate'.

In the context of feeding, understanding this regulation is crucial. Just as you might find that your appetite or energy levels vary depending on how regulated you feel, children experience similar shifts. If your child is feeling overwhelmed, stressed or tired they might struggle to eat, feel less hungry or become more selective in what they want to consume. On the other hand, when a child is in a more regulated state (or 'green zone') feeling calm, comfortable and focused, they can be more likely to come to the table, eat and explore new foods.

Much of the advice throughout this chapter from routines, to managing language and emotions, incorporates factors that aim to support your child, as best as possible, to be regulated at mealtimes.

The challenge with screens at mealtimes is that they can:

✧ Get in the way of your child learning about food – it's much harder to pay attention to others or the food on the table when distracted by a screen.

✧ Slow down the mealtime pace – many parents have to prompt their children through mouthfuls because their children are distracted.

✧ Make it more difficult for children to pay attention to their bodies' hunger and fullness cues because the body is trying to process multiple sensory stimuli. I always use the example of how easy it is to eat a massive pot of popcorn at the cinema – it's not a coincidence!

Removing screen time from mealtimes can be helpful. You can do this by going cold turkey, which I find works effectively for many children, or gradually reducing the time the screen is used at mealtimes, so perhaps by five minutes each day. Either way, it's essential that you also ditch your screens, leaving phones away from the table.

The caveat is that certain groups of children, such as those who are neurodivergent, *may* need a screen to support sufficient dietary intake at mealtimes and/or as a regulatory strategy. Discussing your child's mealtime needs with a qualified professional who understands your child's unique requirements is, therefore, ideal.

Note: Yes, there may be times when we all, me included, turn to screens to support a mealtime – either because it's part of the mealtime plan, such as a family movie and pizza night, or because we just need it that day (for instance, eating out). In the context of any of my recommendations, I'm always talking about what we, as parents, do **most** *of the time.*

Are they sitting comfortably?

Focusing on a task is tough when you are uncomfortable, and this is especially true for children at mealtimes. If your child constantly fidgets, tries to climb out of their chair, sits on their knees or leans on the table, check their seating position.

The best eating position promotes stability and safety, relieves the body of the effort to stay upright and allows your child to focus on using their hands and eating. This position is a 90°–90°–90° angle at the ankles, knees and hips, as illustrated in the diagram below. As adults, we typically have no trouble achieving this on a standard chair, but young children may find themselves in adult chairs or other seating that's not designed for their size. A typical seating 'error' for young children is the lack of foot support (see page 83).

If adjustments to your child's seating position seem necessary, consider these suggestions:

✧ If your child is still using a highchair, adjust the footrest to align with their feet or create a makeshift footrest, such as a resistance band stretched between two highchair legs that can be positioned as needed, or use a securely tied tea towel.

✧ For children sitting in adult chairs, place a cushion behind their back to help them sit forward, allowing their legs to dangle comfortably over the seat's edge. Afterwards, provide a box or step for them to rest their feet on.

✧ Consider using a table and chairs that are appropriately sized for children.

Trust me, you'll see a difference.

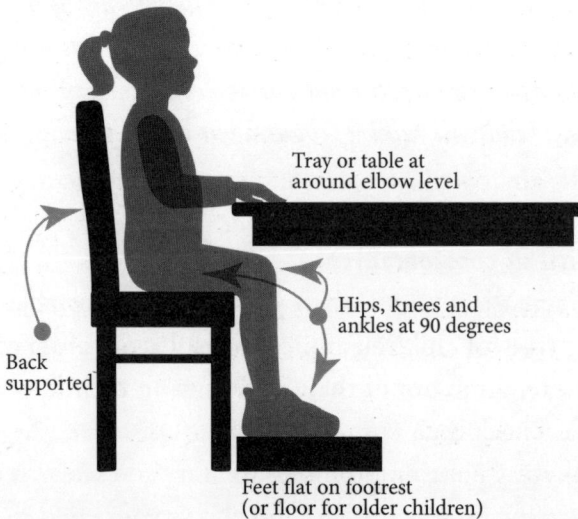

Tray or table at around elbow level

Hips, knees and ankles at 90 degrees

Back supported

Feet flat on footrest (or floor for older children)

Language around food and mealtimes

The impact of verbal and nonverbal communication at mealtimes is easily overlooked but considerably affects how children learn about food and their mealtime experiences.

As an example, if you were offered food such as Bush Tucker to eat, consider whether you'd be more eager to get stuck in if I tried to convince you with language like:

'It's good for you, full of protein.'

'Locals love it, it's a delicacy.'

'It's taken ages to prepare.'

'Just try it.'

'If you don't eat it, you can't have . . .'

When faced with food that feels like a substantial physical and mental challenge to put in your mouth, these persuasions are probably not convincing enough!

Despite this, it's easy to fall into these habits with children at mealtimes. We have all found ourselves asking our children to 'just' do something with food – 'Just try it', 'Just take one bite'. The question to honestly ask yourself is, 'why'? Why do they just need to have one more bite? And who is that one bite for? The reality is, that it's usually for us as adults because *we'd* feel better if they ate a piece of broccoli, or we've made our own rules or expectations about how they should eat.

In some cases, the 'just-one-bite' trap can do more harm than good, with any benefit from a bite of broccoli outweighed by the flood of stress hormones that a child can experience if they are stressed, people-pleasing or feeling under pressure and don't *really* want to eat it. Imagine how keen you'd be to come to the table if someone expected you to eat certain things, even if you didn't want them, every time you were there.

Other language behaviours that can be easy to slip into, that I'd urge you to avoid, include:

✧ **Repeated prompting** – One study exploring parental behaviours during mealtimes found that parents prompt their children to eat an average of 17.5 times per meal, in some cases going up to 30–40 prompts. These prompts often lead to more pressure on a child and mealtime struggles.

✧ **The many languages of persuasion** – Convincing, cajoling, over-encouragement or excessive praise, or any phrases or language embedded in persuading or trying to control your child's eating should be avoided, and studies show that these ultimately <u>increase</u> the likelihood of picky-eating behaviours.

✧ **Health hype** – Parents often tell me they feel pressure for their child to eat the 'right foods' as part of a balanced diet. In clinic I see over-encouragement of vegetables compared to other foods, with their health benefits being plugged in full force! 'But broccoli is good for you.' It's easy to put extra pressure on foods you want children to eat the most. Young children can't yet grasp the nuance around food and health; arguably, they don't need to understand nutrition complexities at this age, and I'd encourage you to keep nutrition education away from the table. It can also remove pleasure from eating. Try to keep all foods on a level playing field – food is just food – and avoid labelling foods as 'good or bad' or over-egging just the vegetables on their plate!

✧ **Constant questions** – It can be easy to start a cascade of questions at mealtimes, such as 'Do you want to try this?', 'What would you like to eat?', 'Is it yummy?' Using questions can increase pressure on the child to respond and engage with the food. Constant questioning can be pretty overwhelming, so it is best avoided. Questions like this can also easily be met with a 'no' and it's difficult to go anywhere from there, except perhaps to negotiation, which I'd also recommend you avoid!

✧ **Labelling your child a fussy or picky eater** – Little ears pick up on comments or inadvertent labels younger than we think! Try to avoid phrases they can hear like 'he won't eat that because he's fussy', as kids can become aware and internalise this, then before you know it you may have a child telling you they won't eat something because they *are* fussy.

So, how *can* we have a natter about food with children? While you may dip in and out of conversation with comments about the food on offer at the table, I'd encourage you to steer clear of a football-style commentary about food and predominantly talk about other things, not just the food.

Here are my top tips for mealtime language.

✧ **Use collaborative and modelling language,** such as 'We are having', 'We can put some peas on our plate', rather than using lots of child-centred language, which for some may increase pressure – 'You need to'.

✧ **Keep positive**, and by this I mean focus on what your child *can* do rather than lots of negative language like 'Don't', 'Stop', and 'If you don't'. For example, instead of 'Don't throw that food', you could say, 'You can put the food here if you don't want it'.

✧ **Remember, your body language counts,** so if you're stressed or anxious, your child is biologically hardwired to pick this up. Take a minute if you need it. Remember what you're modelling – for instance, eating it (or not) – and your facial expressions will be a loud and clear message (positive or negative) about that food for your child.

Ensure your child has some space at the table too, and avoid waving forkfuls of food in front of their mouth. Personal space is important.

If you're talking about the foods at the table in any capacity, check in with the three 'Fs':

◇ **Fun?** Young children learn through play and magical thinking, so meet your child where they are at. Labelling foods with different names that may be relatable, such as 'These orange pieces look like bear ears', can sometimes be a helpful approach. In fact, one study in preschool children found that creative naming of vegetables – power peas and x-ray-vision carrots – increased vegetable consumption. The takeaway is to keep any discussion around food fun, relaxed and relatable to your child's age and how they play and learn.

◇ **Factual?** No, you don't need the food knowledge of Rick Stein, but ask yourself if your description of a food is *actually* telling your child anything about that food that will help them learn about it? For example, 'delicious' or 'yummy' are opinions and don't apply to all foods. Factual or descriptive language, such as 'Peas are green and they grow in pods, this carrot is crunchy and I'm using my back teeth to crunch it,' can support learning about less-familiar foods.

◇ **Fair?** If what or how you're saying <u>anything</u> about the food to your child is laced with emotion about them wanting to eat it or could be perceived as loaded with pressure, try to avoid it. In some cases, avoiding talking about the food altogether is a good start for all parents!

On the next page you'll find some easy swaps to demonstrate language around food, if you're talking about it at all.

2. Encouraging autonomy around food
Imagine having no choice as to when you eat, what you're offered, how

much is on your plate or how long you have to stay at the table – and this is happening up to six times a day. This is the world that children often live in, which is especially tough for toddlers and young children, as development is priming them to take control of their world. I find battles of will are commonplace when discussing mealtime battles with parents of picky eaters, and so often this can reflect when children are being micromanaged around food or at mealtimes.

Swap	For
'Eat your peas, they are good for you.'	'This pea is round and green. Look, I can make it pop and there's a baby pea inside.'
'Two more mouthfuls before you can get down.'	'We can stop when our tummy tells us we are full.'
'Just try it.'	'It's ok, you don't have to eat it' – or ideally say nothing!
'What do you want to eat for breakfast?'	'We are having cereal for breakfast, would you like strawberries or apples with your cereal?'
'Take a bite, you always used to like avocado.'	You model eating avocado.
'Do you want yoghurt instead?'	'I'm afraid yoghurt isn't on the menu tonight. We can pick a day this week to have it instead.'
'Good boy for eating your carrots.'	Nothing! *While it feels counterintuitive, try to avoid excessive praise when your child eats a certain food or amount of food. A big 'song and dance' tells your child what they eat is very important to you, and can add pressure inadvertently.

If you've read through the toddler section, you'll know I've mentioned autonomy already. We all seek and thrive with

autonomy, and a vast review study from 2024 found that auton-
omy-supportive parenting – allowing children to make their
own choices – boosts their happiness and wellbeing. In the
context of mealtimes for children, autonomy refers to their ability to make choices and assert their independence during eating.
It is something I encourage all parents to consider for their
children.

I've already described several ways this can be achieved on pages
88–9, but in the context of picky eating, autonomy can look like:

✧ Supporting your child to feed themselves.

✧ Self-serving at mealtimes; this way they can own what and how
   much comes onto their plate. Studies suggest self-serving can
   enhance children's interest in foods.

✧ Offering a choice between two options that can be included in
   a meal or snack, such as 'would you like crackers or breadsticks
   with your cheese and grapes?'

✧ Involving children in menu planning when age allows.

✧ Offer a choice of plates, cups, placemats or cutlery.

✧ Have dips or 'sprinkles' at the table to include with meals, such
   as yoghurt, sauces, gravy or chopped fruits, seeds/ground nuts,
   grated vegetables.

✧ Family-style serving at mealtimes – more on this below!

Anything that gives a child some choice and agency is likely to be
well received; encouraging autonomy helps children develop confidence in their eating habits, build feeding skills, fosters a positive

relationship with food and, importantly, also recognises that children can and should listen and respond to their hunger and fullness cues.

3. Eating with others and family-style meals
'At the end of the day children follow your example, and not your advice.'

Human beings are social animals, and this is no different at mealtimes. Children rely on observing others to learn a vast number of skills, including eating. As we discussed on page 142, seeing parents and caregivers eat a variety of foods is recognised in the science and in practice to be one of the biggest influences on children's eating habits and food preferences, including when managing picky eating.

I have dedicated a whole section to the benefits of eating with your children, which you can read on page 336, but in the context of picky eating, here's why eating with your child can be so helpful:

✧ Your child sees you eating foods and enjoying them. This helps to build in exposure to a range of foods, but also allows your child to gain confidence with them 'by proxy' – such as how you eat them and how you respond to them. (It also means you stop to eat a meal!)

✧ Modelling eating foods means the focus can shift to *showing* your child what to do (eating the broccoli) rather than *telling* them 'Eat your broccoli'. Modelling to children will always trump telling them!

✧ Socialising, having fun and connecting with your child at mealtimes helps to create a safe and enjoyable environment that they will want to come back to, rather than avoid.

In practical terms, when you are sharing mealtimes or eating opportunities with your child, here are some things to remember:

✧ Include at least one or two of their accepted foods as part of the meal on offer – anyone can eat these; they are not solely your child's food options.

✧ Don't overcomplicate the meal – have the options on offer you were planning, and if your child's accepted foods don't fall within this, just bring them to the mealtime too to offer alongside.

✧ Try out family-style mealtimes, instead of pre-serving. A style of mealtime I'm an advocate for across the board, but especially when managing picky eating, is family-style serving. This is probably what you do at Christmas dinner, where everyone starts with an empty plate, and all options for the meal are available in the middle of the table. Your child can choose what and how much of each food comes to their plate (self-serving where possible), and watch what you bring to yours and what you go on to eat. It's a fantastic approach because it combines the benefits of modelling, exposure to a variety of food and autonomy all at once!

When doing this in practice, I encourage parents not to worry about decanting everything into serving bowls or about the food looking picture perfect. Just bring the options to the middle of the table, keep meals 'deconstructed' (wraps, shredded chicken, cooked onions and peppers, cheese instead of rolled and ready fajitas), then you can allow everyone to choose what they prefer. You can start this with toddlers as young as 14–16 months of age, supporting them by moving serving bowls closer, using smaller serving utensils and guiding their hands.

4. Expectations and emotions

In practice, a considerable aspect of managing picky eating is supporting parents with their expectations and emotions, with a big helping of also removing any blame attached to these. It is often forgotten that feeding children has a bidirectional relationship, and as parents we develop feeding practices in response to how our children eat and the appetite they express. We can also develop our own feelings of comfort and safety based on our children eating 'well' or having a 'full tummy'.

As parents, the challenge can be that it's easy to become attached to beliefs and expectations about how children *should* eat. Our upbringing, social media, family, friends, society and more influence these, alongside our own children's eating habits. Not only this, but how children eat can often stir up big feelings like failure or helplessness for parents. I need you to know that your feelings around your child's eating are valid and you won't be able just to switch them off, but awareness and examination of your own emotions, or 'triggers', when managing picky eating is incredibly supportive in the long run.

I find that many parents' behaviours relating to feeding their child are understandably driven by emotions, expectations and for many, concern. The emotional brain works around 2,000 times faster than the logical brain, so before you can calmly assess the situation (in this case, it might be your child's refused meal), feelings of worry, frustration or even guilt can take over. A rapid emotional response to this can lead to the immediate or reactive behaviours I've discussed throughout this section, like pressuring or persuading your child to eat, or offering rewards. The immediate responses are, understandably, led by the emotional and not the logical part of the brain, but these emotions or expectations can impact the eating and mealtime behaviours of children.

I find a few strategies can be helpful with parents who are finding their emotions leading the way with mealtimes and who may need to check back in with the slower-to-work, but perhaps more reassuring, logical brain. Here are a couple of examples.

Mindset and language shifts

From	To
Mealtimes are for eating.	Mealtimes are an *opportunity* to eat. Mealtimes can be for learning. Mealtimes are for connection.
My child has to eat at meal-times otherwise they will go hungry/not sleep.	I trust my child to listen to their appetite. I know appetite can fluctuate day to day and week to week.
It's my job to make sure they have a balanced diet.	I can role-model eating a balanced diet. A balanced diet is about the bigger picture, not a single meal.
I've offered it 10 times already, they really should be eating it.	My child can decide the right moment to eat something for the first time.

Writing down fears such as 'if my child doesn't eat their dinner every day they will lose weight', then pulling out the facts such as 'my child is growing along their centile', is another approach some parents find helpful, but can often need support from professionals.

What does your child need from you?
At mealtimes, while it's easier said than done, children need what I like to call '4 Cs' from their parents or caregivers. All of these help your child to a place of 'felt safety' at mealtimes:

✧ **Consistency** – With routines, language and how food is offered, as well as an avoidance of unhelpful 'fixing' behaviours, like pressure. Consistency between different caregivers is helpful too – try to avoid 'good-' and 'bad-' cop roles around food!

✧ **Calm** – Children look to caregivers for co-regulation and safety, including at mealtimes. Co-regulation in the context of parenting means when a parent/caregiver steps in to help their child meet their body's needs. It includes emotional support like modelling or 'lending' calm, helping children feel secure, being responsive to communication so their child feels heard and understood and providing structured, consistent routines. At mealtimes, remaining relaxed, offering reassurance, modelling feeding behaviours and supporting the environment to meet your child's needs are all beneficial.

✧ **Connection** – Prioritise building connections during mealtimes by encouraging communication, listening and shared experiences. Create a safe space where your child feels comfortable expressing themselves through words, actions or behaviours.

✧ **Collaboration** – Anything from planning menus together, giving your child an element of choice and autonomy and/or allowing them space to express their preferences and, of course, coming together at mealtimes. Collaborative mealtime experiences empower children, foster independence and strengthen mealtime trust. Ultimately, many children who are social learners will enjoy doing what you're doing and copying you!

Your child's emotions

It can be easy to forget about your child's emotions around food and mealtimes in the thick of managing your own. On tricky days of parenting a picky eater, I often remind parents to return to empathy. Put yourself in your child's shoes; has their routine completely changed at preschool today, so they're using eating habits as a way of gaining back some control? Are they naturally more cautious than their peers, so are the only ones not enamoured with trying the birthday cake (yes – even though it's cake!)? Your child is not trying to manipulate or upset you with their eating habits, the likelihood is they're finding it hard!

Support with managing emotions isn't always easy. At mealtimes, or just with the day-to-day challenges of parenting, our capacity to hold even our own emotions can change from day to day or week to week, which means at times it can be difficult to hold our children's emotions too. Be kind to yourself, and remember there is no blame, you are only human!

Step 2 – Choosing what foods to offer

Oh, finally – the food, I hear you cry!

Here are my golden rules for what to offer your picky eater at mealtimes.

1. Include at least one (or more) accepted/preferred food at every single eating opportunity. Accepted foods are those your child will usually eat when on offer. I avoid calling these 'safe' foods, as this may imply that food they haven't eaten yet is unsafe.

2. Serve other foods as part of the mealtime that your child doesn't accept yet. This 'exposure' gives your child an opportunity to learn about something they don't eat yet. It may just be on the table (if serving food family-style), or on a dish next to their meal, especially if your child is currently unhappy to have unfamiliar foods on their plate.

3. Offer a variety of foods, providing a balanced meal including two or three food groups. Whenever possible, rather than catering solely to your toddler's preferences each mealtime, I encourage you to plan family meals that you enjoy and incorporate your toddler's accepted foods alongside them. It's ok to serve plain crackers with a family meal of curry, rice and vegetables, or mix 'dinner' foods with breakfast options.

Accepted foods

Any advice you've read that suggests you should just withhold your child's preferred or accepted foods to support them to eat something else is dated and, for some children, can be harmful (as they really won't 'just eat' something else). Children who are picky eaters need the reassurance that comes with knowing at least one or more of their accepted/preferred foods is available – *so don't withhold these* – and aim to offer your child one or two accepted foods at each mealtime. When working with families, I will usually start by writing down a list of all the foods a child will accept (including variations on them, for instance, if they will have pasta, write down every shape they eat) split these by food groups on a table like the one on the next page. This can be helpful for two reasons:

1. Spotting any nutritional gaps – if there are whole food groups that a child is avoiding or one that is looking particularly sparse, this means we can explore if any additional vitamin or mineral supplementation is needed and in the long run focus on exposure to these foods. I also find this activity reassures some parents about exactly how many foods their child *will* eat.

2. Food rotation – I encourage parents to use this table to help rotate their child's accepted foods across mealtimes throughout the week. For example, you can ensure that the same food isn't offered every day, at the same meal in the same way. This approach helps prevent 'burnout' with your child's accepted foods, as children often lose interest after repeatedly eating a food at the same meal/s each day (a phenomenon known as food jagging). If you've ever wondered why your child suddenly rejects a food they've eaten daily for months, this is likely the reason!

Top tip: Making small changes to preparing or how you offer familiar foods (or even 'new'/'exposure' foods) can be helpful. For example, try serving carrots in sticks or grated instead of in circles, or offer yoghurt as a savoury dip with a meal rather than with fruit. These simple tweaks help children experience foods in new ways, encouraging flexibility and building confidence with change.

Carbohydrates	Fruit and vegetables	Protein-rich foods	Dairy or fortified alternatives	Misc
bread, rice, cereals, pasta, potato-based foods, noodles	fresh, frozen, dried, juices/ smoothies, pasta sauces	meat, fish, eggs, beans, nuts, seeds	milk, cheese, yoghurt, cream cheese	crisps, chocolate, cakes, biscuits, sauces
Your child's accepted foods here . . .				

Child-appropriate exposure to less familiar foods

Exposure is a necessary puzzle piece to help children learn about foods that they don't currently eat, and **repeated exposure** to foods is one aspect of picky-eating management that's strongly backed by the scientific data. Continuing to offer and expose your child to foods that have been regularly rejected can be something that can feel fatiguing for parents as they watch foods being repeatedly ignored, thrown around or declared 'yucky'. The problem with completely avoiding exposure to all less familiar foods or previously rejected foods is that we remove the opportunity for your child to gain familiarity and learn about them. I always describe this as like learning to ride a bike – it would be impossible if you weren't at the very least shown the bike you needed to learn to ride! It's even better if someone shows you what to do with it.

How this exposure is achieved depends on each child's background. As a starting point, reframing how children learn about new foods and eventually eat them is crucial. For most children, simply putting a less familiar food in front of them and expecting them to eat it isn't fair or realistic. Children learn to eat through exploration with all their senses – looking, smelling, listening, touching and tasting, and their preferred learning method – play!

Allowing your child to have regular opportunities for this exploration, at their own pace and without pressure, can eventually support them to accept a wider range of foods. It can be helpful to reframe progress with exposure as any positive interaction with a less familiar food from acknowledging its existence to licking. I want to reiterate that 'exposure to' does not mean eating!

Exposure may start as serving a meal to the table 'family-style', or eating with your child as I've described above, or placing a small amount of one 'new' food on their plate (this could be too much for some children) or a separate plate near by. In some cases, it might begin by offering a plate of vegetables or options as a 'starter' while preparing a meal.

Food interactions outside of mealtimes also count as important exposure and are something I encourage – shopping, cooking together, growing herbs, reading books about food – all exposure counts and has been shown to support children to gain familiarity with foods, which can lead to acceptance.

Remember, exposure must not be loaded with expectations. If anything, I'd recommend you expect the food to be ignored or rejected initially! Children need to feel safe before they can feel curious.

Exposure is most beneficial when repeated. Depending on the child and the food, it could take 2–200 (or more) exposures to acceptance – hence the long game I mentioned at the start of this chapter! I often encourage parents to consider any type of exposure to food like making small deposits in a savings account, which, when your child decides, may be 'spent' on exploring, tasting or eating a food.

For children with high levels of anxiety or neurodevelopmental diagnoses like autism, exposure may need to be much more carefully considered under the advice of a health professional, as it has the potential to increase anxiety and avoidance around food and mealtimes.

Managing nutritional worries with fussy eaters

In my experience, and this is mirrored in the science, nutrition or growth worries are common among parents of picky eaters. Often, there is a huge sense of responsibility and urgency about ensuring your child is 'getting enough' nutrition. Reassuringly, research shows that in most cases of moderate picky eating, the risk of growth concerns is low, and while there is some risk of lower-than-ideal intake of certain nutrients, like iron, these mirror similar concerns to the general population.

Undercover veggies: Should you hide foods?

Lots of parents ask me about 'hiding' foods for fussy eaters and whether it is a good idea. Blending vegetables into pasta sauce, for example, can give parents peace of mind that their child is getting specific foods or food groups that they may be lacking. While it's great to be creative with incorporating different foods into meals, for long-term acceptance of the 'hidden' foods, your child will need to see and learn about them. For example, if you'd like your child to accept the pepper you blend into a sauce then they will need to see it in other ways e.g. pepper sticks. I would also encourage you to be honest about what's in food. If children become aware of foods being hidden, it can backfire into a mistrust of the meals being offered to them, and you risk increasing food refusal! For children with more complex feeding differences related to neurodivergence, for example, hiding ingredients in their accepted foods may also lead them to reject the food entirely, and onwards from that point, so I tend to advise against this.

I often discuss with parents strategies to help check in on their child's diet and intake, which I find helps to reassure and at times identify when extra steps are necessary to support nutrition.

Here are some usual topics of conversation:

1. The bigger picture – While it can be easy to focus in on foods your child doesn't eat each day, I often spend time with parents reassuring them that nutrition is generally much more about the bigger picture, and that the range of foods a child needs to get the nutrients they need is often much smaller than many parents anticipate.

2. Growth (weight and height) – These measurements can help reassure you that your child's diet is providing them with the energy and protein they need. I'd encourage you to measure your child with a health professional if you are concerned, to ensure accuracy with plotting weight and height measurements. Your child's diet is likely to provide the energy and protein they need if they are growing and tracking well along their weight and height centiles. However, consult a health professional if your child drops two or more weight centile positions.

3. Overall nutritional balance – Young children benefit from a variety of foods from different food groups to get the nutrients required for growth and good health. One (very) simple method to assess their nutritional intake is by completing the food-group review mentioned above. This may help identify any gaps where your child has few or no foods from certain food groups, or reassure you that they actually include foods from all of the main foods groups. Awareness of any gaps can help highlight when additional support, from a professional like a dietitian, may be needed. Remember, as a parent, you're not expected to be a dietitian!

4. Supplementation – While there are obviously some vitamin supplements recommended for all children, depending on their age, additional supplementation of key nutrients 'at risk' in children with more limited diets can support many parents with some peace of mind. In an ideal world supplementation and dosage should be advised by a health professional, however, many parents explore A–Z or complete over-the-counter vitamin and mineral preparations.

What about foods with extras and fussy-eater 'shakes'?

Fortified foods are those that have added nutrients like vitamins and minerals. They can be helpful to consider in the diet of picky eaters. Some foods in the UK are routinely fortified anyway; for example, flour in the UK (non-wholemeal varieties) contains added calcium, iron and from 2026, folate. Here are some common fortified foods that you may find helpful to consider.

Food	Options to consider
Bread	Some 50:50 bread brands are fortified with extra calcium and iron (above that added to normal flour).
Milk	Fortified milk (whole) containing added vitamins A and D and iron. For plant-based alternatives, use 'growing-up' milk alternatives, such as oat or soy-based, which also contain extra vitamins and minerals including iron, zinc, calcium and iodine.
Cereals	A wide range of cereals, including those marketed to children, contain added vitamins and minerals. Exploring these, including being offered dry as a snack, can be helpful for some children. Ready oats are also very well fortified and can be used as cereal but also as a part of flour replacement for foods like pancakes and muffins.

I always urge caution with food products like nutritional shakes marketed for fussy eaters. While they can provide convenience and reassurance, they often come with drawbacks: they can be expensive, high in added sugars and may quickly fill your child up, reducing their appetite for meals and snacks. This can be counterproductive when trying to support a fussy eater!

Health hurdles for fussy eaters

For some children, other things can impact their eating behaviours and interaction with foods. These include constipation, iron deficiency, unmanaged food allergies or intolerances, or even complex medical diagnoses. I would encourage you to make sure these are addressed to support progress with your picky eater, seeking support from your GP as a first port of call.

When will things improve?

This is the million-dollar question for parents of picky eaters. The honest answer is that it takes time and patience. Research shows that fussy eating typically resolves for most children within two years, although for some it can be longer. I recommend seeking professional support if it continues beyond that or becomes more challenging to manage. Two years can feel like twenty when you're cooking multiple meals a day and watching food get sneered at or tossed aside.

It's also important to recognise that acceptance of new foods can vary. Foods similar in taste or texture to what your child already enjoys are usually accepted more quickly than those with challenging flavours or textures. Some foods may take years to accept – and that's perfectly fine. I didn't start eating mushrooms until I was 33, and I know many of you have similar stories.

With this in mind, I always remind parents of some key ways to keep motivated at mealtimes:

✧ Choose foods YOU want to eat at mealtimes and can enjoy – you need to eat too, and choosing foods you enjoy and nourish you will be an ideal modelling opportunity.

✧ Focus on small steps and progress, as a perceived lack of progress is when I often find parents experiencing heightened frustration or slipping back into habits like persuasion. Positive steps could look like:

o You are feeling more relaxed at mealtimes and/or accepting of where your child is now.

o Your child is now happily coming to the table.

o Your child enjoys eating with you.

o Your child is asking questions or showing curiosity around food.

o Your child is starting to acknowledge, touch or smell foods for the first time – it's all progress.

✧ Some families find a progress log (for themselves) helps to keep them grounded, and focused on what's going well.

✧ Find ways to take some pressure off mealtime prep, this can be simple measures such as roasting a tray of different vegetables on a Sunday and keeping it in your fridge ready for the week ahead. This allows you the flexibility to offer multiple different options during the week and will expose your children to new foods with minimal effort.

When is it more than just picky eating?

Not all children with selective-eating habits are fussy eaters. Some have feeding difficulties and differences that go beyond normal age or developmental picky-eating behaviours. But how do you know if this is your child?

Here are some of the telltale differences between fussy eaters and those with more notable feeding difficulties or differences.

Fussy eaters	May indicate 'more than' fussy eater – seek support
Range of foods usually 20+.	Range of foods 15 or under.
Will accept foods across all food and texture groups (except vegetables).	Whole food or texture groups are often refused or excluded.

Evident food preferences – foods/texture groups.	Has very strong likes and dislikes (not just preferences).
Usually resolves within months up to two years, often independently without intensive intervention.	Persists for months to years without improvement or with reducing food range.
Minimal/no impact on weight or growth.	Consistently poor growth and/or appetite concerns (*please note: children can still be, and in my experience often are, within healthy growth parameters but experiencing significant feeding differences*). A healthy weight alone is not an indicator there are no feeding problems.
Tolerant of different brands and packaging of accepted foods.	Can discriminate between brands of foods, and will reject or 'melt down' if the incorrect brand is offered.
May eat differently in different contexts.	Child shares few or none of the same foods as the family and/or may never attend family meals.
May refuse less familiar foods, but the response does not impact the rest of the mealtime.	Child shows significant (and often persistent) physical and/or emotional responses around less-familiar foods, eating or situations involving food such as 'meltdown', gagging/retching, distress. There are signs of anxiety around food or mealtimes, such as complaints of stomach ache at mealtimes, asking to go to the toilet or avoidance of social interactions with food, such as parties.
The child may have preferred routines but will eat without these.	The child needs specific routines or distractions to eat.

May have some sensory sensitivities or preferences, but these do not significantly impact dietary range and/or mealtimes.	Clear evidence of sensory differences that impact mealtimes, such as only being able to tolerate certain colours, smells, textures, shapes and temperature of foods.
No lack of the skills needed to eat.	Difficulty with skills needed to eat, such as chewing, swallowing, using hands.
No previous feeding challenges prior to this stage.	A history of feeding challenges that were present before the toddler years, such as difficulty transitioning with textures or tastes during weaning/stuck on purees.
No notable medical conditions or history affecting eating.	Medical concerns that are affecting feeding, such as vomiting, severe reflux, food allergies, persistent choking, coughing and/or gagging at mealtimes, breathing difficulties.

If your child has any of the 'red flags' on the right-hand side of this table, I recommend you approach your GP for advice and signposting to relevant nutrition and feeding specialists, such as a dietitian, speech-and-language therapist, occupational therapist. Please note that as a parent, if you have any gut feelings or worries about your child's feeding, regardless of the details above, I'd encourage you to seek professional support.

SOS – Common worries about toddler feeding

I'm worried my toddler isn't getting enough protein; they've gone off meat/fish/eggs.

This is an exceptionally common worry from parents, but the good news is that protein intake is rarely a concern in toddlers or children. A recent report of children's eating habits in the UK showed that toddlers often exceed their daily protein needs by up to three to four times the requirement. Toddlers can get protein from more than just meat, fish, eggs or seafood. Dairy, soy, nuts, seeds, grains and carbohydrates all contain protein too.

As an example, a toddler's protein requirement for the day is 14.5g, which could look like:

✧ A small bowl of cereal with milk – 8g protein

✧ A portion of yoghurt or cheese – 4g

✧ Half a slice of wholemeal bread – 2.5g

Total = 14.5g

Going off these foods is also very common during the toddler years, as foods like meat and fish can be far less predictable in terms of texture, taste and presentation, missing the all-important same-ness that lots of toddlers lean towards. If your child is skipping past these foods at the moment, I'd recommend focusing on sources of nutrients they provide, like iron, elsewhere in the diet.

Help! My child won't drink milk – will they get enough nutrients?
When transitioning from formula and/or breast milk, many parents worry their toddler hasn't taken to drinking cups of cow's milk or a fortified milk alternative. Please be reassured that toddlers don't *have* to drink cow's milk/milk alternative to get all the nutrients they need. As long as a toddler is getting on average two to three portions of dairy (or fortified alternatives) in their diet, they can get the nutrients they need.

For reference, a 'portion' of dairy would be:

✧ 20–30g hard cheese or cream cheese

✧ 80–120g yoghurt

✧ 100–120ml milk

My toddler eats anything at nursery/ childcare, but not at home.

First things first, you're not alone, and please don't take this difference in behaviour personally. Parents often find themselves somewhere between laughing and crying when they hear or see that their child has tucked into a five-vegetable Moroccan tagine with couscous at nursery but won't even entertain some cucumber on their plate at home. There can be many reasons why your toddler eats 'better' at nursery, and these include:

✧ **Social eating** – They are surrounded by many small role models, including their peers, who they really relate to!

✧ **Robust routines** – Nursery and childcare settings have that crucial routine around eating times locked in! They probably offer foods at the same time, in the same way, have a clear seating area, have a cue to eating – such as a bell or handwashing – and while this may seem obvious, it comes back to that all-important predictability and felt safety around eating and mealtimes that I've talked about already.

✧ **Allowing autonomy** – Your child likely receives less attention at mealtimes in childcare than at home, as the adults there must share their focus among many kids. While childcare staff care about your child, they're also less likely to react emotionally to food refusals or engage in 'fix-it' behaviours, like offering alternatives, that parents often resort to. In some childcare settings foods may be served in a way where toddlers have more autonomy for food choices.

If this rings true for your toddler, try to replicate some of the environmental factors at childcare at home, such as eating with your toddler or giving them some choice.

Help! My toddler is throwing food.

Many parents assume this is a behaviour reserved for babies, but it can be common in the toddler years too, although often for slightly different reasons. If you're in a food-throwing phase, here are some considerations:

✧ **Avoid big reactions** – Toddler brains can find big reactions from parents or caregivers exciting and can struggle to distinguish between different forms of attention – positive or negative. Try to remain calm and a little nonchalant to the behaviour, as annoying as it is!

✧ **Mealtime check-in** – Consider whether food throwing could be a sign that your toddler is full/has finished eating, or is feeling overwhelmed with the foods being offered – either in the number of foods or the amount of them. Offering smaller portions or allowing them to choose the foods coming to their plate or tray can be helpful. If they repeat the behaviour multiple times during a mealtime you might consider ending the meal with, 'It looks like you're showing me you've finished', then start to remove their food.

✧ **Focus on the positive action** – Rather than just saying no, you can set clear boundaries with your toddler and identify the 'dos' instead of 'don'ts', such as, 'food stays on the table'.

✧ **Try moving them to the table** – From 12+ months you can consider taking the tray off a highchair and bringing your child up to the table. This can help reduce the amount of edge for hurling food over, but it also usually means it's easier to eat together, which can be enough to stop some kids throwing.

My toddler keeps overstuffing their mouth.

Ah, here's another episode of annoying but normal things toddlers can do at mealtimes. There's nothing like watching your toddler try to stuff all of the meal into their mouth at once, then spit it back out because they can't properly chew or swallow it. Toddlers can do this for a variety of reasons, including because they are still very much learning how to eat and overstuffing can help with mouth-mapping, understanding how food feels and how to use their tongue. Some children are also just experimenting and seeking some sensory input, while others are just super hungry that day and take it too fast!

There are a few things you can do to stop this behaviour:

✧ Keep calm.

✧ Don't be afraid to show them how to spit. I know it's not the table manners we are all taught but it's a valuable skill to keep kids safe around food.

✧ Try offering a smaller portion initially, or bring foods to their plate gradually.

✧ Avoid pressure around food; in my experience some children pocket and hold food in their mouths when they don't want to eat/aren't hungry but are also trying to please requests to eat or have another bite.

✧ Model taking bites out of food of different sizes, or prompt or model chewing.

✧ If this behaviour persists, I'd encourage you to seek some support from a health professional like a speech-and-language therapist, especially if there are any other concerns about their sensory needs or biting and chewing (oral motor) skills.

My child often refuses food or eats small amounts of their evening meal. Do I let them go to bed hungry?

As a parent, I can completely empathise with the anxiety of managing any variable that might contribute to night waking or nutrition worries, and anticipation of our child's hunger is one of them! That said, there are a variety of reasons why your toddler might refuse their evening meal. I think it's important to normalise that toddlers can refuse entire meals or only eat a small number of mouthfuls without it being a concern. In my experience, the evening meal may be more likely to be skipped because:

✧ Your toddler has consumed most of the energy their body needs already. In fact, I see many toddlers who 'front load' most of the energy they need earlier in the day and have much less appetite by the afternoon and evening. (Some toddlers can be the opposite.)

✧ Your toddler may be tired at the end of their day and/or less regulated, making eating a more challenging task.

✧ The meal served in the evening may include foods that are less familiar or more challenging for toddlers, such as mixed textures, vegetables or ingredients that you offer less often.

It's understandable to assume your child must be hungry, especially as the evening meal is often the one that as adults we consider to be the 'biggest' meal of the day. There is every chance, though, that your toddler isn't hungry, so it can be helpful to lean back into the advice about trusting their appetite. In general, for typically developing children with no growth concerns, the advice would be to avoid offering alternatives or rescue meals. If you are providing a snack or supper before bed, ensure there is a good length of time between this and the evening meal, and that you are rotating what's on offer, not just picking your child's most preferred foods.

My child wants to get up and down from the table or doesn't like sitting in their chair.

Table time can be a challenge for many parents. Children getting up frequently or being uncomfortable in their seat can be frustrating for various reasons. Here are some things to consider:

✧ Attention span – Toddlers can often only focus on an activity for 2–15 minutes. It's unrealistic to expect them to sit still for as long as adults do.

✧ Busy minds and bodies – Some toddlers may need to leave the table and then return to it. If this is the case, you can set boundaries, such as clearing the food after 30 minutes.

✧ Seating position – If your toddler is still in a highchair, consider removing the tray and bringing them to the table. For those in adult chairs, ensure they are comfortable and properly positioned, using cushions or boxes if needed. (See page 218.)

✧ Movement – Young children need movement to regulate their bodies. If your toddler has been less active than usual, encourage some active play before mealtimes.

✧ Mealtime environment – Eating together, modelling desired behaviours, maintaining a routine and serving manageable portions can also improve the mealtime experience.

How do I manage constant requests for snacks?

Trust me, I've been here too! It's 9:48am and you've already had 11 separate demands from your toddler for a snack. Surely they are not hungry again? Now, it's possible that they are, but they may also be practising their newfound communication skills or exercising their lack of impulse control. Avoiding grazing and having a structure around meals and snacks throughout the day can support your child's appetite regulation, but here are some practical pointers on how to manage these requests.

1. Acknowledge or hear your toddler – respond with 'Mummy can hear that you'd like a snack.'
2. Boundary and reassurance – try telling them, 'It's not snack time right now, but after playtime/swimming/activity, we will have a snack.'
3. Move on or move forward – sometimes toddlers may need a distraction to move on or away from the request, or if it's not long until snack time, you might just want to move it forward.
4. Don't fear the tantrum or use the tantrum fear as a reason to just give the snack – while unpleasant at the best of times, tantrums are a very typical way of a toddler expressing their big emotions.
5. Out of sight – on a practical level, keeping snack foods out of reach of little hands helps to avoid independent snacking (helping themselves!).

Top tip with packaged snacks: The packaging for shop-bought snacks targeted at young children can often be a positive and appealing visual cue for children, potentially increasing their desirability. Famous pigs, dogs and monsters creep onto these foods for a reason, and it's certainly not for your benefit! To help navigate this it can be helpful, where you can, to decant your child's snacks out of the packaging and into a bowl, plate or small container.

Why does my toddler LOVE beige foods?

I always smile at this question because the love of foods that are what I call 'bland and tanned', aka carbohydrates or processed meat/fish products, is common in the toddler years. Carbohydrates or beige-coloured foods can get such negative feelings thrown their way, but please know that they contain valuable nutrients too. As a starting point, toddlers need plenty of carbohydrates as their preferred energy source – meaning they will want to eat these foods. These foods can also provide an array of nutrients from fibre to B vitamins, protein and more.

One of the reasons they can be favoured in the toddler years is their predictability and the 'safety' this brings. Think of it this way – with a cream cracker or brand of cereal, regardless of where or when you buy it, it is likely to be the same shape, colour, texture and taste every single time. It's also easy to recognise and remember. Compare this to something like blueberries – they can be hard, soft, sweet or tart, and so much less predictable.

Can certain foods help my toddler sleep?

I know that having a child who sleeps well is the ultimate win for all parents! Trust me, I've been there, ready to try anything to help my daughter sleep through the night. Unfortunately, the biology of sleep, especially in babies and young children, is complex and influenced by many factors, so I can't promise a silver bullet when it comes to food. However, here are some things to consider.

1. Breast milk – If you're breastfeeding, breast milk is a perfect pre-bed drink as it contains melatonin (the sleepy hormone) towards the end of the day.
2. Tryptophan-rich foods – Tryptophan is an amino acid that the body uses to produce serotonin and melatonin, hormones that help support sleep. Foods high in tryptophan include turkey, eggs, dairy foods (milk, cheese), tofu, oats and other grains, nuts and seeds (especially walnuts and almonds), beans and lentils, and certain fruits like apples, bananas, pineapple, plantain and cherries.
3. Magnesium – This mineral is known to support sleep alongside a wide range of other body functions. I see more and more magnesium supplements promoted for children's sleep, but at

the moment we don't have any good scientific evidence to suggest kids don't get enough magnesium from their diet, or that magnesium supplementation improves children's sleep. Magnesium-rich foods include bananas, wholemeal bread, cereals, avocado, spinach, tofu, nuts and seeds. For context, a one-to three-year-old could meet their magnesium needs for the day just by eating two wheat biscuits (cereal) with some milk and a teaspoon of peanut butter, or one slice of wholemeal bread, a banana and 120g yoghurt.

Some foods or nutrients can negatively affect sleep in children; for example, foods or drinks high in caffeine, like cocoa, hot chocolate and certain beverages can interfere with sleep (though it's unlikely your young child is drinking tea, coffee or cola!). For babies or children affected by reflux, certain triggers, such as acidic foods, chocolate, mint or high-fat meals that take longer to digest, can worsen symptoms of discomfort overnight. It may be best to avoid these foods close to bedtime for some children.

*   *   *

While I could talk about the whirlwind of the toddler years for pages more, it's time to draw this section to a close and think about what's next. The final age section of this book is focused on the preschool years. While much of the advice around nutrition and feeding from this section carries over (phew, I hear you sigh), I wanted to acknowledge these years as another time of transition where nutrition and feeding weave into new skills and experiences ahead, like school. You may also find some of the topics in the next section helpful now, such as information on fibre, salt and sugar.

4

Fuelling Fun

Graduating from the early years, aka preschoolers: 3–5 years

Nutrition and feeding milestones during the preschool years:

✧ Preschoolers grow slower than in their toddler years, gaining about 2–3kg and growing 5–7.5cm per year on average.
✧ By age five, your preschooler's brain is around 90 per cent of its adult size.
✧ Preschool years are crucial for cognitive development, with nutrients like iron and omega 3 fatty acids essential for ongoing brain growth and function.
✧ Your preschooler will become increasingly independent and proficient in eating. They will continue to master cutlery skills, learn to serve themselves and vocalise their food choices and preferences.
✧ Peers will continue to play a significant role in shaping your child's eating habits, as social interactions and mealtime experiences influence their food preferences and eating behaviours.
✧ Regular family meals are an opportunity to model healthy eating habits and encourage positive food behaviours.

✦ **Engaging your child in meal preparation can also boost their interest in different foods and cooking skills.**

You now have a little one rapidly approaching school age and perhaps acting like a preteen instead of a preschooler. While their nutritional needs continue to evolve, I'll let you in on a secret: this age can feel, from a nutrition standpoint, like a bit of a bridge. In the early toddler years there is a feeling of transitioning from baby to toddler feeding, and with this comes lots of change. By the time you reach preschool age you'll be well equipped with what to feed your preschooler, and you may find time to think about more specific areas of their diet, feeding or nutrition. You'll also probably start looking ahead a little into the school years on the horizon.

As you progress through this next section, you'll soon realise that the previous section (on the toddler years) is referenced frequently. It remains accurate and relevant for this age group, albeit with minor tweaks. The advice on how to feed your preschooler is also broadly similar but with some added age-appropriate extras.

For this reason, what I've prioritised in this section is:

✦ A review of what your preschooler needs nutrition-wise (without too much repetition, I promise).

✦ A closer look at a few areas of nutrition that may benefit from some attention during these years, such as fibre, salt and sugar, as habits concerning these can pay forward to future health.

✦ Some age-appropriate extras on how to support and encourage independence and learning about food and eating.

Preschool nutrition 101

✧ **Building balance and nutritional needs – a recap**

✧ **Nutrient spotlight – salt, sugar and fibre**

✧ **Preschool portion sizes**

✧ **Supplements for preschoolers**

✧ **Preschool eating behaviours and feeding development**

Building balance and nutritional needs – a recap

Throughout the preschool years, there is an ongoing need for nutrient-dense foods and nutrition tailored for small bodies growing and developing quickly, albeit at a slightly slower speed than they have been for the last three years. With this in mind, how much your preschooler eats will continue to fluctuate, but the principles of what you offer to provide necessary nutrients for growth and development don't change much. You can find detailed information about building dietary balance for children during the early years from page 178 onwards. By means of a recap, check out the diagram below.

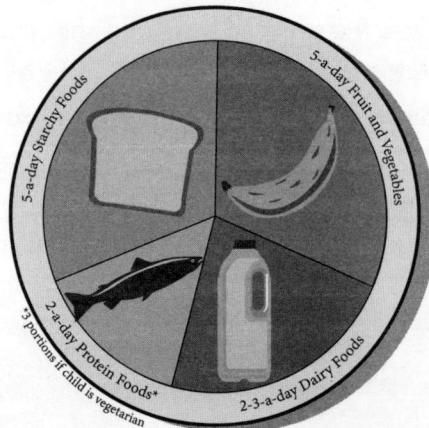

The frequency with which you are offering meals and snacks also remains largely unchanged during these preschool years, however, you will often find that the time between eating opportunities can extend from two to three hours to three to four hours as they get older, and daily routines around preschool or school and bedtimes shift.

From four years of age, the amount of different nutrients needed can shift a little. Many vitamin and mineral requirements increase slightly, but this is not the case across the board. This adjustment is necessary to meet the changing needs of your child's growing body, supporting their development, immune function and overall health as they become more active and continue to grow. Here are just a few examples:

- ✧ **Protein** – increases from 14.5 to 19.7g per day. This extra 5g per day is equivalent to a small egg, 15g of cheese or 60g of cooked beans or lentils.
- ✧ **Calcium** – increases from 350mg to 450mg per day. This is an extra 100mg daily, equivalent to 80ml of milk, 60–80g of yoghurt or two slices of white bread.
- ✧ **Iron** – decreases from 6.9mg to 6.1mg per day. It's not a stark change, but as a nutrient that many young children struggle to get enough of, I wouldn't recommend you take your foot off the gas when prioritising iron-rich foods.
- ✧ **Zinc** – increases from 5mg to 6.5mg per day. This extra 1.5mg daily is equivalent to 30g of chicken thigh, 20g of Cheddar cheese or 50g of cooked lentils.

The good news is that for most children, as long as you prioritise the balance I've discussed throughout this book, your preschooler is unlikely to struggle with keeping up with their requirement changes.

Nutrient spotlight – salt, sugar and fibre

Given that I've already covered the nutrition basics, let's focus on a few nutrients that can be challenging to manage, especially in this age group and beyond. Over recent years, and often due to concerns about children's diets in the UK, these nutrients have gained media attention and interest.

Salt

Salt, also known as sodium chloride, is a nutrient that your child needs, because it's essential for the balance of fluids in the body, for cells and nerves to work correctly, and for other jobs like producing stomach acid.

However, excess salt intake is a concern for much of the UK population, including young children. A recent public health report found that over three-quarters of children aged 18 months to four years consumed more salt than recommended. Too much salt increases the workload for children's developing kidneys and can lead to health issues like high blood pressure, weak bones (osteoporosis) and kidney disease later in life. In the early years, salt intake also has the potential to shape taste preferences later in life.

Salt recommendations for young children are:

<1 year – 1g/day (equivalent to ⅙ of a teaspoon)
1–3 years – 2g/day (equivalent to ⅓ of a teaspoon)
4–6 years – 3g/day (equivalent to ½ a teaspoon)

As with all the nutrients discussed in this book, I encourage a practical approach to managing salt intake. There's no need to track every meal your child eats, and some days will naturally have more salt than others, and that's ok. The tips provided here aim to help you keep salt to a pinch!

✧ Avoid adding salt to food; a lightly salted meal now and again is likely no issue, but if you're in the habit of adding salt to all family meals, consider adding it to your portion at the end or using it as an opportunity to drop your own salt intake.

✧ Try other ways to flavour meals; herbs, spices and fruits like lemon are versatile, cheap and have extra benefits, like feeding friendly gut bacteria.

✧ Swap to low-salt or no-salt stock cubes.

✧ Choose tinned fish or vegetables in spring water instead of brine (salted water).

✧ Grab a glimpse at your food labels when you can – generally, over 1.5g of salt per 100g is considered high.

✧ You don't need to completely eliminate foods that are higher in salt but still offer nutritional benefits, such as cheese. Instead, focus on managing portion sizes and adding variety by including lower-salt alternatives. For cheeses, consider options like mozzarella, ricotta or cream cheese alongside higher-salt choices like Cheddar or Parmesan.

✧ Wherever you can, limit foods that are high in salt, such as processed meats like bacon and sausages, ready meals, jarred sauces, soups, sandwiches and crisps. It's also worth being mindful that many everyday foods like bread and cereals can see the salt content of a child's diet creep up. I always find examples help, so here are a few.

Food	Salt content (approximate)
Two slices of cooked ham	0.6g
Bacon	Some brands get up to 2g/rasher
5 cocktail sausages	0.62g
Corn flakes 30g	0.3g
One slice of bread	Some brands get up to 0.5-0.6g
Large rice cake	Some brands get up to 0.6g
Packet of ready salted crisps (25g)	0.34g
¼ frozen cheese pizza	0.6g
¼ jar of tomato pasta sauce	0.5-0.6g

What about different types of salt?

It always amazes me that even salt can't avoid marketing's fateful eye! You may see all kinds of salt on the market, from Himalayan pink to Celtic salt. You'll be told (sold!) that they are superior to table salt because they contain extra minerals, but I'm afraid the amount you consume to get any benefits from those extra vitamins and minerals is pretty substantial (and *well* above the daily guidance amounts for children).

Sugar

Public health data in the UK shows that 80 per cent of young children consume too much sugar. This is important for several reasons. Firstly, tooth decay is now the leading cause of hospital admissions for children in the UK, and tooth extraction is the most common reason why they undergo general anaesthesia. Excess sugar intake, particularly from sugar-sweetened drinks, can also contribute to excessive energy (calorie) consumption.

Many parents are surprised at how easily sugars creep into their child's diet, and the groups of foods or drinks that seem to contribute the most are:

✧ Sugar-sweetened yoghurts, fromage frais or dairy-based desserts.

✧ Biscuits, buns, cakes and pastries.

❖ Sugar-sweetened drinks, such as squash and carbonated drinks.

❖ Fruit juices and smoothies.

❖ Commercially manufactured foods and drinks explicitly marketed for babies and young children, such as food and drinks in the baby and toddler aisle (this one surprises many people!).

However, many sugar-containing foods can also offer health benefits; yoghurts provide calcium as a dairy source, fortified cereals can provide iron and fibre, and smoothies can offer fibre and count towards a child's daily fruit and vegetable intake. Therefore, I always recommend a balanced and pragmatic approach when managing a child's sugar intake, with the caveat that sugar isn't 'bad' or to be feared, it just needs to be approached mindfully.

I want to share the sugar content of some common foods marketed at young children, some of which you might find surprising:

❖ Toddler 'fruit bars' – 4–5g sugar (1 teaspoon)

❖ Toddler fruit jerky/shapes – 8g sugar (2 teaspoons)

❖ Popular sweetened fromage frais – 4g sugar, *excluding lactose, as this is a naturally occurring milk sugar in yoghurt* (1 teaspoon)

❖ Popular mini chocolate bar – 7g sugar (1¾ teaspoons)

❖ Kids' cake bar – 8g sugar (2 teaspoons)

❖ One plain biscuit (no chocolate) – 2g sugar (½ teaspoon)

❖ 150ml pure apple juice – 14g sugar (3½ teaspoons)

❖ 30g multigrain hoop cereal – 5g sugar (>1 teaspoon)

The UK guidelines for sugar consumption in children under four years advise limiting intake as much as possible. Ideally, no more than 5 per cent of a young child's daily energy should derive from free sugars, which is roughly equivalent to around 1 teaspoon or less a day and as such may be viewed as quite an aspirational target! My key advice is to stay mindful of the free-sugar content in foods and be aware of your child's overall intake. While aiming for strict limits may not always be realistic, making practical adjustments where possible can have a positive impact on their health and wellbeing.

To support you in moderating the free-sugar intake in your child's diet, here are some of my top tips.

✧ If offering foods containing free sugars, aim to include these at mealtimes alongside other foods and avoid your child grazing on these foods at regular intervals across the day.

✧ Get into good teeth-brushing habits – twice a day. I've found that brushing my teeth with my daughter helps her to be much more motivated. Songs, timers and books help too.

Don't fear the fruit

Unfortunately, fruit often gets scooped into the 'sugar-is-bad' conversations as it contains naturally occurring sugars like fructose (fruit sugar). Fruit is not to be feared – it's a valuable source of fibre, vitamins, minerals and antioxidants, which are all great for supporting your child's health.

Part of the reason sugar intake often catches parents off guard is that it comes in many forms. This, combined with halo marketing claims such as 'only natural sugars' or 'no added sugar', can mean it's easy for free-sugar intake to go under the radar. Free sugars are sugars added to foods and drinks or those naturally present in honey, syrups and fruit juices. They do not include the sugars found naturally in whole fruits and vegetables. For example, the sugar naturally occurring in an apple is not free sugar, but the sugar in apple juice, puree or juice concentrate is.

✧ Limit smoothies and juices to 100–150ml maximum or ideally dilute them and aim to consume them with a meal. Avoid sugar-sweetened drinks or fizzy drinks wherever possible. Remember, water and milk are generally the only recommended drinks for toddlers and preschoolers.

✧ Get used to having a quick look at the food labels and don't just go off the front-of-packet claims. Check the section 'of which sugars' under the nutritional information to see the sugar content; >22.5g/100g is considered high in sugar, and <5g/100g is low. Bear in mind that the lactose from milk will be included in the sugar counts of yoghurts and dairy desserts.

✧ Knowing the names of sugar in the ingredients can also help when labelling – look for sugar, syrup, honey, fruit concentrates, fruit paste, sucrose, glucose and dextrose. Food ingredients are listed in order of weight, so if sugar is higher up the list or one of the first few ingredients, it's likely high in sugar.

✧ Be mindful of dried fruit and dried fruit pastes, as these can be more likely to get stuck in your toddler's teeth and accelerate tooth decay. Many dentists recommend avoiding dried fruit until a child is at least five.

✧ Offer sweeter foods alongside the main meal – this doesn't just help manage the impact of the sugar on your child's teeth but it is a helpful strategy to help keep sweeter foods more 'neutral' in their appeal; they are just foods offered alongside other foods: no earning potential, and no excessive focus on them at the table.

Think about making some straightforward food swaps that could help reduce your child's sugar intake, such as:

Swap	For
Sugar-sweetened yoghurts	Plain yoghurts – natural or Greek, with the option of added fruit (whole, grated, stewed) or other toppings like oats, seeds or crushed cereal pieces.
Higher-sugar or coated cereals – chocolate, frosted, honey	Lower-sugar cereal options – wheat biscuits, wholegrain shredded cereals, porridge (or offer a 50/50 mix with a higher-sugar option).
Dried fruit bars or shapes	Fresh whole fruit or a lower-sugar snack.
Tinned fruit in syrup	Tinned fruit in juice.
Juice drinks	Water (optional – added sliced fruit).

Understanding types of sugar

Like salt, sugar also falls prey to marketing halos and misinformation. Words like 'natural' or 'unrefined' mean it's easier to perceive one type of sugar as 'better' than another, when in reality any free sugar – be that white sugar, coconut sugar, agave, fruit juices or syrups, honey or maple syrup will have similar effects in the body and on your child's teeth, despite coming from different sources and processing methods.

As a note, I'm all for pragmatism around higher-sugar foods, and awareness of the fact they can be included in your child's diet now and again. Demonisation of any food or nutrient is often unhelpful, unnecessary and has a ripple effect on food relationships. As always, it's about the bigger picture. I wanted to approach this discussion about sugar to raise awareness and support informed decision-making, but I also want to touch on the fact we do not have to completely demonise nutrients or use a scaremongering approach with sugar to steer young children from overconsuming these foods. Many of the foods I've detailed above have other nutritional benefits, so it can often be a case of considering how to moderate sugar intake in your child's diet as a whole. The other reality is that our children will likely grow up navigating this tricky food environment. Consideration of how we manage our language, relationships and behaviours around sweet or sugar-containing foods, which are so often framed as 'special' or a 'treat', also deserves some attention. I have covered *how* to support a child's food relationship in more detail on page 341.

Fibre

Now's the time to flip the focus to the nutrients that young children need <u>more</u> of. For me, at the top of this list is fibre. In my experience fibre is an overlooked nutrient, often passed off as the nutrient needed to poo! Fibre is a type of carbohydrate found in plants that the body can't easily digest; it remains intact as it passes through the gut.

While its role in digestion and bowel habits is vital, fibre is crucial for overall health, playing a starring role in feeding the community of good bacteria in the gut.

I often think that one of the reasons why discussions about fibre in young children are overlooked is that, historically, much of the messaging focuses on ensuring they don't overeat fibre. While it is true that too much fibre in tiny tummies can be detrimental to nutrients such as energy or iron, getting the right amount and the right variety of fibre is something parents should have more information about – hence I'm including it here!

Role and benefits of fibre in children's diet

✧ Healthy digestion.

✧ Fibre is the preferred food for good bacteria in your child's gut. Ensuring these remain well fed with the right foods (a variety of fibre-rich foods!) supports a healthy and happy gut microbiome. When well fed, these bacteria release beneficial compounds that positively impact other aspects of health beyond the gut, such as brain and immune health.

✧ Childhood constipation is a common and complicated issue. Some children suffer from constipation because they don't get enough fibre. Adding fibre from different foods to your child's diet can help support a healthy gut and may prevent some types of constipation.

✧ Fibre can help stabilise blood-sugar levels, which can help your child have a steadier release of energy throughout the day.

How much fibre do young children need?

Current recommendations for dietary fibre in children are:

0–2 years – There isn't a specific recommendation for children under two years old. They should get fibre from a varied diet once they start solids, and it's likely that as they progress from six months to two years, the amount of fibre will gradually increase towards the recommendation from two years.

2–5 years – 15g per day.

Is all fibre from food the same?

All fibre is beneficial and counts towards this fibre recommendation, however, we know that different fibre types have varying jobs. The terms soluble and insoluble fibre have been used for a long time and are still perfectly acceptable, however, there has been a recent shift towards using descriptions to more clearly capture the specific roles of different types of fibre in the gut and body (poo chat warning ahead).

✧ Fermentable fibre (prebiotic fibre), aka 'the gut gardener', is a type of fibre that is great at feeding good bacteria in the gut.

✧ Bulking fibre, aka 'the stool (poo) sculptor' is a type of fibre that adds bulk and structure to poo, making sure it's well built so that it's easier for the body to push it through the gut.

✧ Water-holding or viscous fibre, aka 'the spongers', soak up water and form a gel-like substance in the gut. They can help to keep things smooth and slippery but are also known to help stabilise blood sugar and be involved in reducing cholesterol (a type of blood fat).

What are the best fibre-rich foods?

Fibre can be found in various foods, including the following list. I've tried to include some fibre 'high-flyers' in each group, but all these types of foods are fantastic!

Foods	Fibre high-flyers
Fruit	Pears, raspberries, blackberries, avocado, guava, mango, figs, apples, pomegranate, kiwi
Vegetables	Broccoli, sweet potato, peas, yams, butternut squash, jicama, beetroot, artichokes

Beans and legumes	Black beans, chickpeas, green and brown lentils, kidney beans, haricot ('navy') beans
Grains	Oats, spelt, quinoa, bulgur wheat
Cereal	Wheat biscuits, shredded wheat, wholegrain loops Note that some cereals can be high in sugar
Nuts and seeds	Almonds, pistachios, hazelnuts, chia seeds, flaxseeds, sesame seeds, sunflower seeds

Here are some examples of how you might get 15g of fibre in a day for your toddler or preschooler:

One wheat biscuit, milk and a small grated pear = 5.9g
One slice of 50/50 toast, half a small tin of beans, cheese = 4.5g
Yoghurt with ½ tablespoon of ground almonds = 1g
Two fish fingers, skin-on potato wedges, 40g peas = 4.8g
Total = 16.2g

Small bowl of oats (30g) with a small banana and ½ teaspoon of chia seeds = 5g
Hummus and grated carrot sandwich with one slice 50/50 bread + satsuma = 5g
Half an apple with one teaspoon smooth peanut butter = 1.8g
Small portion of spaghetti Bolognese = 4g
Total = 15.8g

One slice wholemeal toast, two scrambled eggs, five cherry tomatoes, diced = 3.5g
Small portion of chicken biriyani = 2g
A small packet of raisins = 1g
Chickpea and spinach curry + small wholewheat roti = 9g
Total = 15.5g

My top ways to top up fibre
For the basics, I encourage parents to focus on whole fruit and vegetable

consumption (yes, five-a-day!), incorporating age-appropriate amounts of wholegrains (not everything needs to be the wholemeal variety) and boost the intake of beans and pulses. To take it a step further into small, practical changes, I love the mantra of 'nutrition by addition' as a great way to offer your child more fibre and, in reality, any nutrient. The small adjustments add up over time, so here are some recommendations or fibre 'hacks' I give to the families I work with.

Add ½–1 teaspoon of chia seeds or ground flaxseeds to porridge, baked oats, cereals or yoghurt (start smaller for younger tummies).
Change to a 50/50 bread or alternate between white and wholemeal varieties.
Add a portion of peas or sweetcorn when cooking pasta or rice.
Blend butter beans or white beans into cheese sauce for pasta, or cooked red lentils into tomato sauce.
Swap plain crackers for wholemeal crackers or oat cakes.
Add finely grated fruit (with skin on), such as apple or pear, to yoghurt, porridge or cereals.
Use a mix of white and wholemeal or rye flour for pancakes, muffins and bakes.
Used mashed avocado or hummus as a spread in sandwiches instead of or alongside usual butter or spread.
Add ground unsalted nuts or seeds to yoghurt, bakes, pancakes, cereals, porridge or savoury dishes like curry or stew.
Add a tin or packet of cooked lentils to mince dishes like Bolognese, lasagne, keema, chilli or shepherd's pie.
Consider a 50/50 cereal mix – add shredded wheat or wholegrain cereal to plain cereal such as a rice-based one.
Mash fruit onto toast or sandwich fillings.
Grate vegetables into sandwich fillings, pasta sauce, rice dishes like risotto or biriyani, or dips like tzatziki.
Combine grains – use a mix of rice and buckwheat or couscous and quinoa.
Add vegetables or mashed butter beans to potato toppings or mashed potato, such as parsnips, carrot, squash, broccoli or cauliflower.
Keep skins on potatoes when boiling and mashing or blending, or making chips.

When increasing fibre, I recommend doing this gradually and ensuring your child remains hydrated. In your child's gut, fibre absorbs water, which helps to keep poo soft and easy to pass.

Preschool portion sizes

How much your child eats throughout the preschool years will likely continue to fluctuate, and let me reassure you again, that while this isn't necessarily normal (or noticed) for adults, it is for young children. Appetite will continue to vary from meal to meal, week to week and month to month, and you will likely see periods when your preschooler is eating well before you see a noticeable increase in their growth. As hard as that lack of consistency can feel as a parent, I encourage you to grab a board and surf the waves of appetite, honing in on how wonderful young children are at regulating their appetite.

I would encourage you to allow your preschoolers to remain in the driving seat of how much they want to eat at mealtimes – letting them have agency over this can hold the key to avoiding mealtime battlegrounds and unnecessary stress. You may find that your child is now much more able to converse about their wants and needs regarding food, telling you when they are hungry or full, asking for specific foods or leaving the table when they are done. Offering elements of independence around portion sizes coming to their plate can be great during the preschool years and excellent practice for heading to school.

I've shared more guidance on portion size starting points on page 193, and if you haven't already, I'd encourage you to read back about trusting your child's appetite on page 174 and family-style meals on page 225 and 336.

Supplements for preschoolers

You'll be pleased to know that there are no significant changes to the supplements your child is recommended at this age. Flick back to page 195 for full details on supplements for toddlers, which continue to apply in this age group.

There is a shift from five years of age, however, and general guidelines in the UK recommend supplementing with vitamin D only during the darker months, from September to March. There will be groups of children, however, such as those with darker skin, on certain medications or with more limited sunlight exposure, who will likely continue to benefit from vitamin D supplementation all year round.

Preschool eating behaviours and feeding development

As your preschooler grows and develops, you will likely see ongoing changes in their feeding skills and behaviours. Much of this can be attributed to their increasing independence and abilities, from language to fine motor skills. The advice throughout the toddler section of this book still applies to this age group, so if you're joining here, please flick back and have a read. However, I wanted to touch base with a few additional areas that deserve some airtime, particularly for preschoolers.

Supporting increased independence around food and mealtimes

Around preschool age, children start asserting more independence, including in their eating habits. Your preschooler will likely want more autonomy regarding their food choices and how much they eat and serve themselves. Their language progression means they can also express their food preferences more clearly and might even start negotiating with you about what and when they eat. Children can also commonly experience periods of selectivity around food, interest in certain foods or expression of 'favourite' foods.

It can be easy for a parent to feel intimidated by this increased independence and worry about losing control around mealtimes and the foods offered. For this reason, it's often an age where I remind parents to harness that independence and new skills and let their preschooler's natural curiosity take the lead at mealtimes. Food parenting practices that support a child's autonomy and freedom are generally linked to healthier eating behaviours and preferences in children. So here are some of my top tips for managing eating habits and mealtimes with your preschooler:

1. **Get them involved** – Not only is this a fantastic strategy for exposure to different foods without pressure or expectations around eating, but plenty of science demonstrates the benefits of involving children in food shopping, preparation and serving, including a link to reduced food pickiness. It also seems to help them eat a more balanced diet, enjoy fruits and vegetables, and feel more confident about cooking and making healthy food choices. Some ways in which you could get your pre-schooler involved that don't result in too much chaos include:
   o Washing fruit and vegetables.
   o Chopping foods (with child-friendly safety knives).
   o Stirring mixtures and batters.
   o Picking up and putting foods in the trolley or basket in the supermarket.
   o Setting the table or taking food to the table.
   o Decorating or building dishes, such as pizza, fajitas.
   o Measuring ingredients.

   Practically, kitchen necessities such as a sturdy step or tower, safety knives, an apron, large muslin or coveralls over clothes can help young children get involved in the kitchen.

   Note: Beware of your expectations again, as a parent. I speak to many parents who are baffled by their toddlers and preschoolers who happily get stuck in making a meal, stirring a curry and chopping vegetables but don't eat them. This is normal! From your child's perspective, it's important to remember that the 'task demand' for your child is the activity – cooking – not eating! These tasks are still valuable learning and confidence-building activities around food. Avoid putting any pressure or persuasion on your child to consume the final product or ingredients along the way.

2. **Serving themselves** – If you're not already, incorporating some meal or snack times that start with empty plates and allow your child to serve themselves is a great way of encouraging independence and autonomy around foods. (See page 340). If this

feels like a bit much to begin with, adding dips or sprinkles to meals or having just one element of the meal to self-serve, such as a side of vegetables or topping for pasta, can be a good starting point. Getting involved in packing a lunch or snack bag for when you're outside the house or even helping you with a meal plan for the week can be great options too.

3. **Use their language for learning and exploration** – Preschoolers' newfound language might feel like it works against them at times, with phrases like 'I don't like that', 'It's disgusting', and 'I don't want fish, I want pasta', flying around. This can be hard to navigate as a parent – there's nothing quite like cooking a meal and having it thrown back in your face verbally (or literally!). I've covered lots about language use around food and mealtimes earlier in the book, but I wanted to remind you of a few points here:

   o Your preschooler may not mean, 'I don't like it', but they may use familiar language or phrases like this to express things like, 'I don't like the look of it', 'I'm not hungry', 'It's not what I expected' and more. Remember to avoid persuasion, negotiations or using logic with them at this stage, such as 'But you liked it yesterday', and reassure them that it's ok and they don't have to eat it.

   o Harness their learning and language to explore foods. You can discuss things like the colour or texture of food or involve imaginative play or thinking that support their curiosity and learning around mealtimes (see page 222).

   o Remember to keep discussions about food choices neutral and positive.

4. **Social and emotional learning with food** – Preschoolers are at an age where they become increasingly aware of their peers', social and family routines, interactions and emotions. Social imitation is exceptionally common at this age. While this can throw some fun curve balls (a friend only recently called me to say her preschooler had come home from nursery and greeted her with 'hey babe'), it also means you have a golden opportunity to harness shared social eating

occasions like shared meals and snack times. Awareness of emotional responses and regulation around food can also come into play in this age group. Studies show that preschool-aged children can start associating emotions like sadness and stress with eating. This behaviour is influenced by natural tendencies and their environment, especially when parents model emotional eating.

If you're struggling with mealtimes, fussy eating or supporting positive food relationships, have a read through the sections beginning on pages 211, 200 and 341 for lots more advice.

Transitions ahead – starting school

Nutrition knowhow for the school years, including:

✧ **The importance of breakfast**

✧ **School meals and snacks**

✧ **Communicating dietary requirements**

✧ **Packed lunches**

✧ **Encouraging fluids during the school day**

I'm sure you won't quite believe your tiny human is about to don a uniform and head to school – but it's coming. Many parents tell me it's yet another time of transition; there are new routines, requests and feeding considerations. So, like shopping for new stationery, let's go through a shopping list of nutrition and feeding tips for school that you might find helpful.

The importance of breakfast

I'm not here to insist that breakfast is the 'most important meal of the day'. I understand from the families I work with that it's not every child's favourite meal, and I'm very aware that time adds pressure to breakfast on school mornings. However, extensive research highlights the benefits of children eating breakfast (anything!) before school. Here are a few research-backed reasons why:

✧ Children who consistently eat breakfast have been found to consume more nutrients and have healthier dietary habits than those who frequently skip it.

✧ Children who eat breakfast before school perform better in learning, attention and memory.

✧ Children who eat breakfast have better energy levels.

✧ Skipping breakfast is linked to a higher risk of excess weight gain.

✧ The more consistently children eat breakfast, the more satisfied they are with their lives.

Building a balanced breakfast is ideal, and options that include fibre, wholegrains and protein seem to be beneficial. To help you plan for busy mornings, here are some of my quick and easy or prep-ahead breakfast ideas.

✧ Wholemeal or 50/50 toast with:
  o Peanut butter or almond butter and banana.
  o Cream cheese and mashed blueberries or raspberries.
  o Peanut butter and chia jam.
  o Mashed avocado and sprinkle of seeds.
  o Melted cheese.

- o Beans.
- o Yoghurt and sliced fruit.
- o Tahini and sliced kiwi.
- o Hummus and grated apple.
- o Boiled egg.

✧ Wholegrain cereal with milk/milk alternative, plus:
  - o Chopped or sliced fruit.
  - o Stewed fruit.
  - o Tinned fruit in juice.
  - o Dried fruit and or milled nuts/seeds.

✧ Porridge or overnight oats with milk/milk alternative, plus:
  - o Fruit.
  - o Ground nuts or seeds, such as ground almonds.
  - o Nut or seed butter.
  - o Grated fruit or veg, such as apples, carrots.

✧ Omelette with cheese and vegetables, plus oatcakes.

✧ A sandwich or wrap (any filling).

✧ Pancakes with oats and banana, spelt or blueberry plus yoghurt.

✧ Vegetable fritters, such as carrots, courgettes.

✧ Homemade oat bars.

✧ Dippy egg and toast.

✧ Rice porridge with vegetables and egg.

✧ Leftover evening meals – yes, really, any food can be breakfast food.

✧ Smoothie or smoothie bowl with frozen fruit, yoghurt or oats.

✧ Wholewheat paratha with yoghurt and fruit.

Note: In the UK, breakfast clubs exist in some schools. If you have early starts for work or struggle for resources to support regular breakfasts, please check with your child's school to see if any clubs are available.

School meals and snacks

Handing your child's nutrition to the school can be nerve-wracking, especially with the ongoing discussions about the quality of school meals in the UK. Although clear school food standards exist to ensure that children receive high-quality and nutritious meals, there are still ongoing efforts to improve these and ensure schools adhere to these standards locally. Most schools can provide you with a copy of their menus, which typically follow a regular rotation and you should be able to see the types of foods on offer. Families receiving certain benefits can access free school meals for their children, and efforts are ongoing to extend this to all children over the years to come (I share this without promise).

Across many schools in the UK, children in the first few years of primary school (Years 1 and 2) may be entitled to free milk and fruit, which is often offered as a snack during a school break early in the day. Suitable dairy alternatives are not currently provided for children who are unable to have milk (which I think is a shame), however, some schools allow parents to send this in.

Top tips for getting kids used to school lunches:

✧ Explain how the lunchtime routine might look – lining up, collecting a tray, choosing foods, sitting with friends.

✧ If available, show them the school menus and talk through the foods available.

✧ Try a 'run through' at home where meals are served buffet-style, and your child asks for and indicates what they'd like on their plate.

✧ Ensure your child is happy and confident with using cutlery.

✧ Reassure your child there will be adults around to help them.

✧ Reassure your child that they don't have to eat everything and can choose what and how much they eat. They should not be made to clear their plate.

Communicating dietary requirements

The school must be aware of any dietary requirements your child has in plenty of time before they start. There will usually be processes for this. Communicating food allergies, intolerances or diagnoses like coeliac disease will help ensure food preparation and menu adjustments can be made wherever possible. For children with immediate food allergies, I also encourage you to ensure an up-to-date allergy action plan is in place and additional medications such as antihistamines or auto-adrenaline injections are ready for school, with their prescription labels. Many fantastic patient organisations (listed at the back of this book) have information on starting school and managing food allergies.

Packed lunches

If your child isn't having a cooked school meal, packed lunches will be an option or choice for your child. Over the years, packed lunches have, at times, had a poor reputation. Whether it's the lack of variety, soggy sandwiches being sent home uneaten or worries regarding nutritional balance.

In reality, a packed lunch, packed well, is an ideal opportunity for a child to top up their energy and nutrient intake in the middle of a busy school day. I often describe it to kids as a pitstop in their day to refill the tank and help keep their energy levels up for more thinking and movement in the afternoon. The key to avoiding a hungry, irritable or energy-depleted child at the school gates at the end of a day is building a balanced lunchbox that is easy to prepare and relieves you of that common parent concern: 'Are they getting enough?'

I want to reassure you that, like kids' meals, lunchboxes don't need to be aesthetically pleasing and filled with ten items to be balanced or enjoyable. See the table on the next page for five essential building blocks to a packed lunch and some ideas.

Top tip: From a practical perspective, ensure your child has practised opening their lunchbox! I know it sounds daft, but it's worth familiarising your child with different clips, zips and more before their first day of school.

Encouraging fluids during the school day

I meet a lot of parents who worry about their children not drinking enough during the school day. Alongside, of course, ensuring your child has a good-sized drinking bottle that goes to school every day, I'd recommend:

✧ Ensuring regular drink breaks are factored into your child's school day (this should be the case) especially if drinks are not available during classes.

Food group	Examples	Inspiration
A starchy carbohydrate	Bread, wraps, pitta, rice, pasta, potato, sweet potato, crackers, oat cakes, plantain, chapati, couscous, quinoa, muffins, breadsticks. **Top tip: Wholemeal or 50/50 options will increase the fibre content and help support steady energy release all afternoon.**	Wholemeal wrap with hummus and grated apple or carrot. Yoghurt with berries. Pitta bread pizza with vegetables and shredded chicken, satsuma, yoghurt. Breadsticks with dips, such as cream cheese, hummus. Hardboiled egg, fruit salad.
A protein source	Hummus, beans, tuna, salmon, chicken or turkey, hard-boiled egg, frittata or quiche. **Top tip: These provide vital nutrients for children, including iron and zinc. Protein also helps with satiety and keeps kids full during the afternoon.**	Mini wholemeal pitta bread or flatbread fingers with falafel, tzatziki or hummus and sliced cucumber. Apple slices. Courgette and sweetcorn fritters, mini cheese and a pack of mini breadsticks. Cheese and cucumber sandwich on wholemeal or 50/50 bread, banana, edamame beans, mini muffin.
Fruits and vegetables	Any fruit or veg counts! Pieces of fruit, some tinned fruit in juice, defrosted frozen, grated or stewed fruit in or on yoghurt, slices of avocado, carrot or cucumber sticks or ribbons, vegetable fritters, tinned sweetcorn or corn on the cob, mangetout or sugar-snap peas, mini beetroot, grated or mashed vegetables in fritters or quiche, chopped cherry tomatoes, salad or grated vegetables in sandwiches, pitta or wraps.	Tinned salmon and cream cheese pitta, piece of fruit, plain popcorn (>5 years). Lentil and vegetable-filled dosa, fruit portion and some cheese. Diced meatballs, leftover pasta in sauce, yoghurt with grated apple, raisins and cinnamon. Crackers with slices of cheese and chicken, a piece of fruit, sugar-snap peas.
Dairy or fortified dairy alternatives	Cheese, unsweetened yoghurt, cream cheese in sandwiches, fromage frais or fortified milk alternatives. **Top tip: Dairy foods or those based on soy or pea will also be a source of protein.**	Tuna and sweetcorn wholemeal sandwich, cucumber slices, mixed berries and a small yoghurt drink. Couscous salad with roasted vegetables and chickpeas. Mini cheese cubes, a handful of grapes.

| Fluids | Water, water with chopped or sliced fruits. If offering juice or smoothies, keep to 100–150ml. **Top tip: Keeping hydrated during a school day is essential to support concentration levels, avoid lethargy and help prevent complaints such as constipation.** | |

✧ Make sure your child finds it easy to drink from their bottle and that any straws or spouts don't have a residual soapy taste after washing.

✧ Find ways to encourage fluid intake, such as using bottles that keep water cold throughout the day (or putting the bottle in the freezer the night before) or adding fruit slices for flavour.

✧ Encourage your child to feel confident asking teachers for their drink if they feel thirsty.

✧ Ensure your child feels happy using the toilets at school – I've seen so many cases where, when we get to the crux of poor fluid intake during school, it's down to avoidance of the school toilets!

SOS – common nutrition and feeding worries in the preschool era

As with other aspects of this section, you'll find a fair amount of crossover between this age group and toddlers regarding nutrition and feeding worries. Please skip back to page 240, where you can see an extended range of SOS questions that might also fit the bill for your preschooler.

Help! My child seems to be sugar obsessed.

I have to say I'm hearing this more and more, and the first thing I want to reassure you about is that your toddler almost certainly isn't addicted to sugar. While research into this is ongoing, we don't have conclusive evidence that 'sugar addiction' is a thing, despite what the internet may say. There are many reasons why your child may be drawn to sweeter or higher-sugar foods. These include:

1. **They are normal!** A desire for and enjoyment of sweet foods is expected from a biological standpoint. Energy-dense foods are often sweet, and while we are thousands of years away from the caveman era, this evolutionary safety net around foods still exists – it's just the food environment that's different. Babies are also born with a preference for sweet tastes (breast milk is sweet), and some researchers have also suggested that it's more likely that children remain 'drawn' to sugar because it's a reliable and quick energy source for a rapidly growing body.

2. **High-sugar or sweet foods have been given a halo**. If these foods have been used as bribery or rewards in the past, or children have learned they are special or saved only for special events, then inadvertently they will be more desirable for your child.

3. **Sugary or sweet foods have been demonised or heavily restricted**. Some research has shown that, while parents act with the best intentions, overt restriction of higher-sugar foods may backfire in the long term and increase their desirability. This is sometimes called the 'forbidden-fruit' or 'special-status' effect.

4. **Food manufacturers design foods to be hyper-palatable.** The science behind the perfect textures, fat and sugar ratios and more is big business. Anyone, including a child, who is drawn

to these foods doesn't necessarily have a 'problem' – the foods are made to be desirable.

So, what can you do to neutralise sugar's desirability? Take a read of page 341, where I talk about supporting positive food relationships in children.

Is it true certain foods can make children hyperactive?

In short, this is partly true. In particular, six food colourings are most closely linked to hyperactivity in children:

1. E102 (Tartrazine)
2. E104 (Quinoline Yellow)
3. E110 (Sunset Yellow FCF)
4. E122 (Carmoisine)
5. E124 (Ponceau 4R)
6. E129 (Allura Red)

These colourings are typically found in sweets, soft drinks, snacks, desserts and processed foods. The clue can be these foods' vibrant colour or enhanced appearance. They should also carry the warning: 'May have an adverse effect on activity and attention in children.'

In my personal experience, some children seem more susceptible to the potential effects of these colourings. This is consistent with one study, which found that the impact of consuming these colourings varied among children – some showed no response, while others showed a significant response. For children with ADHD, it is often recommended that they are excluded for at least a period of time to observe impacts on behaviour.

Regarding other foods or food components and hyperactivity, parents often report worries about the following, so let's take a quick look:

Sodium benzoate: Found in some soft drinks, sauces and condiments, sodium benzoate has been linked to hyperactivity in children in some studies.

Caffeine: I doubt you'd be surprised to hear that caffeine, a stimulant, is often reported to affect children's behaviour. While soft drinks like cola are a source of caffeine, other foods such as chocolate and cocoa contain it too.

Sugar: While science has largely debunked the 'sugar-makes-children-hyperactive' narrative, many parents report that their child seems more energetic or hyperactive after eating more sugar than usual. (Although sometimes this can be due to the environment too – parties, celebrations and other children can increase energy levels!)

If you're worried about any of these and the impact on your child's behaviour, trialling a period of exclusion or reduction may be helpful.

My child refuses any foods with mixed textures, such as pasta with sauce, casseroles and mixed rice dishes. How can I offer and encourage these foods?

Parents often raise this concern with me during the toddler and preschool years. Children can often refuse family meals with mixed textures for reasons like feeling unsure of what's in them or the 'unknown'. Wet or saucy foods and 'bits' can also be a texture many children dislike and take some time to get used to. Some of my preferred ways to approach and support children to learn to accept these foods include:

✧ Offering sauce on the side – serve your child's preferred plain pasta with a small cup or bowl of the sauce, such as tomato, pesto or cheese.

✧ Start by using a tiny amount of sauce stirred through a lot of pasta and gradually build up.

✧ Deconstruct meals where you can (it's not possible for all!), but for something like filled wraps, you can have your protein, vegetables, salad, cheese, wraps and sauce separately.

✧ Get your child involved in making these foods with you so they can see what foods are added in and how they change when cooked.

What's next after five?

As promised at the front of this book, all the information shared here will take you up to five years of age. The reality is that, with this alone, I sincerely hope that you'll feel calm, confident and empowered with the foundations for future health and happiness around food and feeding your child. Thank you for trusting me to support you through these first, and incredibly important, five years.

In terms of what next? Nutrition and healthy-eating guidelines from five years of age shift to fit in line with the standard ones in the UK. While these guidelines are not new or particularly sexy, in that they don't warrant lots of social media attention or controversy, they are enforced by years of nutritional research.

And it's here that age-specific advice and support come to an end, but it's not the end of this book. The next three sections are written with even more information-giving, problem-solving, parental perspectives and peace of mind in mind!

5

Healthy Foundations

'What, when and how children eat is more important before age two than at any other time in life.' (UNICEF)

What and how you feed your children in the early years isn't just about keeping them healthy and growing right now, but it also directly shapes their future health and wellbeing.

These early years are a golden window of opportunity. You may remember the phrase 'The First 1,000 Days', which refers to a well-recognised window of opportunity from conception to your child's second birthday, during which substantial physical, cognitive and emotional development occurs. During this time, your child's brain, gut, and immune system develop and grow simultaneously, and how this occurs is foundational for your child's future health.

As a mother, I empathise with how this information can feel like added pressure to 'get it right'. While I've focussed a chapter on under-standing your child's growth and supporting their foundational health, my goal here definitely isn't to overwhelm you; it's to offer advice that is so often not shared, and that I hope goes on to support and empower you with the power nutrition has for your child's health.

Note: Throughout this section, I refer to daily requirements for some nutrients. I am not an advocate of number crunching; these are for awareness only to help you picture what and how much certain foods can help children get what they need. However, I always remind parents to think about nutrient intake over time – weeks and months, rather than daily. There is no need to get the calculator out!

Getting to grips with growth

◇ **Key facts about your child's growth in the first five years**

◇ **Getting to grips with growth charts and your child's growth**

◇ **How often should a child be measured?**

◇ **When to seek support around growth or growth concerns**

Growth is an important indicator of whether a child's diet and feeding habits are meeting their needs. Understanding how young children grow and the role of nutrition in their growth was an important topic for me to include in this book. It could have been woven into every chapter so far, but I felt a section dedicated to understanding how children grow and how this is monitored was important for all parents, if for no other reason than because research shows that 45–60 per cent of parents express concern or worry about their child's growth in the first five years.

Key facts about your child's growth in the first five years

There is a lot of misinformation or misunderstanding about children's growth, so I want to start by sharing a few facts below. Please bear in mind that these are averages and will not apply to every child, as you'll come to understand more as I talk a little more about growth.

✧ Babies and young children grow very fast! However, there are notable changes to just how fast throughout the first five years. One of the best indicators I often reference is children's clothes sizes. Baby clothes move up a size every two to three months (it's expensive!), and then the gaps widen. From one, clothes sizes move to every six months – 12–18 months, 18–24 months – and from two you'll generally find clothes sizes are reflective of a whole year.

✧ Research shows that after the first year, children's growth patterns shift from rapid increases in size to more steady gains in height and weight. This is one of the reasons why we reduce how often we measure children (see below), as we don't expect to see the same big increases in growth, but instead much more steady and consistent growth, which is best monitored over months rather than weeks.

✧ Your child's height potential (how tall they may end up) mainly depends on their genetics, which sets this framework. While good nutrition and a healthy lifestyle can help them reach this potential, they won't exceed the genetic 'limits' set by your heights as parents. Health professionals can calculate mid-parental height (which sets out an expected height range based on the height of both parents) after your child turns two years of age.

Getting to grips with growth charts and your child's growth

Children's growth is monitored and interpreted using growth charts, often called centile (or 'percentile') charts. There are centile lines for weight, length or height, head circumference and, after two years of age, centiles for Body Mass Index (BMI). Growth charts can be found within the personal child health record ('Red Book'), you are given when your baby is born. Boys and girls have different charts, coloured blue and pink respectively. This is because boys tend to be slightly taller and heavier than girls and follow a slightly different growth pattern. Growth charts include a series of lines called centile (or percentile) lines, all based on data about how babies and children grow or are expected to grow according to their age and sex. Specific growth charts also exist for certain groups of children who need closer monitoring or whose growth patterns are known to be different, such as babies born prematurely.

It can be tricky to understand what centiles mean, but over the years, I've found this analogy most helpful with parents:

Imagine a class of 100 children at school. If we measured them all (weight, height), we wouldn't expect them to all be the same. We'd expect a distribution of many sizes within that class. There will inevitably be the smallest in the class, the tallest and everyone in between. So, when we think about centile charts, this is how, very crudely, you might interpret the numbers:

✧ A child who plots the 2nd centile for their height would be the second smallest in their class, with one smaller peer and 98 taller peers. They will appear smaller than their peers, but this doesn't necessarily mean they are not growing well enough.

✧ A child who plots the 75th centile would be the 26th tallest, with 25 taller peers and 74 who were smaller.

No centile line is inherently considered good or bad – **what's most important is how your child's growth tracks over time**. Centile lines simply show the different ways in which children can grow, and it's essential to recognise that each child's growth pattern is unique. The goal isn't to aim for the 'average' centile; for instance, being at the 50th centile or higher isn't necessarily 'better'. Instead, the focus should be on your child growing steadily and proportionally along their centiles.

Our child's genetics largely determine the ideal centile range for their height, and we would anticipate that their weight and head circumference would also be proportional to this centile. This doesn't mean, for example, that weight and height have to be on the same centile lines; they simply need to remain within a healthy range relative to one another.

Remember, one-off measurements don't tell us much! Consistent and appropriate monitoring helps us track your child's overall growth pattern, which is crucial to understanding their health and development over time. We can spot any changes or concerns early by monitoring this pattern and ensuring your child is growing as they should.

When I talk about growth patterns, I also always emphasise that varying patterns lead to different energy and nutritional needs, which, in turn, affect eating habits. Many parents naturally compare their child's eating habits or portions with those of their peers of the same or a similar age, however, these children may plot on very different percentiles for their growth, which is relevant in the context of eating habits.

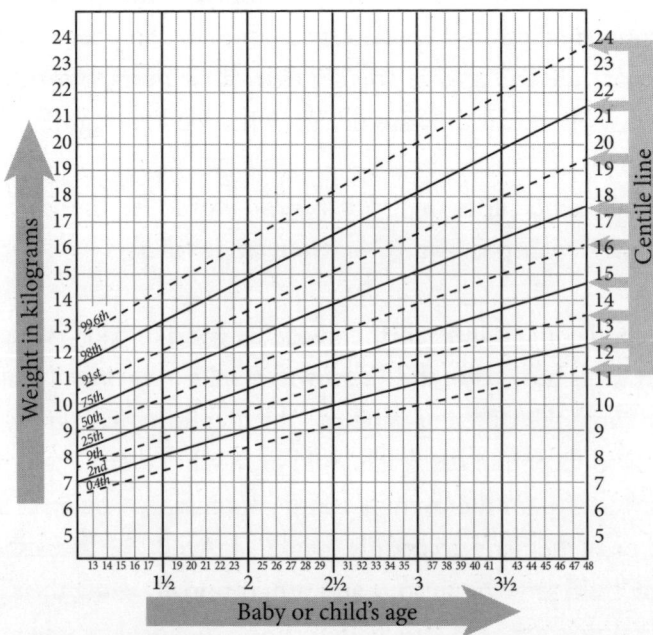

So, for example, a two-year-old girl plotting healthily along the 9th centile will likely need nearly 40 per cent fewer calories to meet her daily energy requirements than her two-year-old male friend who plots healthily along the 91st centile. In real terms, this could look like your child is eating considerably more or less than some of their peers. Understandably, this can often fuel worry, but I hope this reminds you that all children are unique, looping back around to a point I've made multiple times throughout the book so far: trusting your child's appetite is a crucial part of supporting their growth and development as a parent. It may not surprise you that research has shown that parents who perceive their child as 'small', having a smaller appetite or less enthusiasm for eating, are more likely to exert greater pressure on the child to eat. You'll already know from this book that I'd recommend you avoid this as much as possible!

How often should a child be measured?

	0–6 months	6–12 months	1+ years
Weight	At birth, then no more than once a month.	No more than once every two months.	No more than once every three months.
Length – to 2 years **Height – 2+ years**	At birth, then only if there are any concerns about weight, growth or general health. If you'd like your child's length or height checked at any stage, just ask your health visitor.		
Head circumference	At birth, then again at 6–8 weeks.	At any time after 8 weeks if there are any concerns about head size.	

Many health-visiting teams in the UK take the lead in measuring growth for babies and children. This may be via home visits, but outside of this there are usually local drop-in clinics. Other professionals involved in a child's care, such as paediatricians and dietitians, may also monitor growth. If there are any concerns about your child's growth, a health professional will advise on how often their growth should be monitored.

When to seek support around growth or growth concerns

It's typical for your child's weight to 'wiggle' up and down or move gradually from being near one centile to the next, up or down. There are also times when growth can be expected to slow or weight to drop a little, including during or after illness and even when there are giant leaps in development, like starting to walk. There will be specific scenarios when growth pattern becomes a concern or needs to be monitored more often. A health professional should guide this – I cover this in more detail on page 410.

Looking beyond growth

While measurements like weight and height are essential tools for assessing a child's health, it is worth knowing that, while helpful, they can never tell the whole story. Many parents feel unheard or dismissed when raising concerns about their child's feeding or eating habits if they are just told they shouldn't worry 'because their child is growing well'. Growth alone doesn't exclude nutritional concerns; children can grow well but still not get all the nutrients they need. They might also struggle with feeding skills or have difficulties not immediately apparent through growth measurements because children are also brilliant at compensating. If you have any concerns about your child's diet or feeding habits, don't hesitate to revisit these with a healthcare professional.

Brain-Building Nutrients

✧ **Nutrition building blocks for brain growth and development**

✧ **Brain-building and -boosting meal and snack ideas**

Your child's brain development will have been well under way during pregnancy, and from there onwards, through infancy and the early years, nutrition feeds its further development. Here are some mind-blowing facts!

✧ A baby's brain doubles in size during the first year of life.

✧ By three years, your child's brain has reached 80 per cent of its adult size and is around 90 per cent of its adult size by five years of age.

✧ A three-year-old's brain is twice as active as an adult's.

✧ The brain has an almost limitless storage capacity, so your young child will never reach a point where they can't learn more.

✧ A child's brain forms approximately 1 million neural connections every second, especially in the first three years.

The brain keeps growing and developing throughout life, but much of its structure is formed by age three. Important skills like memory, sensing the world and managing emotions also develop early on. Studies indicate that good nutrition in early childhood can have long-lasting benefits to brain health and even later life, affecting the risk of conditions like dementia.

So, what nutrition does this hungry and growing brain need?

Top 10 brain-building foods

1. Oily fish, including salmon, mackerel, sardines
2. Eggs
3. Nuts and seeds
4. Beans and legumes
5. Leafy greens
6. Berries – especially dark-coloured, such as blueberries, blackberries
7. Avocado
8. Wholegrains, including oats, quinoa
9. Sweet potato and other orange fruits and vegetables
10. Yoghurt

Nutrition building blocks for brain growth and development

Brain growth and development are hungry work, requiring enormous energy levels and specific nutrients that contribute to the 'bricks and mortar' of the brain's structure and support cognitive (thinking and understanding) functions for the rest of the lifespan. Below, I've summarised some essential nutrients for brain development and health, including why they are crucial for your child's brain and, most importantly, where you find them.

For babies, please know that all the nutrients I mention below are in breast and formula milk (see the section beginning on page 6).

Energy (calories)

Growing brains are hungry and a significant amount of energy is needed to support your child's brain development. For context, a newborn's brain uses about 60 per cent of its daily energy needs! Your child's high energy needs are best met with nutrient-dense foods. In their early life, milk provides the primary source of energy and nutrition. As your baby starts eating solids, focus on meals and snacks that are rich in nutrients, especially those that support brain development, such as carbohydrates and fats.

Fat

Fat is vital for your child's brain and overall growth – in fact, 60 per cent of the brain consists of fat! While all fats contribute to brain development and the absorption of fat-soluble vitamins like A, D, E and K, some types are particularly significant. As mentioned throughout the book, fat is not a nutrient that should be skimped on for babies and young children, especially those under two years of age. Prioritising healthy fats in your child's diet will support their brain growth and development – you can read more about types of fat on page 186.

Long-chain polyunsaturated fatty acids (PUFAs), particularly omega 3 fatty acids (often recognised as 'good fats'), are particularly important for brain and cognitive development. Omega 3 fatty acids play a vital role in creating and maintaining the protective coating around our brain cells, helping them communicate better and supporting overall brain health. There are three main types of omega 3 fatty acids:

o Docosahexaenoic acid (DHA)
o Alpha-linolenic acid (ALA)
o Eicosapentaenoic acid (EPA)

Of these, docosahexaenoic acid (DHA) is a *powerhouse* nutrient for the brain, making up 15–20 per cent of the brain's fat content, and is recognised as essential to maintain normal brain function. DHA is a vital building block for both the brain and the retina, which is crucial for vision. It plays an important role in sending messages throughout the brain and building new connections, a process known as neurogenesis. This nutrient has a particular impact on the frontal and prefrontal lobes of your child's brain, making it essential for cognitive functions such as memory, learning and problem-solving. Additionally, omega 3 fatty acids are recognised for their anti-inflammatory properties, which help safeguard the brain against various types of stress and inflammation.

In young children, adequate intake of omega 3s, and particularly DHA, are linked to improved cognitive abilities, better attention, memory and even emotional regulation. Since the body cannot make these fatty acids on its own, they must be consumed through diet from food sources or supplements, which I've listed below.

Docosahexaenoic acid (DHA)

✧ Oily fish, including salmon, mackerel, sardines, trout, pilchards (fresh, frozen and tinned options all count).

✧ Fortified or enriched foods – some brands of foods, such as fish fingers, eggs, milk, yoghurt, breads and spreads, contain added or higher-than-normal levels of DHA.

✧ White fish and seafood contain small amounts of DHA.

✧ Breast milk.

✧ Formula milk – DHA is now mandatory in all formula milk.

Eicosapentaenoic acid (EPA) is similarly found in fish and seafood.

If your child cannot or doesn't consume oily fish regularly – at least once a week – then consideration of a supplement containing DHA (and EPA) can be beneficial. For those following a plant-based diet, supplement options based on algae rather than fish oil are ideal. You can read more about choosing an omega 3 supplement below.

Alpha-linolenic acid (ALA)
This type of omega 3 fatty acid is often found in plant foods including:

✧ Flaxseed and flaxseed oil.

✧ Chia seeds.

✧ Walnuts and walnut oil.

✧ Soya, including tofu, soybeans.

✧ Pumpkin seeds.

✧ Some green leafy vegetables, such as Brussels sprouts.

ALA is converted into DHA in the body, but this process isn't particularly efficient and takes some time. Therefore, a supplement may benefit children who don't regularly consume DHA-rich foods, such as those following a vegetarian or vegan diet, or selective eaters.

How much of the different omega 3 fatty acids like DHA do babies and young children need?
The UK doesn't have specific recommendations for the quantities of omega 3 fats such as DHA that young children should be consuming. As a general guide, it's recommended that:

✧ Once solids have been commenced, children have one or two age-appropriate portions of oily fish a week.

✧ If you're choosing a supplement, select an omega 3 supplement instead of cod liver oil and check to ensure there is no extra vitamin A added if your child is already getting that from another supplement.

✧ Choose an age-appropriate supplement, such as an infant or child formulation, instead of an adult formulation.

How much omega-3 should a child have?
The WHO recommends the following omega 3 doses:

6 months–2 years	DHA 10–12mg/kg
2–4 years	EPA + DHA 100–150mg/day
4–6 years	EPA + DHA 150–200 mg/day
6–10 years	EPA + DHA 200–250 mg/day

Choline

Choline, a previously neglected nutrient, is now increasingly recognised, thanks to changing dietary trends, such as lower consumption of animal-based foods. There isn't much research into choline intake in UK children, but a small study in North American children found that over 70 per cent of one-year-olds and 50 per cent of two-year-olds were not meeting the recommended adequate intake. Choline is considered an essential nutrient because the body can only produce a small amount of it, so therefore most must come from food or supplements.

Choline's role in your child's developing brain

✧ Brain and spinal cord development.

✧ Making a brain chemical (acetylcholine) that supports memory, mood, focus and problem-solving.

✧ Building cell membranes, which are essential for brain growth and function.

How much choline do babies and young children need?

There are no explicit requirements for choline in babies and young children in the UK. In America, an adequate intake (AI) of choline is recommended as:

Age	Adequate intake (milligrams/mg) per day
0–6 months	125
7–12 months	150
1–3 years	200
4–6 years	250

Derived from Institute of Medicine. Food and Nutrition Board. Dietary Reference Intakes: Thiamin, Riboflavin, Niacin, Vitamin B6, Folate, Vitamin B12, Pantothenic Acid, Biotin, and Choline. Washington, DC: National Academy Press; 1998

What foods contain choline?

Choline can be found in various foods, including animal-based foods such as meat, poultry, fish, eggs and dairy, as well as cruciferous vegetables, beans, nuts and wholegrains. I've included some food examples alongside the choline content to see how your child's requirement could be met across the day (or week). Check out some meal and snack examples at the end of this section too.

Food	Choline content (milligrams/mg)
One egg	150
85g beef	80–120
85g chicken breast	70
85g cod	70
50g edamame beans	28
50g kidney beans	23
250ml cow's milk	40
100g green peas	25
40g broccoli	15
40g cauliflower	15

100g yoghurt	15
1 medium potato	15
1 medium sweet potato	13
1 tbsp peanut/peanut butter	6
1 tbsp almonds/almond butter	4

Iron

Hello again to a nutrient I have discussed in detail throughout this book! Iron is an essential nutrient in brain development, and iron-deficiency anaemia in early childhood is linked to lower IQ and poorer cognitive and motor development. Unfortunately, iron deficiency is common in young children, but understanding how much your child needs and where to get it can ensure their brain development isn't compromised.

Iron's role in your child's developing brain

✧ Helps to produce myelin, a fatty substance that is wrapped around nerves, which assists electrical signals in moving quickly and efficiently throughout the brain.

✧ A fundamental building block for haemoglobin, which is a protein in red blood cells that transports oxygen around the body, including the brain.

✧ It helps to make neurotransmitters (chemical messengers that can tell the brain and body what to do), such as serotonin (the happy hormone) and adrenaline (fight-or-flight hormone).

✧ Supports cognitive development, which is how the brain learns and how well it learns.

Rather than repeat myself, you can find out how much iron your child needs, where to get it and ways to incorporate it into their meals throughout this book, particularly on pages 105–6 and 402–5.

Iodine

Many parents are unaware that iodine is a vital nutrient that plays a key role in brain and nervous-system development in children and during pregnancy. Iodine deficiency can cause severe developmental issues, including intellectual disabilities. Please be reassured that severe deficiency is rare, but it's important to stress to parents that children are increasingly at risk of poor iodine intake, especially with the UK's rise of plant-based and dairy-free diets.

Iodine's role in your child's developing brain

✧ It makes the thyroid hormones that are needed for the brain to grow and develop, as well as for big brain jobs like learning and memory.

How much iodine do babies and young children need?

Age	Reference nutrient intake (µg/day)
0–3 months	50
3–12 months	60
1–3 years	70
4–6 years	100

Source: Committee on Medical Aspects of Food and Nutrition Policy (COMA), 1991

What foods contain iodine?

The main foods sources of iodine for children in the UK are dairy products and fish – mainly white fish like cod and haddock. Other foods, including eggs, fruits and vegetables, can contribute, but generally in much smaller amounts. I've listed various foods and their iodine content to ensure your child can easily meet their daily needs. Dairy products alone can likely fulfil your child's iodine requirements, and a small serving of cod or haddock can supply more than enough for several days.

In my experience, one of the groups of children who may struggle with iodine intake or need to pay more attention are those with allergies, especially to milk (and even more so if they are also allergic to fish) or those following a plant-based diet without dairy. For this reason, I highly recommend prioritising iodine-fortified milk alternatives if a child follows a milk-free diet.

Food	Iodine content (*g/day*)
Dairy	
Cow's milk 200ml	50–100 (can be higher in winter!)
Yoghurt 150g	50–100 (can be higher in winter!)
Cheese 30g	11
Dairy alternatives (if fortified with iodine) *Check labels carefully as not all are fortified.*	
Milk alternatives, e.g. soya, oat, coconut 100ml	10–40
Yoghurt alternatives 100g	10–30
Cheese alternative 30g	4.5–10.5
Fish and seafood	
Haddock 60g	195
Cod 60g	115
Scampi 85g	80
Pollock 60g	34
Tinned tuna 100g	12
Other options	
One egg	25
One slice of bread	5
Fruit or vegetables 80g	3

Source: Adapted from BDA iodine food factsheet

Zinc

Zinc is a mineral known as a trace element, which means that while it's essential for the body, it is only needed in minimal amounts. Despite being 'small', zinc has some pretty punchy jobs, including supporting brain development. Zinc deficiency in these early years has been found to interfere with growth and the development of cognitive abilities like memory, learning and concentration. Zinc deficiency has also been linked to mood changes, irritability and hyperactivity.

Zinc's role in your child's developing brain

✧ It helps keep neurons (cells in the brain that send and receive messages) growing, healthy and talking to each other effectively.

✧ It helps to make and regulate neurotransmitters (a chemical messenger that tells the brain and body what to do) that can affect learning, memory, mood, attention and behaviours.

✧ As an antioxidant, zinc helps protect brain cells from damage, keeping the brain healthy.

How much zinc do babies and young children need?

Age	Reference nutrient intake (mg/day)
0–6 months	4.0
6–12 months	
1–3 years	5.0
4–6 years	6.5

Source: Committee on Medical Aspects of Food and Nutrition Policy (COMA), 1991

What foods contain zinc?

A range of foods contains zinc, and you'll see that many of these are protein sources within the diet, such as meat, fish, eggs and beans. You'll likely be adding these foods to your child's diet anyway, but here are some example foods and their zinc content to help you compare your child's intake to their requirements.

Food	Zinc content (*mg*)
Meat and fish	
Roast beef – 1 slice (around 45g)	1.9
Pork loin – 50g (half a small pork chop)	1
Turkey – 1 slice (around 45g)	0.75
Half a tin of sardines	0.55
Beans and pulses	
Cooked lentils 50g	0.65
Chickpeas 50g	0.65
Cereals and grains	
Oats – 40g	1
Rice – white 50g	0.15
brown 50g	0.35
1 slice wholemeal bread	0.6
Quinoa 50g	1.1
Dairy	
Cheese 30g	1
Greek yoghurt 120g	0.6
Milk 120ml	0.5
Other options	
One egg	0.6
Pumpkin seeds 1 tbsp	1.1
Peanut butter 1 tbsp	0.6

Vitamin A

This fat-soluble vitamin is essential for brain and eye development, especially in these early years of rapid growth. Vitamin A deficiency can negatively impact brain health and functioning, leading to issues with learning and memory. Significant deficiency can also lead to changes in and loss of sight. Fortunately, it can be found in two different forms:

✧ Preformed vitamin A (aka retinol) – this is found in animal products such as liver, fish and dairy.

✧ Provitamin A (aka beta-carotene) – this is found in plant-based foods like orange vegetables, such as carrots, sweet potatoes and leafy greens. The body converts beta-carotene into retinol, making it an important source of vitamin A for those on a vegetarian or vegan diet.

Vitamin A's role in your child's developing brain

✧ Helps stem cells become healthy brain cells. Stem cells are building-block cells that can change into specific cells the body needs.

✧ Supports neurogenesis – this means helping to create new neurons (brain cells).

How much vitamin A does your child need?

Age	Reference nutrient intake (μg/day)
0–6 months	350
6–12 months	
1–3 years	400
4–6 years	

Source: Committee on Medical Aspects of Food and Nutrition Policy (COMA), 1991

What foods contain vitamin A?

Vitamin A comes from both animal and plant-based sources, providing a range of foods you can include in your child's diet to meet their needs. Here are some examples.

Animal sources		Plant sources	
Food	Approximate vitamin A content (µg)	Food	Approximate vitamin A content (µg)
45g beef liver (give maximum of once per week for young children)	3,300	Half a baked sweet potato	550
1 egg	75	80g carrots	450
65g salmon (½ fillet)	110	80g mango	45
30g Cheddar cheese	75	40g cooked kale	550
45g tinned tuna (in water)	100	80g cantaloupe melon	135

Note: It's recommended that children in the UK aged one to five years are given a supplement containing vitamin A as they might not get enough from diet alone. Never over-supplement with vitamin A.

A nod to brilliant blues and purples for supporting our children's (and our own) brains!

Berries, fruits, beans and vegetables with dark skins, like blueberries, cherries and red cabbbage, are rich in antioxidants called anthocyanins, which help protect brain cells from damage and promote overall brain health. Studies have shown that anthocyanins can support brain function in children by improving memory and learning abilities. For us parents, they may also help prevent cognitive decline and memory loss as we age – I know I feel like I need them by the bucketful since becoming a parent!

Brain-building and -boosting meals and snack ideas

Here are some brain-boosting meal and snack ideas to try at home. Make sure the options are adapted as needed for babies under 12 months of age.

Breakfasts

✧ Scrambled eggs or omelette with chopped spinach and toast.

✧ Plain or Greek yoghurt with mixed fresh or frozen berries and a sprinkle of seeds (such as milled sunflower seeds).

✧ Porridge topped with banana and almond butter.

✧ Avocado on toast or eggy bread with a sprinkle of seeds (ground, if needed).

✧ Smoothie or smoothie bowl made with frozen berries, yoghurt, oats or ground nuts.

✧ Breakfast burrito made with scrambled eggs, beans, cheese and avocado in a wrap.

✧ Pancakes made with wholewheat flour served with fruit and yoghurt or nut butter.

✧ Overnight or baked oats with chia seeds, tinned raspberries and yoghurt.

Lunches or main meals

✧ Pesto salmon pasta with peas.

✧ Chicken or tofu and vegetable stir-fry.

✧ Fish cakes (mix of white and/or oily fish) with broccoli.

✧ Sweet potato and chickpea curry with rice or chapatis.

✧ Black bean and vegetable wraps, tacos or fajitas.

✧ Salmon with sweet potato chips and peas.

✧ Sardine and tomato pasta.

✧ Butternut squash risotto with toasted seeds.

✧ Lentil and vegetable soup with 50/50 bread.

✧ Omega 3-enriched fish fingers with mashed potato and mixed vegetables.

Snacks

✧ Mackerel pate with oatcakes or wholegrain crackers.

✧ Egg cups or tortilla quiches.

✧ Hummus with carrot sticks and wholegrain pitta-bread strips.

✧ Thin apple slices with cheese or nut butter.

✧ Rice or corn cakes with nut butter and mashed fruit or grated carrot.

✧ Fruit fingers, such as melon, pineapple and mango with Greek yoghurt mixed with tahini or nut butter.

Growing a Great Gut Garden

Now it's time to move to the other end of the body to discuss feeding a healthy gut. Despite the distance, the brain and gut are pretty good friends and spend a fair amount of time talking to each other through a 'phone line' known as the gut–brain axis. This connection means that the health of the gut can significantly impact the brain, and vice versa.

✧ **What is the gut microbiome?**

✧ **Why is the gut microbiome so important?**

✧ **What affects the community of 'good' and 'bad' bacteria in the gut?**

✧ **How to help your child grow a great gut garden**

✧ **What about probiotic supplements?**

✧ **Gut-friendly meal and snack ideas**

What is the gut microbiome?

Welcome to a discussion about your child's 'second brain' – the gut. There has never been more focus on the gut, specifically the community it houses and how this can profoundly impact health. It may surprise you that the term microbiome was only coined in the early 2000s, making it relatively new in scientific terms. While our understanding of the gut microbiome has proliferated over the past two decades, we're still only about halfway through mapping all its species, so undoubtedly this section will likely need regular updates as research continues to evolve!

The first three to five years of life are *the* foundation for your child's gut microbiome. The gut microbiome develops rapidly from birth and the early years and is thought to reach an 'adult-like' state by around age three. This means that while the community of gut bacteria can and will still fluctuate throughout life, with notable adjustments during different life events or stages, the community your child has collected during these early years will largely be staying with them for life.

But before diving deeper into growing a great gut garden, let's cover some backstory!

Gut microbiome

The community of trillions of microorganisms, including bacteria, viruses, fungi and single-celled organisms in the gut and everything they produce, is collectively known as the gut microbiome. It is essential for life. I find it helpful to think about this diverse ecosystem as a 'gut garden'. Not only do we want a garden with lots of different and beautiful flowers, but each microorganism also needs specific nutrients and conditions to thrive. Every person's gut microbiome is unique, like a fingerprint.

Most microorganisms in the gut are beneficial and vital for health. They have helpful and much-needed roles, which I'll discuss below. Sometimes harmful bacteria can be present in the gut, and, in large enough amounts, they can cause illness or impact short- and/or long-term health.

Note: We all have microbiomes in other places in the body – the skin microbiome and oral (mouth) microbiome, for example.

Why is the gut microbiome so important?

The gut has long been recognised as the organ responsible for digestion – an essential job. But the metres of gut that your child (and you) have, along with the community of tiny microorganisms it houses, also hold significant power over various aspects of health.

✧ **The gut and immune system are close friends:** Around 70–80 per cent of the body's immune cells call the gut their home, so, really, it's one of your child's most significant immune organs. Unsurprisingly, this means the gut greatly influences how your child's immune system works and develops, and even the risk of developing some immune-related conditions such as allergies or autoimmune conditions. The gut itself can work as a defence system, creating a barrier (the gut's lining) to keep germs and harmful bacteria out while also helping absorb nutrients from food, including those needed for immune health. The community of helpful friends in the gut also help the immune system to recognise and remember which things coming into the body are harmful or safe and release signals so that it can respond appropriately, say, by helping to reduce inflammation. In short, a healthy gut microbiome = a healthy immune system.

✧ **The gut and brain talk:** Even though they are physically distant, the gut and brain communicate back and forth constantly through the gut–brain axis. My favourite way to bring this to life is 'butterflies'. When we are nervous or anxious, we can feel that bubbly, fluttery feeling in our stomach or gut, yet anxious thoughts or worry are something that our brain is responsible for. But what's the relevance for your child? The community of friends in your child's gut has been shown to affect mood, stress levels and how well the brain thinks, learns and remembers. Disruption or miscommunication of this pathway between the gut and the brain has also been linked to conditions such as colic, constipation and irritable bowel syndrome (IBS). Many of these are called 'Disorders of the Gut–Brain Interaction', which you can read more about on page 369. And that's not all; gut bacteria also make neurotransmitters (chemical messengers) which support mood, cognition and learning. In short, a balanced belly of gut bugs = a brilliant brain, and vice versa!

✧ **The gut and nutrition:** Of course, the little friends in the gut are involved in digestion. Gut bacteria are fantastic at digesting complex carbohydrates and fibre (their favourite fuel) to produce nutrients and energy. Plenty of this fuel also helps keep good gut bacteria thriving. Sometimes, we see some (expected) effects of this digestion, such as gas, bloating or changes to poo. Gut bacteria also work hard to help make some nutrients the body needs, like vitamin K and some B vitamins. Research also suggests that the types of bacteria in the gut can influence how the body processes nutrients, including how it stores fat. In short, a healthy gut microbiome = a happy digestive and metabolic system.

✧ **The effect of an imbalance of gut bacteria:** While we're still learning about how these imbalances happen, research increasingly shows that gut dysbiosis – an imbalance where there are more harmful ('bad') bacteria and fewer helpful ('good') bacteria – is linked to various health conditions. Think of it as weeds that have become overgrown in a garden. These can include digestive issues like IBS, immune-related conditions like allergies, as well as broader health problems such as obesity, diabetes and even mood disorders like anxiety and depression.

What affects the community of 'good' and 'bad' bacteria in the gut?

The community of bacteria in your child's gut is shaped by many 'puzzle pieces' and will change over time. While certain factors, like diet and time outdoors, are more within our control as parents, many others aren't. I've outlined these below, recognising that some are simply part of life, like the need for medicine. Gut health has many influences, and thankfully one of the most powerful is diet, which we can control, and which I'll explore next.

Desirable impact	Unfavourable impact
Vaginal birth	Certain drugs, such as antibiotics
Breast milk	Lack of dietary variety
Varied homemade food, and fibre-rich foods	Highly processed, low-fibre diet
Exposure to other children and people	Lack of mixing with other children and people
Exposure to nature, farming and dirt	Excessive exposure to disinfectants and antiseptic agents
Physical activity	Stress
Fermented 'probiotic' foods	Poor sleep

Top 10 foods for gut health

1. Breast milk
2. Beans and pulses
3. Fruits and vegetables
4. Nuts
5. Seeds
6. Wholegrains
7. Herbs and spices
8. Fermented foods, such as yoghurt, pasteurised aged cheese, kefir
9. Prebiotic foods, such as garlic, apples, leeks, oats
10. Extra virgin olive oil

How to help your child grow a great gut garden

The good news is that there are many things you can offer your child to feed those good gut bacteria and help their gut microbiome thrive. For babies, breast milk contains a community of bacteria, plenty of food for the good bacteria, and many factors to support a healthy gut – just flip back to page 11 to understand more.

From the point when your baby has started solids, food begins to significantly change their gut microbiome, with bacteria species found to increase by 60 per cent or more between six and 12 months of age. To support the growth of plenty of good bacteria, my golden rule for gut health will always be to **prioritise plants and dietary variety**. Studies have shown that people with a higher dietary diversity have a more diverse gut microbiota, which is linked to a lower risk of chronic diseases – so the earlier you get started, the better. Let's delve into the dream menu for your child's good gut bacteria.

Fantastic fibre

Fibre is well known to be an important nutrient for digestion and regular poos, but it's also the preferred 'food' for good gut bacteria. When gut bacteria break down fibre, they produce helpful compounds called short-chain fatty acids (SCFAs), which help reduce inflammation and maintain a healthy gut lining. Different types of fibre from various fibre-rich foods will also feed different bacteria, helping nurture a balanced and varied gut garden. Fantastic fibre-rich foods include fruits, vegetables, wholegrains, nuts, seeds, beans and pulses.

The fibre intake of children in the UK is generally below recommendations, suggesting we're 'starving' gut bacteria of their all-important fuel. However, as parents, you're also told to be mindful of how much fibre to offer your young child. I appreciate that balancing fibre intake can be confusing, so I've covered more about exactly how much young children need and practically how to get it into their diet on pages 262–5.

Prebiotic foods

Some plant foods contain a particular type of fibre known as prebiotics. These cannot be digested by the body and are known to be particularly great at helping good bacteria grow. Prebiotics are not the same as probiotics, which are beneficial bacteria found in food or supplements. Foods rich in prebiotics include mushrooms, asparagus, apples, bananas, oats, garlic and onion.

Note: Some children can be sensitive to these difficult-to-digest fibres and experience issues like bloating, excess gas and pain. If you're concerned about any of these symptoms, discuss them with a health professional.

Fermented foods and probiotic foods

Probiotics are often known as 'friendly' or 'good' bacteria, and there is lots of ongoing research looking at their benefits to health, including in children *(Note: probiotic foods may need to be avoided in immunocompromised children).*

In food, 'true' probiotic foods contain specific strains of bacteria that have evidence of surviving digestion and providing specific health benefits. These can include specific 'live' yoghurts or yoghurt drinks. Fermented foods also contain good bacteria, which naturally grow during fermentation and may benefit the community of bacteria in your child's gut. They include foods like kefir (fermented milk), sauerkraut, miso, kimchi, tempeh, some yoghurts (such as Greek) and some cheeses like aged Cheddar and Parmesan.

Some of these foods can be quite salty or have pretty punchy flavours for young children, so they may take some time to get used to or have to be given in small amounts during the early years. In my experience, dairy options, including kefir, yoghurt and aged cheese, tend to be the foods most easily included for kids.

The science surrounding the benefits of probiotic and fermented foods in the diets of young children is still very much growing, with some research highlighting the benefits, particularly of things like yoghurt and kefir, on the diversity of gut bacteria and potential for impact on immune health, including the frequency of respiratory (chest) and gut infections.

Note: Pickled foods are often confused with fermented foods. Pickled foods tend to use an acid, while fermented foods use bacteria that break down sugars and are the ones with most gut-loving benefits.

Hello, herbs and spices

Fresh, dried, frozen – it doesn't matter. Herbs and spices are one of my favourite ways to easily add variety to kids' meals. They can change a dish completely and are a great way of helping to expand young palates! Herbs and spices count as plant-based foods and have the potential to positively impact growing gut bugs. They can also contain antioxidants, vitamins and some compounds that may support a healthy gut microbiome.

Gut-loving extras your child will love too!

◆ **Get your child outside:** Outdoor play and exploring nature (yes, even making mud pies) are repeatedly shown to be great for growing a child's community of gut friends.

◆ **Making furry friends:** Assuming your child isn't allergic, exposure to farms, animals, dogs and cats has been found to positively affect gut bugs.

◆ **Say yes to the playdate:** Socialising has been shown to help build diverse gut bacteria as children are exposed to different microbes from their peers.

What about probiotic supplements?

Understandably, with all the buzz around gut health, there has been a massive surge in the availability of a new type of supplement – probiotics. But what actually are they?

Probiotics are live bacteria ('good bacteria') that, when given in good enough amounts, can benefit the health of the person taking them.

Probiotics sold in the UK currently fall under the umbrella of a 'food supplement', which means they are not regulated as strictly as medicines. For this reason, marketing can take over and it can be difficult to unpick what to use and why it may be beneficial, if at all. Here are some key points to understand about choosing and using probiotic supplements.

What strain (type) of bacteria is in the supplement and does your child need it?	In the realm of beneficial bacteria, there are numerous strains, each with its own unique functions and benefits. Simply put, if you want to address a specific issue in the gut or alleviate certain symptoms, it's important to target the right bacteria for the job. This concept is referred to as *strain specificity* in the world of probiotics. It's worth being aware that more isn't always better when it comes to strains, and ideally robust science should back up their benefits. A health professional is best placed to advise on which strain of bacteria and dose would be needed for your child and your concerns.
How much bacteria is in the supplement, and do they make it to the gut?	There are trillions of bacteria in the gut, so for probiotics to have an impact a pretty good-sized army of bacteria should be proven (by the company) to make it down to the gut alive to be beneficial when it gets there! On probiotic labels you should see 'CFU', which stands for Colony Forming Units. The number should be very high! Robust companies should also provide data that demonstrates the bacteria actually make it to the gut alive.

How long do I need to use them?	In general, it's considered that probiotic supplements should be given for at least four weeks to notice potential benefits, although the exact duration can vary based on individual needs and the specific health issue being addressed. For some conditions, longer-term use may be necessary, while others might see improvement in a shorter timeframe. If you decide to use a probiotic, some children can experience an increase in bloating or gas initially.

I'd advise you to check in on the reputation of a company and probiotic supplement in the same way you would for a food supplement, following the checklist I provided on page 197.

The million-dollar question, though, is whether probiotic supplements are beneficial or supportive of your child's health. I'm afraid the answer isn't particularly clear-cut, and while research suggests that probiotics are generally regarded as safe for healthy babies and children, there is very little data that shows significant benefits. Given their price tag I would always recommend parents focus on food first for good gut health as I'm afraid you can't out-supplement a good diet (at least not yet!).

But what about specific gut troubles or worries in children? This *is* an area that is evolving, and for certain conditions, including colic and antibiotic-associated diarrhoea, for instance, we now have some robust scientific data to start making suggestions for strains and doses of bacteria that may be supportive in symptom management. (You can read more on pages 372 and 393.)

In the meantime, while the research remains ongoing, remember that although there are lots of factors that will influence your child's gut health, there are ways in which you can support it in a positive way, focusing on food first!

Gut-friendly meals and snack ideas

Here are some examples of gut-loving meal and snack ideas to try at home. Make sure all options are adapted as needed for babies under 12 months.

Breakfasts

✧ Greek yoghurt with grated fruit or mashed berries, topped with oats or crushed cereal.

✧ Banana and nut butter smoothie, made with yoghurt, milk or kefir.

✧ Wheat-biscuit cereal with milk and diced, grated or pureed fruit.

✧ Baked eggs (in tinned tomatoes, peppers, spinach) with wholemeal toast.

✧ Porridge with grated carrot, ground almonds and cinnamon.

✧ Banana and oat pancakes with yoghurt and cinnamon.

✧ Eggs, fried plantain and tomatoes.

✧ Stir-fried rice with kimchi and a fried egg and fruit.

✧ Lentil dal and rice.

✧ Mashed avocado and black beans on toast.

Lunches or main meals

✧ Low-salt and -sugar beans on toast with Cheddar cheese.

✧ Sweetcorn and courgette fritters (use gram or wholemeal flour for extra fibre).

✧ Fish pie with potato and parsnip mash and peas.

✧ Red lentil Bolognese with pasta.

✧ Labneh with pitta and vegetables.

✧ Chickpea and spinach curry with roti or rice.

✧ Chicken and vegetable stew with new potatoes.

✧ Butternut squash and butterbean soup with bread.

✧ Chicken, rice and peas.

✧ Salmon and sweet potato fishcakes with broccoli.

✧ Stuffed peppers.

✧ Vegetable stir-fry with tofu, chicken or beef.

✧ Rainbow wraps with grated vegetables and hummus.

✧ Cauliflower mac and cheese.

✧ Wholemeal pitta bread vegetable pizzas.

✧ Mixed beef and bean chilli with jacket potato and cheese.

✧ Broccoli and cheese quiche.

✧ Black bean burger with sweet potato chips.

Snacks

✧ Oatcakes with hummus and sliced fruit or vegetables.

✧ Fruit and yoghurt (plus a sprinkle of seeds).

✧ Thinly sliced apples drizzled with peanut or almond butter, sprinkled with desiccated coconut.

✧ Oat and seed energy balls.

✧ Cucumber, sliced Cheddar cheese and crackers.

✧ Yoghurt and fruit lollies.

✧ Mixed vegetable muffins.

✧ Falafel and yoghurt dip.

So that's the end of a whistle-stop tour of getting excellent gut health started for your little one. Now it's time to move on to one of the gut's close friends, the immune system. Something that as parents we are oh so familiar with, as no parent goes unscathed from the barrage of illnesses in the early years.

Powerful Protection – How to Support Your Child's Immune Health

✧ **Understanding your child's immune system**

✧ **Essential food and nutrients for immune excellence in the early years**

✧ **Can supplements boost your child's immune system?**

✧ **Immune-supporting meals and snack ideas for children**

✧ **The role of food and nutrition in allergy prevention**

Your child's immune system will be one of the most critical aspects of their health for life, and the early years are a prime time for its development. Diet and immunity can be a hot topic for parents as they navigate the treadmill of sickness and illness that the early years inevitably throw children's way. I know first-hand how relentless this can be! While nutrition is one of your best weapons for solid immune health, it's often shrouded in old wives' tales and false promises!

Before I discuss how you can harness diet for your child's immune health, it's probably helpful to give you a brief understanding of the immune system, how it works and what it looks like in the early years.

Understanding your child's immune system

For many, the immune system might feel a bit invisible – after all, many of its cells are hidden away! However, it's a fascinating network of organs (including the skin, gut, spleen and tonsils), cells and proteins. Together, they join forces to defend, protect and keep our bodies alive and well, and during the early years your child's immune system is very much 'in training'.

The immune system has two main parts: the innate immune system and the acquired immune system. I describe these simply as:

✧ **Innate:** This is the immune system your child is born with. It acts as the front line of defence, responding quickly to unwanted invaders, much like the bouncer at a pub door who immediately tries to kick out anything harmful or disruptive.

◇ **Acquired:** This is the immune system your child develops over time based on exposure to different invaders, chemicals, and more. It's why children often get sick frequently in their early years – their immune system is just getting started and learning to recognise and remember various threats. Every new invader is like adding another 'wanted' sign so the bouncer knows to keep them out next time.

While we're here, please know that children are expected to get ill regularly in these early years, especially when exposed to large pools of new potential invaders (hello, childcare!). Many paediatricians I have worked with quote the fact that children under four will contract on average 8–12 illnesses a year. For me, these certainly seemed to bottleneck and overlap during the winter months!

Babies and children will also experience something known as **passive immunity**. This immunity is borrowed from their birth mother, who transfers essential antibodies from the immune system through the placenta during pregnancy and breast milk after their baby arrives. First breast milk, colostrum, is packed with antibodies and other immune cells to help give a baby's immune system a hefty first dose of support when encountering a new world full of threats.

Various factors influence immune-system development during early years and beyond. Of course, exposure to pathogens and bacteria is one aspect, but this exists alongside vaccinations, exposure to beneficial bacteria, nutrition (milk and food), sleep, stress and the environment. All of these factors have a role in shaping or fine-tuning the immune system and how it responds.

The immune system is a robust defence system that's kept us alive for millions of years, but it's not perfect and can be sensitive to changes that mean its responses aren't always correct. Essentially, sometimes, the immune system gets it wrong! Examples of this in the early years include conditions such as food allergies, where proteins that are considered safe are wrongly perceived as a threat by the immune system, similar to other allergic conditions like eczema, asthma and hay fever. For some children, there may also be a conversation between their genes, the environment and their immune system that contributes to the onset of autoimmune conditions such as coeliac disease and type 1 diabetes. Of course, both of these immune conditions also require dietary adjustments for life.

Essential food and nutrients for immune excellence in the early years

The good news for this section is that many of the nutrients integral to immune health are ones that I've mentioned already. From your viewpoint, this is excellent because it emphasises the significance of the nutrients that you're now familiar with. For me, it means I can take a break from typing!

Breast milk – Breast milk contains an impressive array of components that support a baby's immune system, which biology designed for a small and highly vulnerable new human. Beyond vitamins and minerals, it includes antibodies, probiotics, fatty acids, immune cells, enzymes and even natural killer cells that can identify and eliminate cancerous or infected cells. Even breastfeeding for a few days provides significant immune advantages.

Gut-friendly foods – The gut and the immune system are closely connected, with over 70 per cent of the body's immune cells housed in the gut, so foods that support your child's gut health will also bolster the development of a healthy, happy immune system. So, just read a few pages back to understand the best foods for your child's gut health, and you'll be supporting their immune health too – double win.

Vitamin A – Its role in your child's immune health includes:

✦ Involvement in making immune cells (like white blood cells).

✧ Supporting immune cells to work properly.

✧ Helping to maintain and repair protective tissues like the skin or the lining of places like the gut and nose.

✧ Supporting immune responses and reduces inflammation.

In the discussion about nutrients for brain health, you can find out how much vitamin A your child needs and where to get it from on page 301.

Vitamin D – Its role in your child's immune health includes:

✧ Boosting the ability of specific immune cells to fight germs.

✧ Lowering inflammation by helping control the body's response to infections.

✧ Helping to balance how different immune cells work together.

Vitamin D is one of the only supplements I recommend for babies (unless having < 500ml of formula per day) and young children and is recommended by the NHS and other UK health agencies. You can learn more about vitamin D supplementation for your child by checking the supplement section for their age.

Zinc – Its role in your child's immune health includes:

✧ Helping specific immune cells to grow and develop.

✧ Helping to keep protective tissues like the skin or the lining of places like the gut and nose healthy.

✧ Controlling enzymes that affect immune response and inflammation.

You can find out how much zinc your child needs and where to get it from on pages 298–300.

Iron – Its role in your child's immune health includes:

✧ Helping immune cells make chemicals that kill germs.

✧ Supporting enzymes that are important for how immune cells work.

✧ Acting as a fundamental building block for haemoglobin, a protein in red blood cells that transports oxygen around the body, including to the gut and immune cells.

Iron is a nutrient that I've talked about a few times already throughout this book, so you can find lots more information on pages 105–6 and 399–405.

Vitamin C – is often the nutrient most commonly linked to immunity; its role in your child's immunity is essential and includes:

✧ Helping with the production and functioning of white blood cells.

✧ Wound healing.

✧ Being an antioxidant that protects cells from harmful substances that could compromise the immune system.

The good news about vitamin C is that it's generally quite straightforward for your child to get enough of it from their diet. A recent review found that young children in the UK generally get sufficient quantities from food to the extent that previous supplementation advice for vitamin C in the early years is likely to be scrapped.

How much vitamin C do babies and young children need?

Age	Reference nutrient intake (mg/day)
0–6 months	25
6–12 months	
1–3 years	30
4–6 years	

Source: Committee on Medical Aspects of Food and Nutrition Policy (COMA), 1991

What foods contain vitamin C?

Fruits and vegetables are universally known to provide vitamin C in the diet, but there can be some often-surprising sources too, like potatoes.

See the table on the next page for some examples of amounts of vitamin C in children's portion sizes of some foods.

Can supplements boost your child's immune system?

During the winter months, I always notice more parents than usual lurking around the supplement section in supermarkets and pharmacies! I'm unsurprised – the onslaught of winter illnesses can send us all searching for remedies and supplements, hoping they can boost or rev up the immune system. I genuinely wish it were that straightforward, but the truth is there isn't a supplement that universally boosts the immune system whenever your child falls ill.

But what about vitamin C, you might ask? Yes, this is an essential vitamin for the immune system, as mentioned above; however, a major review of vitamin C supplementation and the common cold, including data from thousands of people, found that vitamin C supplementation won't prevent colds or improve symptoms and, at best, may reduce the duration of a cold by about 10 per cent. Most children get enough vitamin C from their diet, with just half a kiwi or a handful of strawberries meeting a young child's daily requirement.

So, you may want to prioritise plenty of vitamin-C-rich foods during illness, but I wouldn't run for the extra supplements.

Amounts of vitamin C (mg) in children's portions of foods					
Fruit		Vegetables		Starchy foods	
Satsuma	35	Broccoli (40g)	35	New potatoes (50g)	10
Strawberries (40g)	25	Red pepper (30g)	45	Half a jacket potato, skin on	9
Kiwi – half	32	Mustard greens (40g)	28	Oven chips (60g)	4
Papaya (40g)	25	4 cherry tomatoes	12		
Guava (40g)	90	Cauliflower (40g)	19		
Mango (40g)	15	Okra (40g)	10		
Frozen mixed berries (40g)	15–20	Brussels sprouts (40g)	25		
Tinned mandarins (40g)	6	Pak choi (20g)	15		

How about other supplements that promote their immune-supporting properties? By now, you may not be surprised to learn that little strong scientific evidence indicates that supplementing with nutrients or fruit extracts will have a meaningful effect on your child's immune system, except in cases where they lack essential nutrients in their diet. While some studies highlight that zinc supplementation may reduce how long a child has a common cold, like vitamin C supplements, there's no suggestion they can impact how often your child will get ill or prevent illness. Of course, prioritising zinc-rich foods from a balanced and varied diet will always be my top recommendation!

As always, there's a caveat here! Supplementation can be helpful for a small group of children who have very selective eating habits, may exclude food groups and are unlikely to get what they need from their diet. I would highly recommend that this be supported by a health professional like a paediatric dietitian, who can tell you how much of key nutrients should be supplemented based on your child's eating habits.

Immune-supporting meals and snack ideas for children

Here are some examples of immune-supporting meals and snack ideas to try at home. Make sure all options are adapted as needed for babies under 12 months.

Breakfasts

✧ Nut butter or tahini on toast with sliced kiwi.

✧ Super green smoothie with banana, avocado, spinach and milk.

✧ Porridge with apple and milled nuts, such as almonds, pecans.

✧ Menemen (Turkish scrambled eggs with tomato).

✧ Baked pear and almond oats.

✧ Buckwheat pancakes with yoghurt and berries.

✧ Mackerel pate on toast.

✧ Fortified cereal with fruit and milk.

✧ Hash browns with mashed black beans and tomato.

Lunches and evening meals

✧ Pasta with spinach, peas and cream cheese.

✧ Omelette with peppers, onions and greens, plus a side of pitta.

✧ Salmon with roasted new potatoes and broccoli.

✧ Chicken and chickpea curry with rice.

✧ Mushroom risotto.

✧ Hummus and roasted pepper sandwich with sliced vegetables.

✧ Tomato and lentil soup with a cheese toastie.

✧ Callaloo and egg scramble with toast.

✧ Meat, egg or tofu with vegetable-fried rice.

✧ Turkey and sweet potato shepherd's pie.

✧ Lamb and spinach curry with roti.

✧ Tofu, beef or chicken with vegetable noodles with satay or tahini dressing.

✧ Chicken and vegetable pie with frozen mixed vegetables.

✧ Mixed bean chilli with avocado, yoghurt and jacket potato.

✧ Mushrooms on toast with spinach, onion and cream cheese.

✧ Coconut cod and mango curry with rice.

✧ Chicken thigh traybake with peppers, sweet potato and tomatoes.

✧ Spanish omelette.

Snacks

✧ Fruit and cheese slices or cubes.

✧ Vegetable sushi balls, made from grated vegetables, mashed avocado and rice.

✧ Tinned mandarins with yoghurt.

✧ Kiwi flapjacks.

✧ Rice or corn cakes with mashed avocado or mashed roasted vegetables and a sprinkle of seeds, such as hemp.

✧ Smoothie bowl with mango, coconut yoghurt, oats and milled seeds.

✧ Crackers with cream cheese and grated carrot.

✧ Banana and oat cookies.

✧ Boiled egg, tomatoes and cucumber.

The role of food and nutrition in allergy prevention

This is a topic close to my heart, and over the last few years science has seen an astounding shift in how we harness food and nutrition to support the immune system in the context of food allergy prevention. I have covered the whys and hows in detail in the chapter on weaning on page 116. From an immune perspective, introducing food allergens to babies once they've started eating solids helps expose them to food proteins through the gut. This early exposure allows the immune system to recognise these proteins as safe, effectively 'training' it to tolerate them. There are other dietary strategies and queries I get on this topic regularly, so here are my key takeaways for you on nutrition and allergy prevention.

1. **Don't delay introducing common food allergens.** Research shows that proactive introduction of allergens from the outset of starting solids can help prevent food allergies from developing.

2. **Once allergens are in, keep giving them often.** Emerging research suggests that one reason the number of children with food allergies isn't decreasing, or at least levelling off, despite the advice in point one now being nearly 10 years old, is that parents don't *keep giving* allergenic foods once introduced. Giving food once or twice might not cut the mustard, so once they are in, try to keep these foods as part of your child's regular diet.

3. **Dietary variety.** Yes, here's another reason why dietary variety is so important. Interestingly, in the context of food allergies, research has shown that for every new food introduced to a child from weaning onwards (and not just allergenic foods), their overall risk of developing food allergy seems to decline. This likely emphasises once again the significance of a balanced and diverse diet for overall health and the thriving community of microbes, which are talking closely to your child's developing immune system.

4. **Probiotic supplements** – I wish I could tell you that specific supplements or bacteria strains could prevent or help children outgrow allergies, but the science isn't there yet. While research shows that gut bacteria can differ between children with allergic diseases and those without, no specific supplement is recognised to treat or prevent this. Ongoing research shows promise for probiotics, but further evidence is needed before recommending specific strains for allergy prevention or management. For now, prioritise food first!

So together, we've explored some of the essential foods and nutrients that support your child's brain, gut and immune system during these crucial early years. But remember, many other lifestyle factors also significantly affect their overall health. Essential elements like sleep, fresh air, time in nature and a nurturing environment are all puzzle pieces for the healthy development of the gut, brain and immune system.

*   *   *

I couldn't discuss foods for future health without acknowledging that nutrition isn't the only reason we eat. In a world where food-related health challenges are often tied to the food environment and our relationship with food, it's important to me to offer guidance on supporting children with healthy food habits and relationships, which you'll find in the next section.

6

Feeding Futures

Here, I'm shifting direction a little away from nutrition but on to something closely linked, and that can't be ignored – feeding your child's future in the context of food habits, behaviours and relationships with food. I'm going to touch on some key topics parents often ask me about or that regularly crop up in my clinic.

Feeding Future Food Habits and Relationships

✧ **Ultra-processed foods – navigating feeding children in the current food environment**

✧ **Family mealtimes – how eating with your children boosts their future health and happiness**

✧ **Future-proofing food relationships**

Ultra-processed foods – navigating feeding children in the current food environment

Undoubtedly, we're all raising our children in a food environment that's not only different from when we were growing up but almost unrecognisable from our grandparents' era. Over recent decades there has been a boom in the availability and consumption of a wide range of manufactured and processed foods, with the term 'Ultra Processed Food', or UPF, now more familiar than ever. While I was writing this book, the most comprehensive study to date found that, on average, toddlers in the UK obtain nearly half of their calories from ultra-processed foods, increasing to almost 60 per cent by the age of seven – figures that certainly sound worrying.

Health professionals are closely monitoring this because as our food environment and intake of UPFs has increased, so have health outcomes, with a sharp rise in poor health, nutritional issues and conditions like type 2 diabetes. While this data is observational – showing a link without proving causation – it still warrants attention. Parents today are asking me more than ever about navigating our current food environment, with many expressing guilt or worry about their child's consumption of UPFs, as well as confusion over what UPFs even are!

Before I discuss this further, I want to remind you that I'm here to reassure and support you, not to judge or become the food police. Not all foods are the enemy, even if social media might make it seem that way sometimes. This topic is incredibly nuanced, so a blend of awareness and practicality is essential, in my opinion!

What are processed and ultra-processed foods?

In simple terms, processed foods are any foods that have been changed from their original form through cooking, canning, freezing or adding preservatives, additives and flavourings. Not all alterations negatively affect food – freezing vegetables actually enhances their nutritional value! Processing has also dramatically expanded the variety of foods available to us throughout the year. However, it may not be surprising that highly processed foods (or UPFs), particularly those with high levels of sugar, salt, additives and unhealthy fats, are likely to contribute to health problems. For perspective, many of these are the same foods that dietary guidelines have advised minimising for everyone, both children and adults, for decades – foods high in fat, salt and sugar (HFSS). In addition to their nutritional content, ultra-processed foods (UPFs) are considered a 'risk' for other reasons. For example, their formulations often prioritise hyper-palatability, influencing the quantity and speed at which these foods may be consumed.

Interestingly, the UK has no formalised or agreed definition of UPFs (yet). They are often described as foods that have undergone significant processing and modification from their original state using industrial techniques and processes. They typically contain ingredients you wouldn't use at home, like sweeteners, preservatives and emulsifiers.

One method of definition used is what's known as the NOVA system, which classifies foods depending on their levels of processing. Within this, many people are surprised to see where some staple foods in a family home sit. A nutrition and health researcher in Brazil put together these classifications, arguing that how much food is processed is more influential on health than its nutritional value. Take a look at the table on the next page for examples.

As you can see, food can move between groups. Peanut butter containing just 100 per cent unsalted peanuts would be group 1, but adding salt, sugar and oils to your peanut butter moves it to group 3, a processed food. The same applies to yoghurt; plain yoghurt, like natural or Greek, is considered group 1, but when sweetened and/or containing additives, it can move to group 3 or 4.

Classification (NOVA)	Meaning	Examples
1 **Unprocessed or minimally processed foods**	Foods that are fresh or have been slightly altered (like cleaning, cutting or drying) but don't have any added substances.	Fruit, vegetables, dried beans, meat, fish, dairy (unsweetened), wholegrains, eggs.
2 **Processed culinary ingredients**	Ingredients that are extracted from foods or nature and are used in cooking to prepare dishes. They are usually processed through methods like pressing, refining, grinding or milling.	Olive oil or other oils extracted from seeds, nuts or fruit, butter, maple syrup, honey, sugar, flour.
3 **Processed foods**	Foods that have been modified to improve shelf life or make them more palatable. This involves adding substances like salt, sugar or oil, and using methods like canning or baking.	Tinned vegetables, cheese, bread, smoked meats, bacon, tomato paste, tinned fish.
4 **Ultra-processed foods (UPFs)**	Foods that go through many industrial processes and have added ingredients that you wouldn't usually use in home cooking, like artificial flavours, colours, emulsifiers or preservatives. They are often hyper-palatable.	Sweets, sweetened drinks/ soft drinks, certain breakfast cereals and bars, pastries, cakes, margarines, pre-prepared pizza, crisps, sweetened yoghurts, pre-prepared poultry or fish nuggets, certain breads.

But, here's why it is crucial to consider the above carefully and critically: it is not perfect, and many health professionals and scientific bodies recognise its flaws.

✧ While this classification system is helpful, especially for researchers and our broad understanding, it risks food being 'labelled' too simplistically: UPF = bad, unprocessed food = good.

✧ When it comes to health impacts, it is very likely to depend on *which* processed foods and ultra-processed foods (UPFs) are being consumed and how frequently they are eaten.

✧ While a diet that prioritises whole foods is recommended and has been within healthy-eating guidelines for decades, not all UPFs are bad. In fact, many can offer an array of nutritional health benefits. Let's use a few examples:

   o Breakfast cereals vary widely in nutritional composition; some contain little salt and sugar, while others have more. In the UK, many cereals provide essential nutrients for children, like fibre and iron, with fortified options contributing about 20 per cent to a child's daily iron needs, according to some research.

   o Many fortified plant-based milk alternatives, such as oat, soya or coconut-based drinks are considered UPFs, yet these are necessary for many children with a milk-free diet to provide key nutrients like calcium and iodine that would usually be obtained from dairy. These foods also allow for dietary inclusion; for example, these children can have pasta and white sauce for dinner too, rather than a totally separate meal.

   o Some children with dietary differences, such as those with Avoidant/Restrictive Food Intake Disorder (ARFID), rely on a significant percentage of UPFs as their daily diet and won't 'simply eat something else' if these are removed from their diet. In such cases, they can be essential sources of nutrition.

   o Financial differences, cooking ability and resource variations mean that many families rely on foods in groups 3 and 4, often through necessity. Simply suggesting a switch overlooks many other variables that need wider support, in order to help with dietary change.

For many of us, a diet containing no processed foods or ultra-processed foods would be a challenge and probably isn't necessary if we focus on getting the balance right the majority of the time. So, with this in mind, I'm going to impart my two pennies' worth into this conversation with some (hopefully) realistic recommendations rather than 'just don't eat any UPFs'.

Suggestions to help you navigate this food environment (with pragmatism in mind)

✧ Where you can, focus on a big part of your child's diet coming from whole foods or minimally processed foods, many of which I've discussed in recommendations across the book – fruits, vegetables, healthy fats, lean proteins, beans, legumes and dairy.

✧ Be mindful of how much and how often you offer UPFs, especially those high in sugar, salt, additives and unhealthy fats like trans-fats. This isn't new information in the nutrition world, but perhaps more important to remember than ever. Ideally, in these early years, keep these foods moderated. You can read more about guidelines for salt and sugar intake on pages 254 and 257.

✧ For foods you see or hear labelled as UPF, be curious and ask yourself things like:
   o Does this contain one additive or lots of additives? Is there a similar option that has fewer?
   o Yes, but is this one of the only ways my child eats dairy (or another food group)?
   o Yes, but does this food contain other essential vitamins, minerals or nutrients my child needs or may struggle to get elsewhere?
   o Yes, but how often does my child/family eat this?
   o Yes, but what portion is my child eating?

✧ Focus on nutrition by addition – is there anything you can add to your child's diet or meal? Can you offer less-processed or whole-food options as a side? Instead of feeling stalled by all the advice about what to exclude, try to think about some new foods to introduce or incorporate into mealtimes.

✧ When you can, check in on the labels of foods you regularly buy, ensure you understand the ingredients, note the salt, sugar and fat content and see if you can make simple swaps.

✧ Remember that you're not a 'bad' parent if your child eats UPFs, and not all UPFs are 'bad'. Food choices shouldn't make you feel blamed or overburdened.

✧ Be mindful of how you talk about different foods around your child. One of my biggest worries associated with the discussion around UPFs is that we seem to be heading again into a time when food is being attached to big, emotive words like 'evil', or oversimplistic labels, which can potentially have a long-term impact on our children's food relationships and eating behaviours.

Remember, one of the biggest contributors to how children eat is their food environment and modelling at home, which beautifully brings us on to how you can harness family mealtimes for your child's future health.

Family mealtimes – how eating with your children boosts their future health and happiness

You might wonder why something as simple as sitting down and eating with your kids is part of this crucial section on setting them up for lifelong health and happiness with food. Honestly, if my hand was forced and I could only give one piece of advice ever again about feeding children, it would be this: eat with them. Over the last 15 years, I have seen this one bit of advice change a child's eating and family dynamics for the better more times than I can count. I also love watching parents' faces when I ask young children who they'd like to have dinner with if they could pick anyone – the majority of children grin and point at their parents (although Peppa Pig, Spiderman and pet dogs have all been contenders!). Even the World Health Organization recognises the importance of eating together as an opportunity for 'learning and love'.

I know that the practicalities of sharing mealtimes with young kids are far from the calm mealtimes we can enjoy as adults. Tonight, I watched my daughter decant her whole bowl of pasta onto the table while rubbing pesto into the wood with awe! Mealtimes *will* be more frantic, with more interruptions, spills and the occasional meltdown – but that doesn't mean they're not valuable.

So, why is eating together so great for kids? The benefits extend far beyond the food. Consider why you enjoy eating out with friends or having loved ones over for a meal. It's not just about the food itself. It's connection, shared enjoyment and the opportunity to commit time to important relationships. Mealtimes offer a chance to explore new food or cuisines together, be nostalgic, share stories, discuss daily experiences and celebrate or support each other through various emotions and life events. It is not much different for children, but let me share some science-backed benefits of eating with your children (some might surprise you).

Benefits of eating together/family mealtimes

Child's social and emotional benefits

✧ Increased self-esteem.

✧ Improved school success.

✧ Improved communication skills.

✧ Social skill development, including empathy, turn-taking.

✧ Increased cultural awareness.

✧ Emotional development and security.

Child's nutrition/feeding benefits

✧ More likely to eat fruits and vegetables daily.

✧ More likely to eat nutrient-dense food and balanced meals.

✧ Decreased likelihood of fussy/picky eating.

✧ Less emotional eating.

✧ More food enjoyment.

✧ Reduced 'challenging' behaviour at mealtimes.

✧ Children are better able to make healthy food choices.

Child's health benefits

✧ Reduced risk of overweight or obesity.

✧ Protection against eating disorders and negative health behaviours as children and into adolescence.

✧ Less likely to engage in high-risk behaviours such as substance misuse and violence.

✧ Reduced risk of psychological difficulties, such as depression.

Parent's benefits

✧ Healthier dietary intake, including consuming more fruits and vegetables.

✧ Improved social and emotional wellbeing.

✧ Reduced stress levels.

✧ Improved parent–child relationships.

✧ Supports work–life balance.

✧ Improved mindful and responsive-parenting practices.

Ways to make eating together easier and achievable

Interestingly, over 80 per cent of parents value family mealtimes and agree they benefit children. However, recent data suggests that eating together has become less and less frequent in recent years (except during the COVID–19 pandemic). The challenge of eating together is almost certainly due to changing working practices, time pressures, routine changes and modern distractions. I get it – for many full-time working households, finding the time and energy to plan, prepare, and sit down to eat together can be really tough! It doesn't happen every day. But rather than admit defeat, I want to give you some tips and suggestions that can make eating with your children easier.

✧ **Set realistic goals:** three meals a day together, seven days a week, may not be achievable for most families. Instead, plan for mealtimes that work for you, such as weekend breakfasts, Sunday lunches or early weeknight dinners. Prioritise quality over quantity!

✧ **Numbers don't matter:** whether it's one parent or both, siblings, dogs or teddies present, what matters is the shared meal experience. If you plan to eat after your child goes to bed, consider having a small amount of their meal with them earlier. They care more about you eating together than the portion size you have.

✧ **Keep meals simple:** they don't need to be picture-perfect! Laying out cereals, milk, and toppings for breakfast is perfectly fine. Picky lunches or dinners work well too.

✧ **Choose meals you enjoy:** this will save time and motivate you at mealtimes while you share food enjoyment with your kids. If you have a picky eater, include one or two of their preferred options, even if it's just crackers or plain pasta alongside your curry.

✧ **Try family-style serving:** this gives children some autonomy over their food choices. Place food options in the middle of the table and let them help themselves with some support. Use dishes and trays and keep hot items away from little hands.

✧ **Focus on connection:** meals may be loud, messy and chaotic. Instead of stressing over 'good' behaviour, concentrate on conversations and fun. Consider using conversation starters like those I've shared below, once your child is old enough.

Things you can ask your child at mealtimes:
✧ What made you laugh today?
✧ Who did you play with today?
✧ Did you sing songs today? Can you sing one for me?
✧ Did anyone help you today, or did you help anyone?
✧ What made you happy this week?
✧ What colours would you use if you drew a picture of your day?
✧ What has been your favourite part of today?
✧ What are you looking forward to tomorrow?

Note: Without a caveat, this book wouldn't be about kids' nutrition and feeding. While family mealtimes and eating around others can benefit many groups of children, some will struggle with this eating environment. For example, some neurodivergent kids may prefer not to eat around others, may need distractions to support their intake or have preferences for eating in different environments.

Future-proofing food relationships

I'd guess many of you reading this book grew up in the same era I did. A time riddled with meal-replacement drinks, 'nothing tastes as good as skinny feels', and constant scrutiny of female and male bodies across the press and, in more recent years, social media. Unfortunately, while times have moved on, the wellness arena means that diet trends or disordered eating often packaged up as 'healthy eating' remain rife. As a parent, navigating this can feel hugely intimidating, including the barrage of information children and young people are now exposed to online. I must be honest; I feel incredibly nervous about handling this with my daughter.

In a book focused on what to feed young children and *how* to feed them, I couldn't ignore the importance of food relationships in shaping future health. You may question why I'm discussing this in a guide for children under five, as isn't it an issue to consider later during their pre-teen or teenage years? Unfortunately, not. Research indicates that children begin crafting their body image and absorbing societal attitudes in early childhood, leading to weight stigma and body dissatisfaction, even as young as three. By this age, children can internalise messages about food from their parents or other adults, for example, categorising foods as 'good' or 'bad.' Studies also reveal that early exposure to dieting and food restrictions heightens children's risk of developing disordered eating patterns as they grow. The truth is that children's understanding of the language and behaviours associated with food starts forming much earlier than we might assume. So, the good news is that these years are yet another opportunity to set positive wheels in motion for future health, and in this case, our children's relationship with food and their bodies.

Here are some evidence-based strategies to support the foundations for positive food relationships, all shared with the support of an experienced child psychologist.

Language around food

What we say to our children and what they hear (or overhear!) can significantly shape their attitudes and beliefs about food, body image and health. I've already discussed language around food throughout this book, but these language tips focus on nourishing positive relationships with food.

- ✧ Avoid labelling foods as 'good' or 'bad', 'healthy' or 'unhealthy', 'rubbish', 'naughty' or 'junk' – you get the gist! Labelling foods this way may lead young children to believe that if they eat them, they themselves are 'good' or 'bad'. This language can lead to confusion, guilt, unnecessary fear or unhelpful attitudes and behaviours towards food. Studies have shown that children feel guilty when eating foods that they are told are 'bad'.

- ✧ In addition to the above, avoid labelling foods with 'halo' terms like 'special' and 'treat'. This increases their desirability and places them on a pedestal above other foods.

- ✧ Remove earning potential from foods. I commonly see parents use certain foods, often 'desirable', preferred or restricted foods such as sweets, cakes and biscuits, to encourage their child to eat other foods or engage in certain behaviours. Saying, for example, 'If you eat your peas, you can have some ice cream', can signal to children that these reward foods have a higher value, ultimately making them more appealing. Research indicates that this practice may lead children to prefer 'reward' foods, eat when they are not hungry, resist mealtimes more frequently and have a reduced enjoyment of food overall.

✧ Don't use wellness washing to encourage food. By this, I mean trying to convince your child to eat something because it's 'healthy' or 'good for them'. Young children cannot understand these concepts with the nuance and critical thinking required. Their brains are not yet developed enough for this type of reasoning. Children can also receive this type of language as pressure to eat that food, which, for many, will reduce their interest in eating it or decrease food enjoyment.

Language around bodies and body size

Language or judgement heard about bodies and body size are picked up by small ears too. Avoid comments about your body or others', or linking food to body size or exercise whenever possible. For example:

✧ 'Gosh, Mummy needs to go for a run because I've eaten three biscuits.'

✧ 'I wish I had a body like his. I need to eat less. I'm so fat.'

✧ 'I've been naughty and eaten all the ice cream. I'll have to diet this week.'

✧ 'I need to go to the gym before I'm allowed that pasta.'

✧ 'They look like they need to eat less of those crisps.'

When children hear this language, they learn that weight, physical appearance and eating behaviours are important and subject to others' scrutiny. Research shows that parental comments about weight, dieting and body shape significantly predict body dissatisfaction and eating disturbances by the teenage years.

Instead, limit body discussions or focus on what your body *can do*, not how it looks, such as 'My legs are strong; they help me run fast around the park with you.' Reinforce that all bodies are good bodies, coming in different shapes and sizes. When discussing food with young children, especially around preschool age, use simple, neutral concepts they can easily understand. For example, say, 'This food gives you energy to play.' They can grasp straightforward ideas but are years away from understanding complex nutritional information!

Note: The way we talk about our bodies and food often comes from the narratives we encountered in childhood and throughout life. If you recognise yourself in the examples I've shared above, please know these suggestions are meant to raise awareness about discussions regarding food and bodies in front of children, not to assign blame.

How to offer food to support a healthy food relationship

It's natural for parents to have numerous questions about how to introduce and discuss various foods while helping their children form a healthy relationship with food. While there's much to consider, here are some key takeaways:

✧ **Keep neutral around food!** Food neutrality means treating all foods equally and putting them on a level playing field. It's based on approaching food without judgement or emotionally charged language. Instead of calling certain foods 'treats' or 'junk', you simply refer to their name – bread, sweets or berries. This helps prevent children from applying unnecessary or unhelpful judgements to food. Food neutrality can include providing a range of foods together, like pairing sweeter options with the main meal, without treating them as rewards or items to earn.

✧ **Modelling** – When teaching children about a healthy, balanced diet, one of the best things you can do is lead by example – by modelling healthy eating habits yourself. Your relationship with food as a parent or caregiver plays a key role in shaping your child's own relationship with food.

✧ **Boundaries vs restrictions** – When children are young, parents generally have control over what foods are offered and how often (especially at home!). It's easy to fall into the trap of thinking you should restrict *all* access to 'bad' foods for their health. However, you can establish age-appropriate healthy boundaries without resorting to over-restriction. For instance, if your child asks for a biscuit, acknowledge their request and let them know you're having a banana or oatcakes for your next snack, but that biscuits will be available another day. Research shows that while some boundaries are beneficial, over-restriction can lead to overeating or unhealthy attitudes towards those foods in the long run.

✧ **Avoid linking foods and behaviours** – If you plan to offer ice cream after dinner, do so regardless of what your child has or hasn't eaten or has or hasn't 'achieved' behaviour-wise. Research shows linking food and behaviours can lead older children or adults to 'reward' or 'punish' themselves with food.

✧ **Look wider than nutrition** – Yes, nutrition is important; I've just written a whole book about it! However, I would encourage you to reflect on what other positive factors food is entwined with. Often, it's nostalgia, traditions, celebrations, comfort, precious time with friends and family, holidays and more. All of these are hugely valuable for health and happiness too.

Getting extended family or friends on board

I know first-hand that this is a tricky one. I speak to many parents who take on the information I've shared above but struggle with consistency from family members or friends. As always, I find empathy is important here, and I always remind parents that previous generations have navigated a very different food environment. Everyone has their own unique experiences and emotions associated with food. The cupboard stocked with your little one's favourite snacks and biscuits waiting at their grandparents' house almost certainly comes from a place of love. Many of the attitudes and language used around food in our society are also deeply entrenched.

When it comes to managing others' approaches to food around your child, I'd encourage an open and honest conversation, acknowledging the care and love that others show for your child, and avoiding language loaded with any blame or judgement. Explain why you're making changes to support positive food relationships and offer some suggestions for alternative food options, ways of offering food, or language to use instead.

Special occasions

Navigating food around special occasions like Eid or Easter is a common query I receive on my social pages during peak times. Parents are often unsure how to navigate having more of certain foods around the house. Here's what I usually suggest:

◆ Accept there will be differences in mealtime routines and foods on offer. Remember, dietary behaviours and nutrition are much more about what happens 80–90 per cent of the time. Four days over a holiday period equates to 1 per cent of the year.

◆ Keep food discussion neutral and maintain an air of nonchalance around additional foods on offer. Avoid making too big a deal out of certain foods compared to others and focus on enjoying the food alongside other festivities. Revisit some of my earlier suggestions, such as simply naming the food what it is.

✧ If your child overeats foods like chocolate or sweets (as many children do at some point) and ends up with a tummy ache or feels sick, this can help them learn to listen to and understand their body's signals. Try to avoid frustration, anger, or blame 'I told you so'. It's important to remember that occasional over-indulgence is a part of children learning moderation in their way. So, while it's understandable to want to prevent this, don't be too hard on yourself or your child. It's all part of the learning process.

✧ Continue offering balanced meals and snacks where possible, incorporating festive foods into mealtimes. Some gradual exposure to foods that may be around more often in the days or weeks leading up to festivities can also work well, to neutralise the 'special' and 'exciting' factor.

✧ Enjoy other aspects of the festivities too – games, time together, films, religious services and more. Remember, these occasions are about joy and togetherness, not just about food.

Acknowledging our own food beliefs and relationships

The elephant in the room is that while all of this advice can be helpful, exploring your own relationship with food may be something that requires consideration. This needs to be approached in an empathetic, kind and compassionate way. Many parents share that they only recognised their struggles with eating habits and attitudes towards food after having children. It takes courage to acknowledge that our beliefs and behaviours as parents can influence how we approach food with our children, and you're not alone in this. If you find this resonates with you and is significantly impacting your day-to-day life, parenting or food relationships, consider seeking support from a suitable health professional or organisation.

SOS:

Solving Common Nutrition and Feeding Dilemmas in the First Five Years

Since establishing an active social media presence, I've hosted a weekly Q&A where parents can share their concerns about their child's nutrition or feeding. Over time, certain topics have come up repeatedly. As a result, I've included a dedicated SOS section in this book to address common nutrition and feeding challenges during the first five years.

Here's what I'll cover:

✧ **Food refusal and poor appetite**

✧ **Food allergies and intolerances**

✧ **Poo problems and tummy troubles**

✧ **Common nutritional deficiencies in early childhood**

✧ **Weight (and growth) worries**

✧ **Vegetarian or vegan diets for babies and children**

Food refusal and poor appetite

Babies and young children can refuse food for various reasons. As a parent, periods of food refusal and poor appetite often push the worry button. It's hard to watch your child repeatedly refuse meals and appear low-energy. In these moments, parents commonly switch into a deep-rooted 'protect-and-direct' mode, looking for any way to get in nutrition. Here are some pointers for managing food refusal in different circumstances.

During illness

Here are some general points, and symptom-specific advice for when your child is unwell:

✧ Parents often find it challenging when a child's appetite decreases during illness. This change can stem from energy conservation, fatigue, pain or altered taste and smell. A child's appetite often disappears first and returns last during illness, which I refer to as an 'appetite hangover'. Understanding that this is normal can often ease some parental worry.

✧ Many children lose weight during periods of poor appetite or repeated illnesses. Adults have more energy reserves, but babies and young children deplete their stores more quickly. Rest assured, most children tend to catch up on growth in the weeks and months after an illness or repeated illnesses. If you're concerned about your child's growth, please consult your health visitor or GP.

✧ Staying hydrated is essential for babies and children when ill, particularly with increased fluid loss due to fever, diarrhoea or vomiting. Here are some ways to encourage fluid intake:
  o For babies under six months, offer additional milk feeds.

o For babies over six months, provide extra milk feeds and water.
o For children over one year, offer small sips of water through-out the day and ongoing milk feeds if breastfeeding.
o Include fluid-rich foods like fruits, vegetables, yoghurt, ice lollies, smoothies and soups.

Signs of dehydration in your baby or young child

✧ For babies, the 'soft spot' on the top of their head may sink (dipped fontanelle).
✧ Dry and/or cracked lips, tongue and/or mouth.
✧ Lack of tears when crying.
✧ Passing less urine or not at all.
✧ Very dark urine.
✧ Deep-set or sunken appearance of eyes.
✧ Tiredness, drowsiness or irritability.
✧ Being more thirsty.

✧ Consider using an age-appropriate rehydration solution for gastro-intestinal illnesses ('tummy bugs') like gastroenteritis. Interestingly, research indicates that a 50:50 diluted apple juice can be as effective as oral-rehydration solutions and is often preferred by children over six months old, due to its more pleasant taste.

✧ Mealtime routines often falter during illnesses. Some children may refuse meals, spend less time at the table or seek comfort, like sitting on your lap. Offering smaller amounts of food more often is fine. Once your child shows improvement, return to regular mealtime and snack routines to prevent grazing from becoming the norm. Children frequently prefer uncomplicated, familiar foods when unwell.

✧ Adding energy and nutrients to food can be helpful for children with persistently poor appetites due to illness. Some of my favourite options include:

    o Toast with plenty of toppings; try butter or spread on both sides of the bread plus avocado, cream cheese, hummus, nut butter, jam or mashed banana and peanut butter.

    o Soups packed with vegetables, noodles, rice or pasta and protein, such as blended beans or shredded chicken and a drizzle of extra oil.

    o Smoothies with fruit, avocado, yoghurt, milk/kefir, oats, nuts or seeds can pack quite a punch from a nutrition perspective!

    o Snack plates with options such as cracker sandwiches with cheese spread or nut butter, dry cereal, oat bars, pancakes, grated cheese or other easy-to-eat options.

    o Eggy bread – add in mashed fruit, cream cheese and/or nut butter for an eggy-bread sandwich.

    o Oats or cereals with added extras, such as ground nuts, stewed or mashed fruit, coconut, chia jam or yoghurt.

When teething

Teething commonly affects appetite in babies and children – if you remember getting your wisdom teeth as an adult, you'll empathise. Some children may prefer soft foods like milky cereals, risotto, stews, rice, lentils and ripe fruit. Others prefer crunchy or cold foods to gnaw on, like chilled veggies, fruit sticks, breadsticks or lollies made from breast milk, yoghurt and/or fruit. This phase is temporary, and appetite usually returns once the teething discomfort fades.

Illness-specific feeding considerations

Type of illness	Food considerations
Fever/high temperature	**Fluid-rich foods,** such as yoghurt, rice pudding or kheer, frozen lollies, fruits, vegetables, smoothies, soups or broths.
Sore throat	**Soft, easy-to-manage options,** such as porridge, well-soaked cereals, scrambled eggs, macaroni cheese, rice and dal, soups, lollies, yoghurt, rice pudding.
Diarrhoea and/or vomiting *Note: Symptoms of vomiting can often resolve before diarrhoea. It is common for looser poos (which may also be paler in colour) to persist for a few days (or weeks) after illness. If ongoing, speak with your doctor to rule out conditions such as temporary lactose intolerance.*	**Fluids are a top priority** – offer regularly alongside rehydration options that are suitable for your baby or child. **Plain, easier-to-digest foods** (lower in fat and fibre) can be helpful for some children. Typical examples are toast, rice, potatoes, soups and noodles. Foods like concentrated fruit juice, smoothies and fruits like pears or plums may exacerbate symptoms of diarrhoea. Reintroducing a varied diet, alongside fermented foods (see page 311), can be helpful to help restore good gut bacteria after illness like this.

During weaning

Worrying about your baby's food intake during weaning is normal – many parents share the same concerns, so you're not alone! Babies are still learning to eat and developing experience with food, so a lack of acceptance or minimal intake may not reflect an issue but be typical progress as a baby learns to eat. In my experience, many parents describe that their baby starts to 'click' with food between 9 and 11 months after they've had time to practise and try a variety of foods. (See page 112 for more on why babies may refuse food and what to do.)

Picky eating

Picky or fussy eating is a common worry for parents in the early years, and it deserved a more extended section all of its own, which you can find on page 200.

Feeding differences in neurodivergent children e.g. Autism, Attention Deficit Hyperactivity Disorder (ADHD)

Food refusal and a limited dietary range can be linked to other diagnoses for some children. Feeding differences are prevalent in neurodivergent children, with research indicating that they affect 80–90 per cent of children with autism, for example.

Feeding differences in this group can be incorrectly labelled as fussy eating, which is inappropriate given that differences often reflect factors such as (but not limited to):

✧ Sensory-processing differences – such as being more or less sensitive to sensory input such as sound, touch, taste and smell.

✧ Preference for predictability and routine, particularly around foods, mealtimes and environments.

✧ Oral motor delays, meaning they lack the skills needed to eat a range of foods.

✧ Anxiety levels around food or mealtimes.

✧ Lack of interest in eating.

When it comes to eating and food, this group of children may:

✧ Accept a minimal range of 'same' foods (I prefer 'same' instead of 'safe' foods).

✧ Refuse foods from food groups altogether.

✧ Have specific routines or preferences about the eating environment, such as which cutlery or crockery they use, or they may struggle with eating in specific environments, such as the school canteen.

✧ Experience significant difficulty with exposure to unfamiliar foods, which may be evident as gagging, distress, crying or running away.

✧ Prefer to eat foods with specific sensory qualities, such as dry and crunchy, salty, plain or sweet-tasting, soft or pureed.

✧ Lose foods from their accepted range and never get them back.

✧ Appear to prefer 'processed' foods that are the same every time.

✧ Only accept specific brands of the same foods.

✧ Reject their 'same' foods if the packaging or food looks different.

✧ Reject their 'same' foods if the ingredients change, affecting taste, smell or texture.

✧ Require distraction to eat or regulate (be in the right body state) to eat.

✧ Have difficulty being around others while they are eating.

✧ Refuse to, or be unable to, feed themselves or rely on caregivers to support this.

✧ Be on certain medications that reduce their appetite.

I frequently meet parents at feeding clinic who experience significant stress and burnout over their child's eating habits. This reaction is entirely understandable. Seeking help to support a child's dietary and feeding needs can be beneficial, but be mindful of who this comes from. I often see people online claiming they can 'fix' a neurodivergent child's eating or wrongly asserting neurodivergence is caused by factors such as an imbalance of gut bacteria (to give just one example). Reassuringly, in more supportive and evidence-based circles, I've noticed a positive shift in recent years towards embracing neurodiversity and recognising the unique eating differences that come with it. This means avoiding the urge to 'fix' these habits using neurotypical methods or expecting a neurodivergent child to eat like their neurotypical peers. Various health professionals, such as occupational and speech therapists, psychologists and dietitians, are well equipped to understand feeding differences in neurodivergent children. They can provide support with a holistic approach, individualised to a child's needs.

It's important to note that variations in feeding habits among this group may increase the risk of growth issues and nutritional deficiencies, which can significantly impact their health. If your child follows a highly restrictive diet, I recommend consulting a paediatric dietitian, who can perform a thorough nutritional assessment and guide support strategies, including dietary supplements. Additionally, it's vital to stress (and feel free to share this with anyone who disagrees) that monitoring growth is not enough on its own to determine if your child is receiving all the essential nutrients.

Food refusal – the bigger picture

There can be a vast number of reasons why children refuse to eat, and I have covered key indicators that food refusal may be more than common young-child eating behaviours or picky eating on page 238. Many parents with children with more significant food refusal or feeding differences are keen to seek a more appropriate diagnosis that better represents their child's eating habits and behaviours around food, such as Avoidant Restrictive Food Intake Disorder (ARFID). However, it's important to remember that assessment by appropriately skilled health professionals is essential to support such diagnoses. You can find more information about ARFID and other eating differences from the references at the back of this book.

Food allergies and intolerances

Over the past five years, I've received more enquiries than ever about food allergies and intolerances in children. These conditions are understandably concerning for parents, especially given recent UK statistics indicating that food allergies have doubled between 2008 and 2018. The rates are also particularly high in preschoolers, affecting four out of every 100 children, and food allergies are among the most prevalent chronic-health issues in the UK.

A food allergy occurs when the immune system mistakenly identifies a normally safe substance, such as a protein in food (like milk protein), as harmful, triggering an inappropriate immune response.

Parents often ask about food allergies when starting to introduce solids. For this reason, I covered some key questions about food allergies in the section beginning on page 117, including what food allergies are and common symptoms to look out for. However, there are many more questions that parents have, so I've covered some common ones below.

I have a food allergy; will my child inherit it too?

Parents with food allergies are often eager to learn how to prevent their children developing similar conditions. Although children do not directly inherit specific allergies from their parents, a genetic predisposition to allergic conditions exists. A child is more likely to have a food allergy if they already have an atopic disease (like eczema) or if there's a family history of atopy (the genetic tendency, associated with 'overactive/incorrect' immune responses, to develop allergic diseases, including hay fever, asthma, eczema and food allergies). This risk is further heightened if both parents have atopic conditions. The link between food allergies and eczema is strongest. Evidence shows that babies with eczema in their first months of life or severe eczema are 30–50 times more likely to develop food allergies. Environmental factors may also influence the microbiome and food allergy susceptibility, such as antibiotic exposure, birth method, milk-feeding history, dietary habits and living conditions. Research continues to explore these links.

Can you test for food allergies and intolerances?

As parents, it's understandable that you'd want a clear diagnosis of food allergies or intolerances for your child, especially if struggling with tricky symptoms. Testing depends on a child's specific symptoms and background, so here is a quick rundown of what is available and advisable.

For immediate type (IgE–mediated) food allergies (symptoms appear within minutes to two hours after eating a food)

A doctor or allergy specialist will gather your child's history of reactions to potential allergens, including food intake, symptoms and timing. This is called an allergy-focused history. They will also ask about your child's medical, family and feeding history. Based on this information, the doctor may recommend allergy tests like Skin Prick Testing (SPT) or Specific IgE blood tests. These tests detect IgE antibodies produced by the immune system in response to allergens during immediate reactions.

In certain situations, more detailed testing known as component testing can be performed to pinpoint specific proteins in an allergen. If the diagnosis remains unclear, a supervised food challenge might be recommended in a hospital setting to monitor any reactions when small quantities of the allergen are eaten.

Here are some critical points about immediate-type food-allergy testing:

1. **Avoid large panels**: Allergy professionals do not recommend testing for a wide range of allergens 'just in case', as it can lead to confusion and misinterpretation of results.
2. **Specific allergen testing**: Testing for specific allergens, like peanuts or milk, is more effective than testing for broad categories like 'common food mix', which can complicate understanding the results.
3. **Interpreting results**: A higher test result indicates a higher likelihood of an allergy but *does not predict the severity of any reactions.*
4. **False positives**: IgE tests can have false positives, especially in children with eczema, which is why understanding your child's symptoms and allergy history are essential.

For delayed-type food allergies (symptoms appear two to 72 hours after eating a food)

Diagnosing delayed-type food allergy requires a detailed history of your child's symptoms and the intake of suspected allergens. Unlike immediate allergies, specific tests for delayed reactions <u>do not exist</u>, as usual tests check for IgE antibodies, which are not involved for this type of reaction. I describe to parents that using these tests for delayed food allergies is like fishing in an empty pond! I'm also frequently asked about patch testing for delayed allergies, but unfortunately, these tests are not validated to diagnose delayed allergy either.

Our understanding of the immune response to delayed allergies is still evolving, so diagnosis requires a process of removing and reintroducing the suspected allergen, guided by a trained health professional like a paediatric dietitian or allergy doctor.

Diagnosis of delayed food allergy – the 4 Rs

1. **Record**: If you are unsure about potential allergens, keep a food-and-symptom diary to track what your child eats and any related symptoms.

2. **Remove**: Eliminate the suspected allergen from your child's diet. For instance, if cow's milk is suspected, all milk-containing foods should be removed. Breastfeeding mothers may need to avoid milk, and formula-fed babies may require a specialised formula prescribed by a GP. Monitor symptoms during this period; symptoms should improve if it's an allergy.

3. **Replace**: Dietary replacements may be necessary for specific food groups, like milk, to ensure your child gets the nutrients they need.

4. **Reintroduce**: After two to four weeks, gradually reintroduce the removed allergen. This step can be challenging, especially if symptoms have improved, but it's necessary to confirm the allergy. If symptoms return during reintroduction, it helps confirm a diagnosis.

Intolerance testing

Intolerance testing is rife with misinformation and pseudoscience. Unfortunately, there are few testing options for food intolerances, and most are focused primarily on lactose (milk sugar) intolerance. For lactose intolerance, although a scientific breath test exists to confirm the diagnosis, simply eliminating lactose from a child's diet can often suffice for diagnosis. For other intolerances, the 4 Rs strategy mentioned above can aid in the diagnostic process.

Allergy and intolerance tests to avoid

I understand why parents seek answers, especially with long wait times for appointments with professionals. However, one of the biggest scams out there is the generic 'food allergy and intolerance' tests marketed online and in stores. These tests often promise easy answers from simple blood spots or hair samples but lack robust scientific support for diagnosing allergies or intolerances. Many parents come to me after using these tests, having eliminated numerous foods from their child's diet, only to find no improvement in symptoms. This can lead to nutritional deficiencies and even the risk of developing food allergies. Remember, if these tests worked, we'd use them routinely in healthcare too. Save your money and seek professional advice instead.

Food allergy and intolerance 'tests' to avoid

✧ IgG testing – I understand this one is particularly convincing because we *do* use IgE testing for children with immediate-type food allergies, *but* IgG antibodies indicate a normal immune response to food. High levels just suggest a food or food protein was recently consumed.

✧ Vega testing.

✧ Kinesiology (muscle analysis).

✧ Hair analysis.

✧ Pulse testing.

✧ Provocation, neutralisation testing.

✧ The ATCAT (Antigen Leukocyte Cellular Antibody Test).

Do food allergies cause eczema?

Eczema, or atopic dermatitis, affects about one in five children in the UK, causing dry, inflamed and itchy skin. Symptoms often appear in early life and result from excess water loss due to a compromised skin barrier. Think of skin cells as bricks; in children with eczema, the mortar is weak, allowing moisture to escape and making the skin prone to irritation and infection. Studies indicate a genetic predisposition to eczema, with research showing that alterations in the Filaggrin gene heighten the likelihood of developing eczema. Unfortunately, there's no known cure, though many children outgrow it by school age.

Managing eczema can be challenging for parents, especially when children have itchy, weeping skin. Many parents wonder if food allergies cause their child's eczema. While eczema may be linked to an increased risk of food allergies, and certain foods can worsen it for some children, **they don't directly cause eczema.**

I empathise with why parents are keen to find the root cause of their child's eczema. Unfortunately, many online 'experts' exploit this issue to sell diet plans and supplements, but I promise if there were solid evidence these worked, we'd use them! Here are vital points my colleagues, such as GPs, dermatologists and allergists, typically discuss regarding eczema management that you might find helpful.

✧ **Skin treatment:** Eczema requires consistent and effective skincare. Regular emollients (moisturisers) are essential, and sometimes stronger creams like topical steroids (which have varying strengths) may be recommended (usually in short bursts) to reduce inflammation. Based on emerging science, I would highly discourage you from using moisturisers containing food components such as oats, coconut and nuts on eczema, unless your child is already regularly eating these foods. This is because we understand that exposure to these food proteins via the damaged skin barrier can increase the risk of sensitising to these foods, potentially leading to food allergies. This is another reason why washing your hands and using a scoop in pots of cream is important.

✧ **Identify triggers:** Each child's eczema triggers are unique and can include environmental factors like temperature, dust mites, animals and chemicals. Keeping a skin diary can help identify triggers and support any changes needed.

✧ **Food triggers:** If you suspect food triggers like milk or eggs, follow the 4 Rs approach <u>under a dietitian or doctor's supervision.</u> Avoid removing multiple foods at once; methodically exclude and reintroduce suspect foods to minimise unnecessary exclusions. Be mindful that prolonged removal of food from a child's diet can lead to loss of tolerance and potentially cause allergy, so reintroduction for confirmation is essential. Allergy testing may not be helpful, and broad screening tests are generally not recommended. Many children with eczema have elevated levels of specific allergic proteins in their blood, but this doesn't always indicate a true food allergy.

✧ **Nutritional considerations:** From a nutritional perspective, while diet as a whole is important for skin health, there are two nutrients I often speak to families about.

o *Vitamin D* – Some scientific evidence suggests that low vitamin D levels may be linked to worse eczema symptoms, and in children with eczema who have low vitamin D, supplementation may help improve their condition. While more research is needed, ensuring your child has regular supplementation of vitamin D would be recommended.

o *Zinc* – In practice, I often find that children with eczema (especially severe eczema) have low zinc levels, and this is mirrored in some research. Zinc-rich foods can be beneficial to include regularly for your child's skin and overall health. They include meat, shellfish, nuts and seeds (well-ground or butter form for young children), cocoa powder, eggs and dairy. Specific supplementation may be recommended if your child's zinc levels are very low.

What are the most common food allergies, and how are they managed?

The most common foods to be allergic to in the UK are known as the 'top nine'; these include cow's milk, egg, peanut, wheat, soya, sesame, tree nuts (like almonds, hazelnuts, cashew nuts), fish and shellfish. If your child is allergic to one or multiple foods, they must exclude them from their diet. If entire food groups, such as dairy, are eliminated, appropriate alternatives should be used to ensure your child's diet remains balanced and they get all the nutrients they need. Depending on the type of food allergy, your child may be able to reintroduce the allergen into their diet under the advice of a health-care professional. This often uses a 'ladder' approach for delayed allergies like milk, soya, wheat and egg. A ladder is progressive rein-troduction to a food allergen, working through stages where more of the allergen is offered, and/or in a form where the immune system is more likely to recognise it. Many ladders start with baked or well-cooked foods, as heat can change the shape of food proteins like milk or egg, making the immune system less likely to recognise them.

Children with immediate allergies may be rechallenged using an adapted ladder or supervised hospital trial.

Over recent years, oral immunotherapy has become available for some children with specific allergies, such as to peanuts. This is an exciting time for the allergy world, with the hope that these thera-pies will allow more children to build tolerance and potentially outgrow their allergies. As research continues, we may see more advancements in treatment options, offering new possibilities for managing and overcoming food allergies.

Cow's Milk Protein Allergy (CMPA)

CMPA is a common food allergy in the early years, and it is often diagnosed in babies under the age of one. Here, a baby's immune system incorrectly labels cow's milk protein as a danger and consequently kicks into action every time a baby consumes milk protein. For formula-fed babies this exposure is via their milk. For breastfed babies, some mothers may have to remove milk from their own diet, but some babies will only react when milk protein is introduced during weaning, as exposure to cow's milk proteins via breast milk differs from direct exposure to foods or formula (see page 118).

Delayed type CMPA, in particular, can be exceptionally difficult to diagnose, as symptoms cross over with familiar baby 'complaints' like reflux, eczema and poo changes. Studies show that parents will often visit their doctor five times or more before diagnosis. You can read more about food-allergy symptoms on page 118. If you suspect CMPA, please speak to a health professional who can advise on the next steps, including a possible trial of specialised formula or a milk-free diet for mothers if breastfeeding.

Can my child be allergic to fruit and vegetables?

Yes, a child can be allergic to anything, but true fruit and vegetable allergies are rare. In the UK, the most common immediate fruit allergies are to bananas and kiwi. Here are more common reactions to fruit and vegetables you may experience:

Contact reactions or irritation – These reactions are not limited to babies during weaning but can occur during childhood. Symptoms include a red and/or blotchy rash around the mouth, face and possibly hands shortly after consuming food, usually where the food has made contact with the skin. It will not spread or cause your child any discomfort. It is generally caused by acidic foods, such as citrus fruits, tomatoes or fruits and vegetables high in histamine, like avocado, spinach, aubergine and strawberries. Foods like hummus, snacks with certain coatings and salty foods can also cause a similar reaction. While these contact reactions may look concerning, they are generally mild and usually resolve on their own without further complications. **This type of reaction is not a food allergy.**

Pollen Food Syndrome (PFS), aka Oral Allergy syndrome – I have personal experience with this! It's most commonly seen in children with hay fever, and typically doesn't develop until at least their second pollen season. For this type of reaction, a child may develop immediate symptoms after consuming raw fruits, vegetables or nuts containing proteins similar to the pollen they're allergic to. Essentially, the immune system gets confused and reacts to these foods due to similarities in the proteins, as if they were pollen. Symptoms can include itching, tingling or mild mouth, lip or tongue swelling. Occasionally, sneezing, watery eyes and nasal congestion can also occur. Cooking these foods often means they can be consumed without symptoms for those with PFS.

PFS is not common in under fives and classically develops in the late-primary-school/early-secondary-school age group. It is therefore important to speak to a professional to ensure a true food allergy is not missed, especially in the case of foods like nuts.

How can I tell if my child is intolerant to gluten?
Poor old gluten has taken quite a beating in recent years, thanks to wellness trends and diets that advocate strict gluten avoidance. When tummy troubles or skin issues arise, gluten is often the first to be

blamed, but this judgement isn't always justified! I find it beneficial for parents to understand the most common diagnoses associated with gluten or wheat consumption, as these are often confused and there is some crossover between conditions. If you suspect any of these, I'd highly encourage you to speak with your child's GP.

> **Pitstop first** – Gluten and wheat are not the same thing! Gluten is a protein found in wheat, rye and barley. It's what makes bread bouncy and it gives dough its elasticity. Wheat is a grain that contains gluten but also includes other proteins and components like starches and fibre. All wheat contains gluten, but not all gluten comes from wheat. This is a really important distinction, especially when it comes to understanding and managing gluten sensitivities or coeliac disease.

Coeliac disease

This is a common autoimmune condition thought to affect around 1 in 100 people in the UK. Specific genes have been identified to be associated with coeliac disease. Therefore, if a first-degree relative has coeliac disease, the likelihood of developing it increases to 1 in 10.

Coeliac disease differs from a food allergy or intolerance. When individuals with coeliac disease consume gluten their immune system attacks tissue, especially in the small intestine. This reaction leads to the symptoms outlined below, and the resulting gut damage can prevent adequate absorption of essential nutrients.

Children can be diagnosed at any age, however, they have to be eating gluten to confirm a diagnosis. If you or your child's other parent has coeliac disease, there is currently no scientific evidence to suggest you approach the introduction of gluten any differently when starting solids.

If coeliac disease is suspected, first-line testing to help get a diagnosis is usually a specific set of blood tests that look for specific signs that the immune system is raising a response to gluten. Children have to have been eating gluten regularly – daily, in good amounts for at least six weeks – before this blood test. Sometimes other investigations may be needed, such as a biopsy (small sample of tissue) from the small intestine.

Management of coeliac disease needs strict lifelong avoidance of gluten. There is no current cure available. To support your child on a gluten-free diet and have support with managing increased nutritional requirements associated with coeliac disease, all children with it are recommended to be under the care of a paediatric dietitian.

Symptoms of coeliac disease in children

✧ Diarrhoea
✧ Constipation
✧ Excess wind or flatulence
✧ Nausea and/or vomiting
✧ Mouth ulcers
✧ Unexplained tiredness and fatigue
✧ Weight loss, faltering growth
✧ Distended abdomen
✧ Nutritional deficiencies, such as iron, vitamin B12 and folate
✧ Neurological symptoms or ataxia – disturbance to coordination, balance, movement, speech

Note: If your child has any of these symptoms, or you suspect coeliac disease, please see their GP.

Wheat allergy

Wheat allergy occurs when the body's immune system mistakes one or more of the proteins found in wheat as a threat, causing a series of symptoms related to food allergy. It is thought to affect around 2 per cent of children. Allergic reactions to wheat can be immediate (symptoms occur quickly, within minutes to two hours) or delayed (2–72 hours later). Children allergic to wheat must exclude all foods containing wheat from their diet.

Wheat intolerance

Some children may experience bloating, gas, discomfort or pain after consuming wheat, especially if they eat more than usual. If no other symptoms are present and other diagnoses have been excluded, it could be due to fructans, a carbohydrate in these grains that are also found in onions, garlic, leeks, bananas and watermelon. Fructans are poorly absorbed in the small intestine and may ferment in the large intestine, causing these symptoms. If you suspect this issue, I'd recommend you consult a paediatric dietitian for further evaluation.

Poo problems and tummy troubles

Anyone familiar with the dietetic profession won't be surprised that this book includes a section dedicated to understanding tummy troubles and exploring children's bowel movements. More than one in four parents express concerns about tummy troubles in children, and I often see the stress and worry they can cause.

Throughout this section, I'm going to cover normal poo and toileting habits briefly, and discuss lots of specific tummy and poo scenarios, starting with those more common in babies and moving through early childhood. Many of these diagnoses, including colic, reflux and constipation, fall under a group of conditions known to medical professionals as 'Disorders of the Gut–Brain Interaction'. These conditions are diagnosed based on your child's symptoms and after ruling out other medical causes. As the name suggests, these conditions are believed to occur, at least in part, because of miscommunication between the gut and the brain. For all of these conditions, one of the most frustrating things I empathise with parents about is not having an apparent reason, or 'root cause', or being told it's 'just colic/reflux/constipation' because it's common in babies or young children. Research is ongoing to understand these complex conditions better. However, this doesn't mean we're powerless.

Colic

'My baby is constantly crying, but I don't know why. At 5pm, it's like witching hour begins, and it can go on for hours.'
Typical age range: 2–20 weeks, peaking around six weeks of age.
Affects: Around one in five babies
Symptoms:

✧ Your baby is under five months of age when these symptoms occur.

✧ Your baby has no other symptoms, such as faltering growth, fever or illness.

✧ Your baby has repeated and prolonged periods of crying, fussing and irritability with no apparent cause. You cannot prevent these periods of crying from happening, and they can't be resolved by other caregivers either.

✧ Your baby may go red in the face, clench their fists, draw their legs up or arch their back.

✧ Your baby many have rumbly tummy noises or a lot of wind.

Why does this happen?

We don't fully understand why colic occurs, which can be frustrating for parents dealing with a crying baby for hours and looking for answers. Research shows that colic affects both breastfed and formula-fed babies equally. Many theories exist regarding its causes, including gas, feeding difficulties, food allergies and digestion issues. Various factors, including genetics, early life experiences and nervous-system regulation, are also likely to contribute to colic.

What can you do?

Firstly, I want to acknowledge that parenting a colicky baby is hard, and you're not alone. I think it's important to acknowledge that it can be exceptionally tough watching your baby inconsolable or in discomfort, and for many parents it takes a significant toll on their mental health. It can also often feel lonely, with lots of advice akin to 'wait it out'.

It's widely encouraged (including by me!) that you seek the support of others where you can. Take turns comforting your baby, giving yourself some reprieve and rest. Finding pockets of time or space to try to refill what I call your 'calm cup' can be helpful, as it's very common for parents themselves to feel dysregulated and over-whelmed with a crying baby. You'll likely be doing this intuitively already, but advice also suggests soothing your baby with options like white noise, a change of scenery or fresh air, positioning (I remember this is when we first found 'tiger-in-a-tree' hold!), a warm bath (or co-bathing), skin to skin and plenty of comfort and cuddles. If you suspect or query any concerns about your baby's feeding, I'd highly encourage you to seek support, as I see feeding factors contributing to colic symptoms regularly.

But what about all the 'remedies' for colic that you can buy? Here's a quick rundown of what they are, how it is suggested they work and if there is any science behind them. Remember that if you're using something that works for *your* baby, despite what the science says, that's great!

What	How is it reported to work?	The science
Simethicone (Infacol, Dentinox drops)	By breaking up gas bubbles in the stomach and intestines. It reduces the surface tension of these gas bubbles, causing them to combine into larger bubbles that are reportedly easier to pass through burping or flatulence.	Large-scale, robust scientific evidence does not strongly support effectiveness.
Lactase enzymes (Colief)	These enzymes help digest the sugar (lactose) in breast or formula milk.	Large-scale, robust evidence does not strongly support effectiveness.
Gripe water – a mixture of water and various herbs like fennel, ginger, dill or chamomile	The herbs within gripe water are reported to have a soothing, calming and gas-relieving effect.	The effectiveness of gripe water is not well supported by scientific evidence, and its use should ideally be discussed with your GP or health visitor, especially for very young infants.
Probiotics – 'live friendly bacteria'	By balancing gut bacteria, reducing inflammation and improving digestion.	There is some evidence that probiotics providing the strains of bacteria *Lactobacillus reuteri DSM 17938* or *B-lactis BB-12*, may help reduce crying in colicky infants, particularly breast-fed babies*. The recommended dose is 1×10^8 CFUs daily for 21–28 days in an infant with suspected colic, with improvements typically seen within 2–4 weeks.

Note – some breastfeeding parents prefer not to consider probiotics for their babies given breast milk already contains a community of bacteria of its own and many other factors to support healthy gut microbiome development.

Gastro-oesophageal reflux
'My baby is spitting up/sick/uncomfortable after feeds'

Gastro-oesophageal reflux (known simply as reflux) refers to the backward flow of stomach contents, either milk or food, into the oesophagus (food pipe).

Babies with reflux can be separated into two distinct groups: those with reflux typical of infancy and those with gastro-oesophageal reflux disease. The vast majority of babies fall into the first group. They have symptoms such as vomiting and regurgitation and are often known as 'happy spitters'. A smaller number of babies have a more pathological condition known as gastro-oesophageal reflux disease (GORD), which causes more challenging symptoms, such as pain, persistent discomfort, poor weight gain, feeding difficulties, sleep disturbances and other complications.

Typical age range: First year of life, more common under six months

Affects: Regurgitation and uncomplicated reflux can affect up to 40 per cent of babies under one year of age. GORD is thought to affect 2–8 per cent of babies and young children

Symptoms: In babies, reflux often occurs after feeding and may result in:

✦ Regurgitation (bringing milk back up into the throat or mouth without forceful action of vomiting).

✦ Posseting (small amounts of sick or 'spit up').

✦ Vomiting.

✦ Pain and discomfort.

✦ Coughing or hiccupping during or after feeds.

✧ Distress or crying during or after feeds.

✧ Swallowing or gulping after feeding.

✧ Difficulty with weight gain if vomiting frequently.

✧ Frequent ear infections.

Sometimes babies may have signs of reflux but will not bring up milk or be sick, sometimes called 'silent reflux'. They may still have other signs above, like pain, discomfort or a hoarse cough – sometimes called 'silent reflux'.

Why does this happen?
There are a number of contributing factors to reflux and GORD.

Reflux

✧ Low muscle tone.

✧ The lower oesophageal sphincter, the muscle that keeps stomach contents from flowing back into the oesophagus (food pipe), is still immature.

✧ Lots of time spent lying down.

✧ A liquid (milk) diet.

✧ Babies have small stomachs and feed frequently.

✧ Feeding challenges, including tongue-tie, breastfeeding difficulties such as oversupply, shallow latch.

GORD commonly co-occurs with:

✧ Developmental delay.

✧ Cow's Milk Protein Allergy, as well as other food allergies or intolerances.

✧ Other medical conditions, such as laryngomalacia or a hiatal hernia.

What can you do?

Reflux

For most babies (9 out of 10), symptoms improve by the time they are one.

Before discussing reflux-management strategies, I wanted to reassure you that very few babies lose weight from reflux-related milk loss. I speak to many parents concerned about how much milk they see down muslins, their baby and themselves. However, there can often be a difference in perceived volumes versus how much is lost! To help visualise this, try splashing 10ml or 30ml of water or milk on your kitchen counter – it often looks like so much more!

From a practical point of view, here are some things you can do to minimise reflux symptoms for your baby:

✧ Keep your baby upright after feeds – gravity helps! (Sling use can also be helpful for lots of babies.)

✧ Feed your baby responsively.

✧ If breastfeeding, consider checking in on:
  o Latch (shallow latch may cause air swallowing, which can exacerbate reflux).

o Positioning during feeds – koala (baby held in an upright position while feeding) or laidback feeding (mother reclined with baby positioned on their stomach against her) can be helpful.

o Breast-milk supply – oversupply of breast milk may cause or exacerbate reflux.

❖ Let your baby lead with the volume taken, and avoid encouraging them to finish specific feed volumes or targets.

❖ For bottle-fed babies, trial smaller, more frequent feeds.

❖ If bottle feeding, try a paced bottle-feeding technique (see page 51) and/or an elevated side-lying position for feeds.

❖ Some babies may benefit from feed thickeners or thickened formula milk, but these should only be considered after other strategies have been tried, and on the advice of a healthcare professional. Feed thickeners should be avoided in pre-term babies due to increased risk of a serious intestinal condition called Necrotising Enterocolitis (NEC).

GORD

In addition to the strategies mentioned above, there are additional treatment options for GORD. In some cases, medication may be recommended, but these should only be prescribed by a doctor.

Reflux suppressants, such as Gaviscon. These contain alginic acid, which is made from seaweed. They work by forming a protective layer (or barrier) on top of the stomach contents that helps to prevent stomach acid flowing back into the food pipe.

In my experience, constipation can be a side effect of these medications, which is worth being aware of, especially because constipation may make reflux worse for some babies. In practice, it's also worth mentioning that these are not usually a practical option for breastfed babies!

Medicines to reduce acid production, such as Omeprazole. These medications block the proton pump in the stomach that produces stomach acid. This reduces how much gastric acid is produced, helping to relieve symptoms associated with acid reflux and GORD – the pain and irritation to the food pipe. These medications should be the last line of treatment and have limited scientific studies behind them in babies and children. There are known side effects, including the fact these medications can impact the absorption of vitamins and minerals, so if your child is on them for several months or years, it can be helpful to discuss this regularly with a dietitian.

The ideal scenario for babies and young children with reflux or GORD is that when seeking support you're able to begin with non-medical assessments and treatment, such as input from an infant feeding specialist, speech-and-language therapist (SLT) and/ or dietitian, then progress through to more medical intervention if needed, guided by a GP or paediatrician.

For some babies, a review by a paediatric dietitian can be beneficial, particularly if they are struggling with managing reflux through weaning, if reflux is affecting intake and, therefore, growth, and/or if you suspect a possible food allergy is a contributing factor to reflux.

What about weaning and foods to avoid?

Many parents ask me if there are specific considerations for starting solids when their baby has reflux. Here are some of my key points to consider.

✧ Ideally, ensure reflux is as well managed before weaning, including support with milk feeds.

✧ Be aware that early weaning isn't a magic bullet for all babies with reflux. While health professionals may occasionally recommend weaning after individual assessment, starting too early with a baby who isn't developmentally ready for food can, in my experience, make reflux worse and feeding a whole lot more stressful.

✧ Some foods can worsen or trigger reflux symptoms, so they may be best avoided or at least limited or moderately portioned for some children. You'd often expect acidic foods such as tomatoes, citrus fruits or spicy foods to be the culprit, as they may irritate your baby's food pipe. In older children, it can be other foods, such as carbonated drinks, chocolate and mint. The other thing worth considering at all ages is the fat content of a little one's meal. As I've talked about, fat is an essential nutrient for young children, so it shouldn't be skimped on, however, higher-fat meals can delay gastric emptying (the time it takes for food to leave the stomach). This can worsen reflux symptoms for some children, especially if the meal is given before bed or is shortly followed by a milk feed.

✧ Please avoid reflux-management approaches that recommend avoidance of huge lists of foods, as these are not grounded in science and often prey on your parental worry. Unnecessarily restricting a baby or young child's diet has implications for their feeding development, food relationship, nutrition, growth and the gut microbiome.

Understanding normal poo and pooing habits in babies and children

Before I go into tummy worries, I thought it would be helpful to take a pitstop in the often-unpopular world of poo. If you're squeamish, put down your chocolate digestive for this one.

Understanding what's expected or 'typical', especially for babies and children, can help you know when something might be wrong. How often your child poos, its colour and consistency can tell us a lot about what's going on with their feeding and overall health.

1	**Looks like:** Rabbit droppings. Separate hard lumps, like nuts (hard to pass). **Notes:** Likely to be constipation in babies and children – seek support.
2	**Looks like:** Bunch of grapes. Sausage-shaped but lumpy. **Notes:** Suggestive of constipation – seek support.
3	**Looks like:** Corn on cob. Like a sausage but with cracks on its surface. **Notes:** May suggest risk of constipation or constipation, but may be within a spectrum of normal poo for some formula-fed babies and those starting or established on solids.
4	**Looks like:** A sausage or snake, smooth and soft. **Notes:** The ideal poo texture for babies for children established on solids, and formula fed babies. For children in nappies, this may be squashed!
5	**Looks like:** Chicken nuggets. Soft blobs with clear-cut edges (passed easily). **Notes:** Can be normal poo for breastfed babies, those on certain formula milks and children who are well but with a higher fibre intake and/or those on laxatives.
6	**Looks like:** Porridge. Fluffy pieces with ragged edges, a mushy stool. **Notes:** Can be normal poo for breastfed babies and children who are well but with a higher fibre intake and/or those on laxatives.
7	**Looks like:** Gravy. Watery, no solid pieces, entirely liquid. **Notes:** This could be diarrhoea or overflow diarrhoea – seek support. For children in nappies – likely to soak into a nappy, similar to urine.

The Bristol Stool Chart, shown above, is a widely recognised tool for assessing poo (stools) based on consistency and shape. This visual guide helps identify potential concerns, such as constipation or diarrhoea, and what an 'ideal' stool should look like. Alongside the chart, I've included notes for babies and toddlers who are not potty trained, as their stool habits can differ, especially for those on breast milk. Efforts are under way to adapt this chart for younger children because poo can appear different in a nappy versus a potty or toilet!

What colour should children's poo be?
Varying shades of brown are typical for healthy poo. However, not all poo is brown!

✧ Breastfed babies typically have more yellow or lighter-brown poo.

✧ Babies transitioning to solids can have a mixture of different shades of yellow, brown and green.

✧ Babies on formula milk may have a darker brown or greener poo.

✧ Once established on solids, poo will usually be darker and stronger smelling! Colour can also change depending on what your child has eaten.

How many poos?
The number of poos your baby or child has daily will depend on their age and whether they are breastfed and/or formula-fed. The time it takes for milk or food to move through the gut (transit time) tends to be quicker in babies and young children. You will find transit time reduces in the first few months of your baby's life. Babies can go from pooing 12 times a day to three (or fewer) times a day, for example.

Here's a very general guide to how many poos your child may have daily or weekly.

Chid's age	Average number of poos per week	Average number of poos per day
0-3 months bread fed	5-40	2.9
0-3 months forumla fed	5-28	2.0
6-12 months	5-28	2.0
1-3 years	4-21	1.4
3 years older	3-14	1

Source: ERIC bowel and bladder charity, 2024

Infant dyschezia
'Help, my baby strains and goes very red in the face when trying to poo, and when they do poo, it's soft!'
Typical age range: 0–9 months of age, but typically 0–3 months
Symptoms:

✧ When your baby poos, their poo is soft (they are not constipated), but your baby can experience times where they are visibly straining and crying for at least 10 minutes before they poo (in some cases, they will not poo).

✧ These episodes can occur frequently – daily or multiple times per day.

Why does this happen?
Put simply; infant dyschezia is uncoordinated pooing in young babies. It happens because they are still learning to coordinate the muscle movements needed for effective pooing. Having a bowel movement requires relaxing the pelvic floor while increasing

abdominal pressure. When both actions work together, it's easier. However, your baby may not have mastered this coordination yet, leading to straining, grunting and discomfort before passing stool.

What can you do?
Infant dyschezia is usually short-lived and often resolves on its own within weeks or months. However, I empathise with how distressing and worrisome it can be for parents to watch their baby go through these episodes. Many parents find gentle positioning, such as keeping baby upright or cycling leg movements, helpful.

Constipation
'My child isn't pooing often, has pebble poos and seems in pain.'
Typical age range: Any age during infancy and childhood
Affects: Up to 25 per cent of children
Symptoms:

✧ Your child poos three or fewer times per week.

✧ Your child's poo is large and hard.

✧ Your child's poo looks like rabbit droppings or pellets.

✧ Your child is straining or in pain when they poo.

✧ Your child has bleeding during or after a poo because the poo is large and hard.

✧ Your child's appetite or milk intake decreases, then improves after they poo.

✧ Your child (if old enough) has soiled pants.

✧ Your child is having very loose, watery poo (diarrhoea/type 7 on the poo chart above) – this is called overflow diarrhoea and happens when runny poo leaks around hard poo in your child's intestine.

✧ If your child has reflux, constipation can make it worse by increasing pressure in their abdomen (tummy).

✧ Constipation can significantly impact your child's mood, and engagement with activities, including eating, can drop.

Speak urgently to your GP if your child has the symptoms above and any of the following – delayed passing of meconium (over more than 48 hours), is one month old or younger, there is a family history of Hirschsprung's disease, they have ribbon-looking stools, there is fresh blood in their stools or stools are black (if not on iron supplements) or white, you're worried about their growth, they are vomiting or they have severe tummy bloating.

Why does this happen?
Constipation can have many causes in children, so it's important to first chat with your child's GP to explore their history. Most children have what is known as 'functional constipation', which means there is no underlying medical cause. As I mentioned in the introduction, we are still trying to understand why some children develop conditions like constipation, and there is lots of work going into understanding how the brain and gut talk to each other.

Constipation can be prevalent at specific points in early life where there are changes in diet or toileting behaviours. These include:

✧ Changing milks, for example from breast milk to formula milk, from breast or formula milk to cow's milk at one year old, plus.

✧ Once starting solids (weaning).

✧ When potty training.

Some common reasons young children may develop constipation include:

✧ Not eating enough fibre, including fruits and vegetables.

✧ Not drinking enough fluids, including when children may be more dehydrated, such as during illness.

✧ Drinking too much cow's milk.

✧ When worried or anxious, such as in times of transition like starting childcare or school, moving house, when a sibling arrives.

✧ Getting used to potty training and toilet use, including feeling nervous or pressured or withholding (which can often get worse if poos are painful to pass).

✧ Developmental, learning or neurodevelopmental differences which seem to coincide with tummy troubles like constipation more often (this is likely to be for reasons from dietary intake to sensory differences, for example).

What can you do?
There are a variety of strategies to support children with constipation. Optimising fluid and fibre intake is helpful for some children. However, many will still be recommended medications to help them poo. For some groups of children, such as highly selective eaters, dietary changes may be difficult too. I know many parents can feel daunted or disappointed that their child needs medication, but I often reassure them that medications are not to be feared. Some children need to use them for a short period, and others may

need them for longer, but promptly getting on top of your child's symptoms can help in the long term.

Fluids

Getting enough fluid helps children to poo. Fluid is needed to help make poo soft and easier to move through the bowel. Fluids can come from drinks and fluid-rich foods such as fruits, vegetables, smoothies, lollies, soups and yoghurt. In previous sections, I have covered how much fluids babies and children need, alongside tips to encourage drinking.

Food and fibre

The foods your child eats, including how much fibre, can have a big impact on their poo. Fibre is important for healthy bowel movements for several reasons. It helps bulk up stools, helping them move more easily through the intestines, and it supports gut health by feeding helpful gut bacteria. Too little or too much fibre can contribute to constipation. However, research suggests that up to 90 per cent of young children in the UK don't get enough fibre. You'll find detailed fibre recommendations and practical tips to help boost your child's fibre intake on pages 264–5.

There are several foods that I, and the science, find can be helpful to include or limit to manage constipation.

Foods to help with constipation

There are lots of fibre-rich foods that may support constipation management, but here are some of my favourites:

◆ Kiwi – Yes, this often-overlooked little green fruit can be very helpful for constipation, according to several studies. Kiwi is excellent at attracting water into the bowel (gut), helping poo move through more easily. It also contains a substance called actinidin, which is an enzyme that helps break down proteins and supports digestion.

✧ 'P–fruits', including prunes, peaches, pears, papaya and plums – Many parents are familiar with these fruits as a constipation 'cure'. They can be effective because they contain higher amounts of certain natural sugars, like sorbitol, which help draw water into the bowel, making stools softer and easier to pass. They're also a good source of fibre.

✧ Beans and lentils, such as red lentils, dal, black beans, kidney beans and baked beans – These are packed with fibre, which adds bulk to stools and supports the movement of poo through the gut. They also contain certain types of carbohydrates that help feed healthy gut bacteria.

✧ Certain vegetables – Studies have found that non-starchy vegetables that are dark green, red or orange in colour can be particularly helpful for constipation management. Of these, tomatoes were strongly associated with a reduced risk of constipation.

✧ Wholegrains and oats – Both are rich in dietary fibre, containing types of fibre that not only help bulk up poo but also make it softer and easier to pass.

✧ Seeds, such as flaxseeds and chia seeds – These great for children's digestive health. Chia and flax are known for their stool-bulking effect and for helping to keep stools soft and easy to pass. They are very high in fibre, so I always recommend starting small and increasing gradually in young children, for example, ¼ teaspoon initially. I'd also recommend soaking or adding chia seeds to a dish containing fluid, such as porridge or yoghurt.

Remember, the rule with fibre is always to increase it gradually, ensuring good fluid intake alongside it.

Advice online often recommends limiting certain foods like rice, potatoes, dairy and bread to prevent constipation. It's not that these foods cause constipation directly, but consuming them in large amounts may displace the intake of other foods that promote healthy digestion and regular poos or affect transit time. For children over one, checking in on their total cow's milk intake can be important too, as excess milk intake can mean your child doesn't get enough of lots of different nutrients, fibre included. Check out page 164 for more about milk intake in young children.

Activity – Movement is a great way to get the gut going. Physical activity helps to 'wake up' the muscles in the intestines, which may help with regular pooing. Young children need lots of activity (at least three hours a day!), so help your child stay active through play, walking and age-appropriate physical activities.

For babies or young children who are not walking yet, I find that time upright, for example, seated (if old enough), time in a sling, or gentle, supportive movements such as cycling legs and baby massage can greatly help with constipation.

Toileting habits – If your child is at the age where they are starting to use a potty or toilet, here are some considerations:

1. ***Poo positioning*** – The ideal position for pooing is actually when the feet are supported and the knees are slightly higher than the hips, similar to a squatting position. You'll have probably seen your child intuitively squat when they poo before you start toilet training. For this reason, a 'traditional' potty instead of a mini toilet can support better positioning when potty training; if your child is using a toilet (with an adapted seat), don't forget to provide a step on which they can rest their feet.

2. ***Poo timing*** – I'd recommend you encourage your child to sit on the potty or toilet in the morning and for five to 15 minutes after eating. This is because it can be a more common time to poo thanks to something known as the gastro-colic reflex.

3. ***Pressure-free pooing*** – Try to keep times on the potty or toilet pressure-free for your child. Reading books, talking and reassuring your child can help manage feelings of worry or anxiety that can make pooing more difficult. A task like blowing bubbles can also help children relax their pelvic floor and engage the muscles they need to poo.

Medication – For many children with constipation, a doctor or nurse will prescribe laxatives to help them poo. Laxatives work in different ways, but when used consistently they can help children to poo more regularly and comfortably. It's important to follow the advice on how to use laxatives correctly. Avoid suddenly stopping and restarting them if your child hasn't had a bowel movement, instead working towards a regular dose that supports your child to have regular poo.

Different laxatives work in different ways – so here's a quick rundown.

Type of laxative	How they work
Osmotic laxatives – 'The water attracter' **Examples** Lactulose – a sticky liquid Movicol, Laxido – a powder to make up with water	• Bring and keep water in the large intestine. • Keep poo soft. • By expanding in the gut, they can give the gut a gentle nudge to contract (squeeze) regularly.
Bulk-forming laxatives – 'The filler' **Examples** Fybogel Methylcellulose Psyllium	• Increase size and weight of poo. • Hold more water in the poo. • Keep poo soft. • Remind the gut to contract regularly.

Stimulant laxative – 'The mover' **Examples** Senna Sodium picosulfate Bisacodyl (sold as Dulcolax)	• Prompt the muscles in the gut to move poo along the intestine. • Some 'wake up' or 'nudge' nerves in the colon or rectum (both are parts of the large intestine). • Some help poo stay soft.

Probiotics – There is lots of research going on to see if probiotics (live bacteria) can help manage constipation in babies and children. Differences in gut bacteria have been found in some children with constipation, but the impact of this is not yet fully understood. At the moment there is not strong enough scientific evidence to recommend any probiotic strains for babies or children with constipation.

Toddler diarrhoea
'My toddler seems to have regular loose or watery poo and I don't know why.'
One of the most common causes of long-term loose stools in young children is 'toddler diarrhoea'.
Typical age range: 1–5 years of age
Affects: Up to 15 per cent of toddlers, more common in boys
Symptoms:

✧ Loose, watery and often pale-coloured poo, occurring at least two to three times per day but can be up to 10+ times a day.

✧ Poos that frequently contain undigested pieces of food and have a more pungent smell than usual.

✧ Symptoms that last at least three weeks or more.

✧ Your child is otherwise well, not ill, and has no other symptoms of concern, such as weight loss, pain, temperature or vomiting.

Why does this happen?
The cause of toddler diarrhoea is not fully understood. Medical professionals agree that it's likely to be down to one or more of the following reasons:

✧ Toddlers can have fast gut transit time (sometimes known as intestinal flurry), which means food moves more quickly through their bowel. I explain to kids that their 'food is in a hurry!'

✧ An imbalance of fluid, fibre and undigested sugars that reach a toddler's large bowel.

What can you do?
These symptoms can understandably cause parents much concern. I encourage parents to speak with their child's GP if they're worried, especially if diarrhoea is accompanied by weight loss, pain, nutritional deficiencies, a history of constipation or is significantly impacting the child's or family's quality of life.

The good news is that a few dietary shifts following the 'four Fs' can usually help improve toddler diarrhoea.

Fat – One of the benefits of fat is that it can slow down digestion and how quickly food moves through the gut. For this reason, a low-fat diet seems to worsen toddler diarrhoea, so ensuring plenty of healthy fats are in your toddler's diet is essential. Aim to include a healthy fat source regularly in meals and snacks, for example, nut butter, full-fat dairy, oily fish, avocado and oils.

Fibre – A low- or high-fibre diet can make toddler diarrhoea worse. Looking at how much your toddler is getting and the types and amounts of fibre can be helpful. I talk about fibre in more detail in the section beginning on page 261.

Fruit juice and fruit – Certain fruits, large portions of fruit, fruit juices, purees and smoothies can lead to a high intake of fructose and sorbitol. Both are naturally occurring sugars in fruit. This can contribute to or worsen symptoms of toddler diarrhoea as these sugars attract water into the bowel, contributing to loose poo. Aim to limit fruit juice and smoothies to 100–150ml and once per day. Consider being mindful of fruit portions, spreading them throughout the day and pairing them with fat- or protein-containing foods.

Fluids – Excessive drinking can also contribute to toddler diarrhoea. Spread your toddler's drinks throughout the day, and refer to page 199 for more details about fluid intake for toddlers.

Lactose intolerance
'My child has ongoing loose, watery poo and tummy pain after a diarrhoea and vomiting bug.'
Typical age range: Can occur at any age during infancy and childhood
Symptoms:

✧ Your child has loose, watery poo/diarrhoea, usually multiple times per day. Symptoms worsen after eating higher-lactose foods like milk, certain yoghurts, soft cheese, creamy foods and ice cream, or after milk feeds (in babies).

✧ Your child may have excess wind, flatulence or bloating.

✧ Your child may have gripey abdominal (tummy) pain or cramping.

Why does this happen?
After a gastrointestinal illness (tummy bug) with symptoms of diarrhoea or vomiting, the enzyme lactase, which helps digest lactose (milk sugar) in milk and milk-containing foods, can be

temporarily reduced, or 'wiped'. This means undigested lactose reaches the large intestine, draws in water and is fermented by bacteria, leading to symptoms like diarrhoea and bloating.

Rarely, children can have lactose intolerance for other reasons, including:

✧ Developmental lactase deficiency, which occurs when a child's lactase enzyme production is lower than normal. This is often due to immature enzyme development in babies, which usually improves as they grow. It can be more common in preterm babies.

✧ Inherited lactose intolerance or primary lactose intolerance, which is a rare form of lactose intolerance. In this case, a child inherits a condition where the body produces little to no lactase enzyme. Usually, one or both parents will also be lactose intolerant. These children will be lactose intolerant for life.

What can you do?
Lactose intolerance is managed by removing the lactose from a baby's or child's diet. This is usually only needed temporarily while the lactase enzyme 'regroups' to normal levels in your child's gut. Breastfed babies can continue to breastfeed (*note: you cannot change the lactose content of breast milk*), while those on formula milk may change to lactose-free formula milk, which the GP can prescribe. For babies on solids, lactose-free dairy products such as milk, yoghurt and cream cheese will be needed. Lactose can usually be introduced back into the diet (or normal formula milk resumed) within six to eight weeks.

Lactose intolerance is not the same as Cow's Milk Protein Allergy, which is discussed on page 365.

Antibiotic-associated diarrhoea (AAD)

'My child is on antibiotics and having frequent loose poos.'

Typical age range: Can occur at any age during infancy and childhood

Symptoms:

✧ Your child is having antibiotics, or has just finished a course of antibiotics and is experiencing loose or watery stools (diarrhoea) usually three or more times a day.

✧ Your child has abdominal (tummy) pain or cramping, nausea and/or wind.

Why does this happen?

AAD is thought to affect around 20 per cent of children on antibiotics, with symptoms more common in children under two years of age. It occurs because the antibiotics your child is taking, which kill harmful bacteria that cause infection, also disrupt the balance of bacteria in your child's gut.

What can you do?

Most AAD will resolve without any specific treatment. You must not stop the course of antibiotics prescribed early due to these symptoms. Ensure your child remains well hydrated, and when their appetite returns try to resume their normal diet, including plenty of gut-friendly foods (see section beginning on page 315). There is some research that shows certain strains of probiotics can help reduce the symptoms of antibiotic-associated diarrhoea. These strains include *Saccharomyces boulardii* and *Lactobacillus rhamnosus GG*, which should be given at a dose of at least 5 billion Colony Forming Units (CFU) per day and started alongside antibiotic treatment (allowing a gap between giving the medication and probiotic).

A small percentage of children may experience a secondary

lactose intolerance due to antibiotics and associated gut side effects, especially if on repeated courses of antibiotics. You can read more about lactose intolerance earlier in this chapter.

Quick-fire poo questions

Yes, I'm afraid there's more poo chat! Here are some of the most common poo questions parents come to me with, which tend to start with 'Is it normal if . . .?'

My child often poos during or after a feed or meal

This is normal for many babies and children and is usually related to the gastro-colic reflex, which is a natural communication strategy in the body where feeding or eating triggers the stomach to tell the large intestine (specifically the colon) via the brain that it's time to make room because more food is arriving! These signals cause the colon to contract (squeeze) to start making room, which means that a baby or child may pass a stool during or shortly after eating or feeding.

It's worth mentioning that urgency after eating, accompanied by other symptoms such as pain and discomfort, loose stools or diarrhoea, is worth checking with your doctor, especially if it occurs frequently.

There is mucus in my baby/child's poo.

Seeing mucus in your baby or child's poo can be a worry for many parents. Mucus can occur in small streaks within poo or, in some cases, be passed in more significant amounts. I always start discussions about mucus in poo by reassuring parents that a little can be normal, as mucus is found in the lining of the intestine. There, it has essential jobs such as lubricating the intestines to help poo pass through and protecting the gut lining from 'bad' bacteria and other harmful substances.

Some mucus can occur within stools at various points during the early years, for example:

✧ During periods of illness.

✧ When babies are teething. (Many parents report this, though there isn't much scientific evidence to support it.)

However, if you notice a significant increase in mucus, or if it's accompanied by other symptoms like blood in the stool, diarrhoea or signs of illness (such as fever, vomiting or irritability), please consult a healthcare professional. These could be signs of an underlying condition such as an infection, food allergy or inflammatory bowel disease.

My child has undigested food in their poo.

Pieces of undigested food can be present in poo, and these tend to be foods high in fibre that are hard to digest (and sometimes chew!), such as those with tough outer skins, like seeds, nuts, sweetcorn and husks or fibrous pieces of fruit or vegetables. It can be more common in younger children who haven't yet developed all their molars or fully developed their rotary chewing, both of which help grind these foods. Seeing undigested food more regularly in your child's poo can also be a sign that food is passing through their intestine quickly. In the medical world, we sometimes call this 'intestinal flurry', or food in a hurry, and it can be more common in younger children. Sometimes this can be associated with conditions such as toddler diarrhoea (covered above), but if it occurs alongside any of the red-flag symptoms detailed below, please contact your child's GP.

Fun fact: The sweetcorn test is sometimes recommended to monitor bowel habits. Understanding how quickly food moves through the digestive system (called transit time) can help us identify conditions like constipation.

My child's poo is green.

Green poo can often be a worry for parents, however, there are several reasons why this can happen.

Breastfed babies – It is not uncommon for breastfed babies to have the occasional green poo. This can often indicate that they are getting more lactose-rich milk at the start of feeds, which may be due to factors such as an oversupply, fast let down or short feeding sessions.

Formula-fed babies – Specific formula milks can cause poo to go green, including those containing proteins that are partially or extensively hydrolysed (broken down) or amino acid-based formula milk.

Babies and children on solids – Children on solid foods, particularly those eating dark greens like spinach or kale, might have a greener tint in their stool afterwards.

Babies or children on iron supplements – Iron supplements may cause stools to appear green, dark brown or black.

Babies and children may also experience greener stools when unwell with a bacterial or viral illness. In some cases, green stools can be associated with food-allergy symptoms, but this will typically be alongside other food-allergy symptoms rather than a standalone symptom.

RED FLAGS – Poo or tummy troubles to talk to your doctor about straight away.

✧ **Blood in poo** – Blood in poo, which may present as anything from specks to more prominent streaks or more, is *always* something to discuss with your doctor. There can be multiple causes for blood in stools, including infection, a small tear (fissure) in the anus, or a Cow's Milk Protein Allergy.

✧ **White, chalky poo** – This can be a sign of liver problems in children, so discuss with your GP immediately.

✧ **Black Poo** – Very dark or black-looking poo can sometimes be a sign of blood loss higher up in the bowel. Discuss with your GP immediately (note that certain supplements and medicines, such as those that contain iron, can turn poo a much darker/ black colour).

✧ **Any poo or poo habits that are associated with recurrent pain, discomfort, weight loss, fever, feeding difficulties or that interfere with daily life and are concerning you.**

Common nutritional deficiencies in early childhood

While I hope you won't need this, young children can struggle to meet their vitamin and mineral requirements, often due to their high nutrient needs relative to their size. A nutrient deficiency occurs when the body lacks specific vitamins or minerals for optimal health. Visible signs may develop over time, but some deficiencies can exist without apparent symptoms.

Based on research and clinical experience, I'll cover four common nutrient deficiencies in young children. Children at higher risk of more significant nutritional deficiencies include selective eaters, those with feeding differences like ARFID and those with food allergies or coeliac disease. A personalised dietary review with a paediatric dietitian is recommended for these groups of children.

Vitamin D deficiency

If you've made it this far, you might be tired of hearing me talk about vitamin D! I've purposely given it plenty of attention throughout the book because this deficiency is exceptionally common in children – thought to affect around 20 per cent of them, equivalent to 2.5 million in the UK. Getting enough vitamin D from food alone is difficult, as the body mainly makes it from sunlight exposure. Considering the UK's limited sunlight, particularly during winter, coupled with our careful stance on sun exposure for children, it's easy to see why deficiencies may arise.

Vitamin D is a fat-soluble vitamin essential for many body functions. It supports the absorption and use of other bone-friendly nutrients, including calcium, magnesium and phosphate. It also has a role in muscle contractions, immune health and much more.

Symptoms of vitamin D deficiency

Symptoms of vitamin D deficiency can be quite general or vague but included within them are unexplained tiredness and fatigue, growth difficulties, recurrent illnesses, weakness, developmental delay and bone pain or changes. Severe deficiency in children can cause rickets, a bone condition associated with 'softer' bones and bowing of bones in the legs. Children can also experience leg pain, muscle weakness, cramps and, very occasionally, seizures.

While all children in the UK are at risk of vitamin D deficiency, some are at higher risk, including children who:

✧ Have darker skin – This is because darker skin has more melanin, which reduces the skin's ability to produce vitamin D from sunlight.

✧ Take certain medicines, such as anti-epilepsy medications – These can affect how the body processes vitamin D, potentially leading to lower levels in the blood.

✧ Spend limited time outdoors – Limited sun exposure can decrease vitamin D production.

✧ Certain medical conditions – Conditions like coeliac disease or cystic fibrosis can affect how the body absorbs vitamin D from food or supplements.

How much vitamin D does your child need per day?
0–1 year: 8.5–10µg
1–5 years: 10µg

How is vitamin D deficiency diagnosed?
A blood test completed by your child's doctor.

How can you make sure your child gets enough vitamin D?
The most important step to prevent vitamin D deficiency in babies and children is to provide the recommended supplementation. At the end of each age section of this book I cover the general recommendations about what supplements are needed and how much to give. Remember, you can help your child get the best out of their vitamin D supplement by giving them a feed, meal or snack containing fat and ensuring their diet includes other nutrients that work with vitamin D, like magnesium.

Vitamin D-containing foods are perfectly safe to include alongside supplementation. These include egg yolks, oily fish, fortified cereals, fortified milk and milk alternatives and mushrooms. (Fun fact: if you leave your mushrooms in sunlight, their vitamin D content increases.)

Iron deficiency
Iron deficiency is a common nutrient deficiency (in fact, the most common worldwide) and affects up to one in five young children. The importance of this nutrient won't surprise you – there is not a chapter of this book which doesn't at least mention iron. Iron is an essential nutrient that supports a child's rapid growth and development, especially brain development.

Iron deficiency can occur for several reasons, but in many children it often stems from inadequate iron intake relative to their needs. Additional factors may raise a child's risk of iron deficiency, such as:

✧ Mum having low iron levels during pregnancy.

✧ Preterm delivery.

✧ Delayed or slow introduction of solids.

✧ Excess intake of other foods or drinks, such as cow's milk.

✧ Medications that interfere with iron absorption.

✧ Diagnoses that affect how much iron can be absorbed, such as coeliac disease.

Symptoms of iron deficiency
There can be tell-tale signs that a child's iron levels may be low, however, some symptoms are subtle or easily mistaken for other conditions. Common symptoms include:

✧ Poor appetite.

✧ Unexplained fatigue.

✧ Difficulty concentrating.

✧ Pallor (pale skin).

✧ Headaches.

✧ Dizziness.

✧ Racing heart or heart palpitations.

✧ Shortness of breath during activity or active play.

✧ Some children may try to eat non-food items (this is called pica), including dirt or paint.

✧ Irritability and low mood.

In very severe cases, iron deficiency can contribute to developmental delays and behavioural differences or disturbances.

How much iron does your child need per day?
0–3 months – 1.7mg
3–6 months – 4.3mg
7–12 months – 7.8mg
1–3 years – 6.8mg
4–6 years – 6.1mg

How is iron deficiency diagnosed?
A doctor completes a blood test, and iron deficiency or iron deficiency anaemia may be diagnosed depending on the results. The difference between these conditions is that iron deficiency is when a child's iron stores are low but do not yet affect the production of red blood cells. Iron deficiency anaemia occurs when a significant lack of iron begins to affect the body's capacity to produce healthy red blood cells. In simple terms, iron deficiency is an early stage of iron depletion, and if it's not addressed, it can progress to anaemia.

How is iron deficiency treated?
If a child is diagnosed with iron deficiency or anaemia, a doctor will prescribe iron supplementation. They will advise on how much and how often to give this, but a typical routine is a dose of iron three times a day. This usually continues for around three months, at which point a repeat blood test is completed to check iron levels have been restored. Iron supplements can have side effects, including darker stools, tummy pain, diarrhoea and/or constipation. If your

child experiences these symptoms, it's helpful to discuss them with a doctor to explore other options.

If your child is diagnosed with iron deficiency, keep iron medications out of reach and in a safe place. Excess iron intake can have severe consequences for children.

Alongside this, it can be helpful to check in on dietary iron intake or manage other factors that may have contributed to the deficiency to help prevent it from occurring again.

How can you make sure your child gets enough iron?
The best way to prevent iron deficiency is to ensure your child has a regular intake of iron-rich foods in their diet, aiming to include iron-rich sources at least two to three times a day across meals and snacks.

Which foods contain iron?
Dietary iron is available in two different forms – animal-based iron (haem iron) and plant-based iron (non-haem iron).

Haem iron: Haem is typically considered the easiest type of iron to absorb. Haem iron can be found in animal products such as:

✧ Red meat such as beef, lamb and pork.

✧ Offal, like liver and kidney.

✧ Fish – oily fish, like salmon, sardines and mackerel are higher in iron.

✧ Pate or fish paste.

✧ Chicken or turkey – the darker meat is higher in iron.

Non-haem iron: Non-haem iron is typically found in plant-based foods and can be slightly more difficult for our bodies to absorb. Non-haem iron sources include:

✧ Wholemeal/wholegrain breads and cereals, chapati.

✧ Peas, beans and legumes, such as lentils, baked beans, kidney beans or foods like hummus.

✧ Peanuts and tree nuts (well ground or in butter form for young children).

✧ Seeds, such as sesame seeds/tahini.

✧ Leafy green vegetables, such as spinach, kale, broccoli, watercress.

✧ Eggs.

✧ Tofu.

✧ Dried fruit, such as apricots.

✧ Iron-fortified breakfast cereals – check the label to see if iron is added.

Other foods fortified with (added) iron include breads, smoothies, cow's milk and plant-based milk alternatives.

Carefully planning your child's diet to include iron-rich foods regularly will help ensure they get enough. As a general guide, I often encourage parents to aim to give a good iron source during at least three meals or snack times during the day, regardless of what dietary pattern a child follows.

Here are some examples to help you visualise how a young child might meet their requirements across a day.

Breakfast: One wheat cereal biscuit with whole milk and fruit (2.3mg)
Lunch: Baked beans (two tablespoons) on one slice of wholemeal bread (2mg)

Evening meal: Beef chilli (one large tablespoon) with rice and avocado (2.5mg)
Snack: Two crackers with one tablespoon peanut butter (0.7mg)
Total – 7.5mg

Breakfast: One small bowl of porridge with ½ a sliced banana (2.0mg)
Lunch: Chickpea and vegetable curry (one large tablespoon) with a small piece of chapati (2.5mg)
Evening meal: Lamb kebab (one small piece) with a small portion of couscous and steamed carrots (2.8mg)
Snack: One small slice of apple with one tablespoon almond butter (0.8mg)
Total: 8.1mg

Breakfast: One small bowl of millet porridge with a sprinkle of dried fruit (1.7mg)
Lunch: Hummus and cucumber small pitta (2.0mg)
Evening meal: Turkey meatballs (two small meatballs) with pasta and tomato sauce (2.6mg)
Snacks: One small bowl of dried apricots and two small wholegrain crackers (0.9mg)
Total: 7.2mg

Breakfast: One small slice of wholegrain toast with one tablespoon mashed avocado and one boiled egg (1.4mg)
Lunch: Vegetable dal (lentil curry) with a small portion of brown rice (2.2mg)
Evening meal: Grilled chicken (one small piece) with quinoa and roasted bell peppers (2.5mg)
Before-bed snack: Small bowl of fortified cereal with milk (2mg)
Total: 8.1mg

Alongside iron intake, considering foods or nutrients in your child's diet that help or hinder iron absorption can be helpful too! In the table on the following pages you can find some key considerations.

Folate (B9) deficiency

You might not have come across this vitamin very much, but it's part of the B-vitamin family and a nutrient I am seeing more and more children deficient in. Research agrees that while it's not as common as iron or vitamin D deficiency, we are seeing more children deficient in folate. You'll have been well aware of the importance of folate during pregnancy, but in babies and young children, folate is essential for growth and development, making DNA, red blood cells and enabling cell division.

Nutrients to *help* iron absorption	Examples	Suggestions
Vitamin-C-rich foods *Vitamin C is also known as ascorbic acid*	Citrus fruits, strawberries, kiwi, berries, papaya, blackcurrants, guava, soursop, mango. Bell peppers, broccoli, cabbage, okra, spinach, tomatoes, cassava leaves, pak choi. Potatoes – especially with skins on!	Aim to include vitamin C-rich foods alongside every iron-rich meal or snack. Often a portion of fruit or vegetables is enough!

Nutrients that <u>can hinder</u> iron absorption	Examples	Suggestions
Tannins and polyphenols *Naturally occurring compounds found in various plant-based foods and drink*	Tea and coffee.	These compounds can attach to iron, reducing its absorption. Your little one shouldn't be delving into these drinks, so you won't have to think too much about these! They can be a consideration for breastfeeding mums though.
Calcium	Milk, yoghurt, cheese, cream cheese and fortified milk alternatives.	In simple terms, research shows that calcium can compete with iron for absorption in the gut. However, most studies focus on calcium supplements rather than dietary calcium and over the long term, the total amount of calcium consumed overall seems to be more important than how much is consumed at each meal From a parenting and meal-planning perspective, I therefore recommend:. • Being pragmatic – iron and calcium-rich foods will be offered together in the diet and that's ok. • Being mindful of how much cow's milk, calcium-fortified milk alternative or other dairy products are consumed throughout the day (aim to stick around recommended amounts and proportions – see page 164). • considering offering some iron-rich foods separate from calcium-'heavy' meals or snacks • Focusing on iron intake overall and regular iron opportunities throughout the day..

How much folate does your child need per day?
0–12 months – 50µg
1–3 years – 70µg
4–6 years – 150µg

Symptoms of folate deficiency
Like other common nutrient deficiencies, signs that your child's folate levels are low can creep up gradually and be difficult to spot. Here are some common ones:

✧ Heart palpitations.

✧ Unexplained weakness, tiredness and fatigue.

✧ Mouth ulcers, sore or red tongue.

✧ Slow or poor growth.

✧ Diarrhoea.

✧ Headaches.

✧ Vision problems or changes.

Children usually have low levels of folate because they are not consuming enough from their diet or via supplementation. Some groups of children are at higher risk of folate deficiency, including those with malabsorption conditions like coeliac disease or IBD. Children taking certain medications, such as anti-seizure medications, are also at higher risk, as these medicine can interfere with the absorption of folate in the body.

How is folate deficiency diagnosed?
Folate deficiency can be identified through a blood test completed by your child's GP.

How is folate deficiency treated?
If your child's folate levels are low, their GP will usually prescribe a course of folate supplementation.

Prioritising folate-rich foods in your child's diet is essential for preventing folate deficiency and is ongoing after supplementation if a child is deficient. Folate-rich foods include:

✧ Fortified cereals.

✧ Liver.

✧ Poultry, like chicken and turkey.

✧ Eggs.

✧ Green, leafy vegetables (such as spinach, kale, broccoli, mustard greens).

✧ Beans, lentils and peas.

✧ Avocado.

✧ Fish and seafood.

✧ Citrus fruits like oranges and lemons.

While I was writing this book, the government also announced that folic acid will be added to non-wholemeal flour in the UK (alongside calcium and iron which are already added) from 2026.

Fibre 'deficiency'

Based on recent data, 75–90 per cent of young children in the UK don't meet daily fibre intake recommendations. There is evidently a huge fibre gap in children's diets, and overlooking this important nutrient can have both short- and long-term effects on your child's health.

Signs of fibre deficiency

Unlike the smaller nutrients I've discussed above, low intake of fibre in your child's diet may not be very obvious. Signs could include:

✧ Constipation, and associated bloating and/or abdominal pain.

✧ Poor appetite control, satiety after meals or snacks.

✧ Differences in the community of gut bacteria (which of course you can't see or test for).

I cover fibre intake in young children in detail on pages 262–5, including practical examples of how to ensure the right amount and balance of fibre in your child's diet. You can also read about the importance of fibre on children's gut health on pages 310.

Weight (and growth) worries

✧ **Faltering growth (a slower rate of weight gain than expected for age and sex)**

✧ **Excess weight gain in children**

Weight and growth concerns are common reasons for me to see children in clinic. As a parent, learning that your child isn't growing as expected can be daunting, often leading to feelings of guilt or inadequacy. It's important to understand that as parents, you are doing your best – there is no failure here! This is why the term 'failure to thrive' was replaced; it inaccurately suggests shortcomings on the part of the parent or the child. Growth issues can stem from various medical, nutritional and developmental factors, so taking a comprehensive approach to assessing a child is essential.

It's important to note that growth, like nutrition, is complex. The information here provides a general overview, but individual advice is necessary for specific growth concerns.

What is faltering growth, and why does it happen?

Faltering growth refers to a situation where a child's growth pattern deviates from the expected trajectory; typically a child's weight, but perhaps also their height, is not developing as anticipated for their age, sex, developmental stage or background. The most common causes of faltering growth are not consuming enough calories, not absorbing nutrients properly and having a higher need for calories or burning more calories than usual. There can be many more reasons, as detailed in the box on the next page.

How is faltering growth diagnosed?

A qualified medical professional specialising in treating babies and children is the best person to diagnose faltering growth. Accurate weight and length/height measurements must be taken, as even slight variations can show significant differences in centile positions for young children. Diagnosing faltering growth requires more than just a single weight and height measurement; it involves examining a child's growth and growth rate over a period, using centile lines on the growth charts.

Based on current UK guidelines, faltering growth should be assessed for in any of the following circumstances.

Weight

✧ During the first few days of life, if weight loss is more than 10 per cent of birth weight, or weight does not return to birth weight by three weeks of age.

✧ After the first days and weeks of life, if a baby or child has fallen or drifted down by:
   o One weight centile space, if their birth weight was below the 9th centile.
   o Two weight centile spaces, if their birth weight was between the 9–91st centiles.
   o Three weight centile spaces, if their birth weight was above the 91st centile.

✧ If a child's weight is below the 2nd centile, regardless of birth weight.*

Common reasons for slowed growth in children

✧ **Feeding difficulties** – Which make it hard for children to consume enough nutrition. This can include early-life feeding difficulties, such as challenges with establishing breastfeeding.
✧ **Medical conditions** – That affect a child's feeding ability, skills, nutritional requirements, food options (such as allergies) or ability to absorb the nutrients they need.
✧ **Illness** – Short- or long-term illnesses or recurrent periods of illness can affect appetite, ability to eat or the amount of nutrition a child needs.

- ✧ **Developmental differences** – May affect feeding skill development or cause delays in learning how to eat a variety of foods.
- ✧ **Nutritional deficiencies** – That impact a child's appetite (such as iron) or may have side effects that make eating difficult, such as fatigue.
- ✧ **Poor appetite** – Caused by nutritional differences, pain or discomfort when feeding, constipation or lack of interest in food.
- ✧ **Emotional or environmental factors** – Stress, anxiety or negative experiences with feeding or eating.
- ✧ **Limited access to nutritious foods** – Not having enough suitable milk or food options due to financial or other reasons.

Please note that some babies and children may plot on or below the 2nd centile for their weight and/or height, and in many cases this can still be normal and healthy for them. This is often seen in specific groups, such as certain ethnic populations, where data that helped produce the growth charts might not fully account for all variations in healthy growth across different populations. While it's generally recommended to have these children assessed to ensure their growth is on track, it isn't always something to worry about.

Height

Once over two, a child's height can be compared to their parents', using a measurement called mid-parental height. If a child's height centile is more than two centile spaces below the mid-parental centile, this may indicate undernutrition or a growth disorder.

I would also recommend getting a drop in height-centile positions checked out. However, it's important to note that this can often be due to inaccurate measurements, which is actually quite common as length and height measurements can be difficult to take accurately.

Body Mass Index (BMI)

BMI may be used to assess growth in children over two years of age. Unlike adults, children's BMI ranges are plotted on centile charts specific to their age and sex. While BMI is definitely not a perfect measure of health or growth, it may be an additional measurement, alongside those I've mentioned above, to evaluate growth by combining weight and height measurements.

When it comes to assessing for faltering growth it's recognised that:

✧ A BMI below the 2nd centile *may* indicate undernutrition or a small build.

✧ A BMI below the 0.4th centile can benefit from further assessment.

How is faltering growth treated?

Treatment for faltering growth will vary from child to child, depending on why their growth isn't tracking as expected. One or multiple health professionals should be involved, including a paediatric dietitian and possibly a paediatrician. A child may have investigations like blood tests, urine samples or stool samples to help rule out or understand if any medical reasons are contributing, such as thyroid problems, diabetes, nutritional deficiencies or signs that the body isn't absorbing nutrients properly.

Nutritional advice ensures a child gets enough energy and nutrients to support their growth. Ways to support extra energy and nutrient intake may include, depending on the age of the child:

✧ Breastfeeding assessment and support.

✧ Adjusting concentration of infant formula milk or using prescribed high-energy formula milk (only under the direction of a medical professional).

✧ Food fortification – this is where foods that provide extra energy and/or nutrients are added to the foods a child eats to help boost the amount of nutrition.

✧ Use of specialised high-energy drinks (known as oral nutritional supplements). A GP prescribes these; they are not shakes you can buy over the counter.

✧ While rare, in some cases, babies or children may require a short or long period of time to receive nutrition via a tube into their nose or tummy.

Feeding support may also be needed if a child shows signs of struggling with the skills needed to feed or eat what they need to grow, such as biting, chewing, swallowing and self-feeding skills.

All of the above should be under the advice of a medical professional.

How can extra energy be added to a child's diet?

There is a wide range of ways you can add extra energy and nutrients into your child's diet if their growth is a concern. I encourage families to think about little additions, often throughout the day. Here are some of my favourites:

✧ **Toast toppings** – Add butter or spread it on both sides of the toast. Use double toppings like butter, then nut butter or jam, or jam and cream cheese.

✧ **Oil** – Use a small amount of oil and add it to pasta, rice, potatoes, pasta sauces, curry, pie, dressings and vegetables.

✧ **Change cooking methods** – Consider roasting vegetables or frying suitable foods in oil rather than baking.

✧ **Avocado** – Add to smoothies, blend through a pasta sauce or pesto, use mashed as a spread onto read or on toast, use for lollies or 'chocolate puddings'.

✧ **Consider swaps** – Such as tuna or tinned fish in oil instead of spring water, higher-fat yoghurts, such as 5 or 10%-fat Greek yoghurt.

✧ **Smoothies** – Blend full-fat milk or yoghurt with fruits, vegetables and add-ins like oats, nut butter or seeds.

✧ **Cheese** – Add grated or cream cheese to dishes like casseroles, scrambled eggs and sandwiches or sprinkle over vegetables and pasta.

✧ **Nuts and seeds** – Use well-ground nuts or nut butter added to yoghurt, over porridge or cereal, in smoothies, into baked recipes like muffins, spread on toast or pancakes, added into savoury dishes like a stir-fry sauce or curry.

✧ **Eggs** – Cook eggs in various ways, such as scrambled, omelettes or frittatas, adding vegetables and tinned oily fish or cheese.

✧ **Full-fat dairy** – Use full-fat milk, cream or yoghurt in cooking, baking or as snacks.

✧ **Hummus** – Serve with pitta bread, vegetable sticks, use as a spread in sandwiches or as an easy pasta sauce.

✧ **Coconut milk or cream of coconut** – Use in cooking, baking or as a base for smoothies.

✧ **Baked goods** – For extra nutrients, add ground or milled nuts, seeds or dried fruit to muffins, pancakes or breads.

Note: The above is not a substitute for personalised advice. If you have any concerns about your child's growth, please contact your GP to discuss initially.

Excess weight gain in children

Excess weight gain has the potential to affect children's health and is increasingly common in the Western world. In the UK, one in eight toddlers is obese, and over 20 per cent of children starting primary school are now overweight. Understanding and discussing weight gain in children is a complex and delicate subject. I've often observed that the stigma surrounding weight and related discussions poses a significant challenge, frequently placing undue blame on parents and caregivers. Excess weight gain is complex and influenced by diet, lifestyle, genetics, medical history and environmental factors. A balanced approach is essential, focusing on support and positive actions instead of blame, but also with realistic expectations. We're all familiar with how weight concerns are often discussed at a societal level, where much of the support should begin. However, in my experience, it often feels like these issues are treated solely as an individual's problem.

When discussing this topic with families, I always stress that their child's health is my primary focus, not simply numbers on a scale or body size. Data shows that excess weight gain in children under five years of age can be associated with an increased risk of developing health conditions, including type 2 diabetes and heart and liver problems. Notably, the impact goes beyond physical health, as emotional and social health are known to be affected too. Children who are overweight tend to experience lower self-esteem, social isolation and an increased risk of bullying or discrimination.

What worries me, and other children's health professionals, is how excess weight has the potential to affect a child's health and overall wellbeing.

When to consider support with weight gain in children?

Firstly, it's important to remember that periods of weight gain are a normal part of young children's growth and development, and not all weight gain is a cause for concern. Methods to assess a child's weight and size versus health status are also flawed, and it is well acknowledged that the Body Mass Index is far from perfect as a measure of health.

Current guidelines for young children, especially those under two years old, are more limited. As a general guide, recommendations for seeking advice would include:

✧ A child's (older than one year) weight consistently increasing across centiles (for example, moving up two or more centiles) without a history of faltering growth or low weight.

✧ Children over two years of age, BMI* is above the 91st or 98th centile (especially if this hasn't historically been the case).

✧ A significant difference between weight and height centiles, such as when weight falls more than two or three centiles above the height centile (especially if this hasn't historically been the case).

But, it's worth knowing that these are just criteria for assessment, and may not indicate any reason for health concern when a child is reviewed by a health professional individually.

As discussed, it's essential to look beyond just the numbers and consider a child's overall health and wellbeing. So, other factors that may indicate a need for support include:

✧ Difficulty engaging in active play, walking or sport.

✧ A preoccupation with food, including stealing it and eating it repeatedly off the floor or out of bins.

✧ Diagnoses that can impact feeding behaviours or nutritional status (not necessarily weight), such as learning disabilities or neurodevelopmental conditions, such as autism.

✧ Signs of emotional distress related to eating, such as anxiety or comments about foods or body image (more likely in preschool years and beyond).

✧ Difficulty with social interactions or reluctance to participate in group activities that might be linked to self-esteem issues or weight-related concerns.

✧ A noticeable decline in engagement with learning, play and activities or behavioural changes that could be associated with physical health issues.

These guidelines are here just to help you decide when to seek support, but they may not capture all individual factors. If you have any concerns about your child's weight, growth or health, please speak to your GP.

It is acknowledged that BMI isn't a perfect method for assessing health risks in children, but as yet, more robust assessment criteria aren't available for young children. Other methods, such as comparing waist-to-height ratios, are currently being explored as alternative measures in older children (aged five plus).

How can weight-gain-related health concerns be managed?
It's important to seek individual advice for weight concerns and be aware that weight loss is generally not recommended in young children. Children must still get all the nutrients they need for growth and development. Some principles that may be discussed include:

✧ A family-focused approach, considering dietary or lifestyle adjustments for the whole family.

✧ Dietary balance overall. This may include increasing certain food groups or nutrients, such as fruits and vegetables, fibre-rich foods and reducing higher-energy but low-nutrient foods, such as sugar-sweetened drinks.

✧ Meal and snack routines.

✧ Family eating opportunities and routines.

✧ Physical activity, including active play. Young children need a lot of physical activity, with a minimum of three hours recommended per day, of which one hour should be moderate to vigorous activity.

✧ Managing sedentary time, such as time in front of screens.

✧ Supporting dietary or lifestyle changes for health, without blame or stigma and with an approach that is body inclusive, and safeguards a child's long-term food relationship.

If you have any concerns or questions about your child's growth and development, please initially contact your child's GP or health visitor.

Vegetarian or vegan diets for babies and children

An increasing number of families are adopting plant-based diets for health, sustainability or ethical reasons. The notion that plant-based, vegetarian or vegan diets are unsafe for young children is a myth. A well-planned vegetarian or vegan diet and targeted supplementation can promote healthy growth and development in babies and young children. Although this topic is a book of its own, here are some essential points to keep in mind if you're thinking about raising a plant-based little one.

Variety is key

As I've shared below, a plant-based, vegetarian or vegan diet can provide the necessary balance of nutrients to support your child's growth and development across all essential food and nutrient groups. And as mentioned earlier in the book, the advice about how often to offer these foods remains the same. However, it's recommended that protein-rich foods be offered three times a day.

Fruits and vegetables	As for all babies and young children, a variety of different fruits and vegetables can be offered.
Carbohydrates	As for all babies and young children, a variety of different starchy foods and grains like potato, oats, rice, pasta, noodles, plantain, breads/flour-based produce, yam, buckwheat and quinoa can be offered.
Protein	Plant-based protein sources include beans, lentils, legumes, tofu (and other soy foods e.g. soy mince) and nuts or seeds. Wholegrains and pseudograins like quinoa also contain protein. For vegetarians, dairy and eggs are also sources of protein.
Dairy or fortified alternatives	For vegans, unsweetened and fortified soy, pea, oat or coconut milk and yoghurt alternatives can replace dairy. For vegetarian families, dairy remains included.

Healthy fats	While these are not a food group, young children need fat, and with plant-based diets often being higher in fibre, and potentially lower in energy, inclusion of fats, such as avocado, oils (like olive or rapeseed), nuts, seeds and coconut, at meals is encouraged.

Key nutrients to consider

If following a plant-based, vegetarian or vegan diet, here are some nutrients I commonly discuss with families in more detail and why:

◇ **Energy:** Young children have high energy requirements but have small stomachs. Some meals high in plant foods can be higher in fibre and lower in energy; therefore, it's essential to include energy-rich foods like carbohydrates and fats at each mealtime.

◇ **Protein:** Many parents worry about plant-based children meeting their protein requirements; however, this is easily achieved with the inclusion of beans, lentils, nuts and seeds, soy-based foods, wholegrains and, of course, dairy and eggs for vegetarians.

◇ **Iron:** Prioritise plant-based sources of iron like beans, lentils, tofu and fortified cereals at each mealtime. Combining these with vitamin C-rich foods like fruits and certain vegetables can help with iron absorption.

◇ **Omega 3 fatty acids:** Oily fish is a key source of specific omega 3 fats, like DHA, which are important for brain development. However, these are not included in vegetarian or vegan diets. While plant-based sources of omega 3s, such as ALA, are found in foods like chia seeds, flaxseeds and walnuts, algae-based DHA supplements are generally recommended for children following a plant-based diet to ensure they get the necessary nutrients for brain health.

✧ **Calcium:** For children on a vegan diet, calcium must be obtained from non-dairy sources like fortified plant-based milk alternatives, calcium-set tofu, tahini, leafy greens and fortified bread or cereals.

✧ **Vitamin B12:** This is usually found in animal products, so it is rarely a concern for vegetarian children consuming dairy. However, if following a vegan diet, B12 supplementation is recommended once a child is established on solids.

✧ **Iodine:** As a nutrient consumed mainly from dairy and white fish, iodine intake needs careful consideration, particularly for children on a vegan diet or those who exclude dairy. Including iodine-fortified plant-based milk alternatives is recommended; for many vegan children, an iodine supplement may also be necessary once established on solids.

✧ **Vitamin D:** As mentioned throughout this book, supplementation is advised for all young children. Many supplements use vitamin D from animal sources, but vegan-friendly options are available.

In summary, a well-planned plant-based diet can be healthy for children, especially when supplemented appropriately. Families often find it helpful to seek guidance from a paediatric dietitian to get more tailored advice for their child.

A Final Note from Me to You

I sincerely hope that this book, whether it's been bought, borrowed or kindly gifted, has been a guiding force and a source of reassurance for you when navigating these first five years feeding your little one. Parenthood, and especially the journey (or obstacle course) of nourishing your child can feel overwhelming at times and the goal of this book was always to be a trusted source of information, reassurance and direction.

As I bring this book to a close, I want to finish on a few reminders:

✧ Nutrition is nuanced, and not all advice in this book will necessarily fit your child or family – and that's ok. There is no one 'right' way to feed your child, and health can look different for everyone. If you need additional advice and support that is specific to your circumstances, do reach out to a health professional.

✧ Nutrition and feeding kids often comes with the added weight of perfection. There is no such thing, and what's most important with much of what I've shared across this book is what you do most of the time!

✧ You can do everything 'right' and 'by the book' when it comes to feeding, but your child's journey will probably still have bumps and detours. I always remind parents we are feeding little humans, not little robots.

✧ Feeding your child is not just about nutrition; it's about connection, traditions, culture, nurturing and love. Don't let nutrition perfection get in the way of connection.

✧ You're doing a great job.

Thank you for allowing and trusting me to be a part of this chapter in your parenting journey.

With warmth and encouragement,

Lucy

Appendices

When and where to seek professional advice?

Throughout this book I've covered many common nutrition and feeding worries, but it must be recognised that individualised support is exceptionally important in many of these circumstances, and as a parent you shouldn't have to navigate big concerns on your own. Primary-care services such as your GP or health visitor are likely to be the first port of call for many concerns, however, onward referral to specialists in specific areas may be needed based on your child's history.

Below I've highlighted some key scenarios that warrant discussion with a health professional, with some additional considerations alongside. At the back of this book there is also a list of resources and recommendations for patient charities, independent advice or professionals and more.

Concern	Who to contact	Comments and considerations
Breastfeeding support or concerns	Midwife, health visitor or lactation consultant (IBCLC)	There may be local infant feeding teams available to you; your midwife and health visitor should be aware of these

Parents may also choose to seek out independent support with breast and/or bottle feeding from an IBCLC

Referral on to additional professionals such as a tongue-tie practitioner, paediatric dietitian (if allergy suspected or for growth concerns) or paedi-atrician may be recommended |
| Combination or formula-feeding concerns | Midwife, health visitor or lactation consultant (IBCLC) | |
| Lack of progress with solids (weaning) or specific feeding concerns such as difficulty swallowing, coughing or splutter-ing repeatedly with food, persisting gagging with food that doesn't improve | Contact health visitor or GP initially | Referrals to specialists, such as a paediatric dietitian and/or speech-and-language therapist may be recommended |

Growth concerns, such as not gaining weight	For babies, contact your midwife, health visitor or feeding team or professional For children older than one you can contact your GP and/or health visitor	Concerns about growth may need a referral to a paediatric dietitian. A health visitor or GP will be aware of how to refer into dietetic services local to you
Food allergy or intolerance A food-and-symptom diary, plus pictures of skin, nappies or symptoms you're worried about can be helpful	Your child's GP – some GPs may be able to provide first-line information and support **For any immediate food-allergy reactions causing red-flag concern such as breathing difficulties, floppiness or collapse please call 999**	Onward referral is likely to be required to a paediatric dietitian. Referrals into allergy teams can vary based on your location and referral criteria. All children with suspected immediate-type allergies should be referred to a children's allergy team or doctor
Tummy troubles – colic or reflux	For babies – health visitor, GP or lactation consultant For young children – GP	Referrals to specialists, such as a paediatrician, gastro-enterologist (gut specialist) or paediatric dietitian may be necessary
Tummy troubles – constipation	For babies – health visitor, GP or lactation consultant For young children – GP	Referrals to specialists, such as a paediatrician gastro-enterologist (gut specialist) or paediatric dietitian may be necessary

Tummy troubles – diarrhoea, blood in stools, abdominal pain, symptoms associated with fever or weight loss	Child's GP	Referrals to specialists, such as a paediatrician, gastro-enterologist (gut specialist) or paediatric dietitian may be necessary
Food refusal and/or selective eating	Contact GP initially, especially if: • Ongoing over several weeks or months • Associated with concerns such as weight loss or nutritional deficiencies • Associated with persisting illness or worrisome symptoms, such as tummy pain, diarrhoea • Associated with other concerns about your child's development **For suspected fussy eating, your health visitor may be able to offer some first-line advice**	Referrals to specialists, such as a paediatrician, gastro-enterologist (gut specialists), speech-and-language therapist or paediatric dietitian may be necessary Many local NHS dietetic teams are unable to accept referrals for fussy eating without associated complications. You can often access fussy-eating support from some independent health professionals, like dietitians, online
Nutritional deficiencies, such as worries about iron deficiency	Contact GP initially. They will usually be able to complete or refer onwards for testing (such as bloods) if considered necessary	Referrals to specialists, such as a paediatrician, gastro-enterologist (gut specialist) or paediatric dietitian may be necessary

Parent mantras for days when feeding your children feels HARD

Sometimes mealtimes can be tough and feel relentless as a parent – there's no day off from feeding your kids. It's natural to have peaks of frustration, helplessness, anger and more. Feel these emotions, and don't hold guilt for them. Parenting around food, especially in the early years, can be difficult. I'm sharing these affirmations to turn to on tricky days and to practice regularly, to help you keep a calm and positive mindset during meals, promoting a healthy and stress-free atmosphere for you and your child.

✧ I am a good parent and I am trying my best.

✧ My parenting or self-worth is not defined by what my child does or doesn't eat.

✧ My child's eating habits are not a reflection of my parenting and are not my fault.

✧ Mealtimes are an opportunity for my child to eat, not an expectation that they will or should.

✧ My child is learning to eat different foods – it takes time.

✧ Over-encouraging a single of bite of food in a moment isn't worth the long-term impact on my child's stress levels or enjoyment of mealtimes.

✧ Patience is key; progress takes time.

✧ My child's growth and health are about the long term, not just one meal.

✧ I trust my child to listen to their body, including their hunger and fullness cues.

✧ We are building a healthy relationship with food, step by step.

✧ It's ok if my child doesn't eat a balanced meal every mealtime.

✧ Small wins are still wins.

✧ I can celebrate food exploration, not just eating.

✧ Offering love and support is more important than a perfect diet.

✧ I am not alone; many parents face these challenges.

✧ Taking care of myself is important too.

✧ Nutrition is about the bigger picture, not just a single meal.

Know your nutrients

These tables won't be for everyone (nor do they need to be), and I am sharing with the caveat that you don't need the nutrition knowledge of a dietitian or nutritionist or an in-depth understanding of these to support your child to be a healthy happy eater. They are shared for reference only, to provide context or information for those who might find it helpful.

Vitamins

Nutrient	What does it do?	Foods found in?	Additional notes
Vitamin A (Retinol)	Supports eyesight, immune function, reproduction, skin health, growth and development.	Dairy, eggs, oily fish, fortified products, liver. Plant-based sources (carotenoids) can be found in orange, yellow and red fruits and vegetables as well as dark, leafy greens.	Liver should be given a maximum of once a week to babies and children (from six months of age) in small quantities. Plant sources (carotenoids) do not cause toxicity.
Vitamin D (Calciferol)	Supports bone and teeth health, immune system, muscle function and mood regulation.	Sunlight, oily fish, egg yolk, meat, offal, fortified foods, UV-exposed mushrooms.	Supplementation is recommended for babies and young children, as long as they are not having >500ml of formula milk per day
Vitamin E (Tocopherol)	Supports healthy skin and eyes, and immune system.	Vegetable oils, nuts, seeds, dark, leafy greens, fortified products.	
Vitamin K	Supports bone health and blood clotting.	K1: Dark, leafy greens, vegetable oils, cereals, some fruits. K2: Animal products, fermented foods, gut bacteria.	Most babies have a vitamin K injection after birth.

Vitamin B1 (Thiamine)	Helps make energy, supports nervous system. Important for children's growth and neurological development.	Wholegrain bread, pork, liver, black beans, nuts, fortified cereals, fruits.	
Vitamin B2 (Riboflavin)	Helps release energy from food, supports nervous system, maintains healthy skin and eyes.	Lean meats, dairy, eggs, mushrooms, fortified cereals.	
Vitamin B3 (Niacin)	Involved in energy production, keeps nervous system and skin healthy, supports growth and development.	Meat, fish, wholegrains, eggs, peanuts, fortified cereals.	
Vitamin B5 (Pantothenic Acid)	Helps release energy from food, supports brain and nervous-system function.	Meat, liver, kidneys, eggs, mushrooms, wholegrains, avocados, dairy, nuts, seeds, fortified cereals.	
Vitamin B6 (Pyridoxine)	Supports energy production, immune system, red-blood-cell production, growth, brain development.	Pork, poultry, fish, potatoes, bananas, peanuts, soya beans, oats, milk, fortified cereals.	Gut bacteria also produce vitamin B6.
Vitamin B7 (Biotin)	Helps turn food into energy, supports hair, skin, nails, nervous system.	Meat, fish, eggs, nuts, seeds, vegetables.	Gut bacteria also produce biotin.

Vitamin B9 (Folate)	Supports DNA synthesis, cell division and growth. Essential for foetal development.	Vegetables, legumes, liver, fortified cereals.	Crucial during the first trimester of pregnancy. Supplementation recommended for those trying to conceive or pregnant.
Vitamin B12 (Cobalamin)	Supports nervous system, DNA synthesis, energy release and helps use vitamin B9. Prevents megaloblastic anaemia.	Meat, fish, dairy, eggs.	Not found in plant foods – vegans may require supplementation or fortified products.
Vitamin C (Ascorbic Acid)	Supports immune system, foetal development, aids iron absorption.	Fruits and vegetables (peppers, kiwi, citrus fruits, strawberries, tomatoes, broccoli).	

Minerals and trace elements

Calcium	Supports bone and teeth development, muscle function, nerve transmission, blood clotting.	Dairy, small fish with bones, sesame, tofu, leafy greens, almonds, fortified foods like milk alternatives	
Phosphorus	Works with calcium to maintain strong bones and teeth, energy production, cell repair.	Meat, fish, eggs, dairy, tofu, nuts, legumes, wholegrains, vegetables.	

Magnesium	Supports bone health, muscle and nerve function, energy production, blood-pressure regulation.	Nuts, seeds, whole-grains, leafy green vegetables, legumes, dairy, fortified products.	
Sodium	Maintains fluid balance, muscle contractions and nerve function.	Processed foods, hard cheese, soy sauce, gravy	**Sodium (salt) should be limited in the diet of babies and young children**
Potassium	Maintains fluid balance, muscle and nerve function, supports kidney and heart health.	Fruits, vegetables, legumes, nuts, animal products.	Excess potassium intake should be avoided in certain medical conditions like kidney disease.
Iron	Helps produce haemoglobin, supports the immune system, growth and brain development.	Haem iron: Red meat, poultry, seafood, eggs Non-haem iron: Legumes, fortified cereals, spinach, nuts, seeds, dried fruits.	
Zinc	Maintains taste and smell, supports DNA/protein production, immune function, growth.	Meat, seafood, dairy, eggs, legumes, whole-grains, seeds, nuts, fortified cereals.	
Copper	Helps produce energy, red blood cells, proteins; supports immune system and brain development.	Liver, shellfish, nuts, seeds, whole-grains, legumes, leafy greens, fruits.	Excess copper is rare but can be harmful.

Iodine	Crucial for thyroid hormones, regulating energy use and supporting growth and brain development.	Dairy, white fish, seafood, seaweed, iodised salt.	Too much iodine from certain types of seaweed can be harmful. Those on a vegan diet may need additional supplementation
Selenium	Supports DNA production, skin/hair/nail health, immune system and thyroid function.	Nuts, seafood, meat, eggs, wholegrains, dairy, legumes, some vegetables.	
Choline	Supports brain function, gene regulation and cell health.	Meat, dairy, eggs, legumes, nuts, seeds, cruciferous vegetables.	

Budget-friendly foods

Throughout this book, there is a lot of information about foods for your baby and young child, highlighting their role in a balanced diet for these age groups. With the cost of food higher than ever, I am aware that some of the foods detailed may not always feel like budget-friendly or obtainable options for all families. For this reason, I wanted to highlight some of my favourite budget-friendly foods advice.

General advice
✧ Fruits or vegetables in season are likely to be cheaper; often these are sold at the front of the fruit and vegetable aisles. Wonky fruit and vegetable options and boxes can also be good value for money.

✧ Check out local food markets; often fruits and vegetables are cheaper and locally sourced!

✧ Batch cooking, or considering meals you can cook once and eat twice can help keep costs down.

✧ Meal planning is a great way to prevent waste and ensure you just buy what you need for the week.

✧ Choose store own brands over branded items; often there's little difference!

✧ Consider budget-friendly staples like frozen vegetables, tinned beans and pulses, dried lentils, large bags of pasta and rice.

Here are some of my best budget suggestions for different food groups:

Fruit

✧ **Berries** – Swap fresh for frozen berries or tinned options in juice.

✧ **Bananas** – These are usually affordable and can be frozen easily if getting ignored. Perfect to add to smoothies or baking at a later date.

✧ **Dried** – Buy larger bags and decant into pots or reusable bags for snacks. No need for branded options!

✧ **Tropical fruits** – Fruits like mango and pineapple can be found cheaper frozen or tinned in juice.

✧ **Apples** – These tend to have a long shelf life. Check the cost of loose versus pre-bagged.

Vegetables

✧ **Frozen vegetables** – These include peas, sweetcorn, corn on the cob, butternut squash, spinach, broccoli, cauliflower, beans.

✧ **Tinned vegetables** – Opt for sweetcorn, tomatoes and other vegetables in unsalted water.

✧ **Root vegetables** – Opt for fresh carrots, swedes, potatoes and parsnips – these tend to have a longer shelf life.

Herbs and spices

✧ Buy bagged, dried herbs and spices like those from the world-food aisle, instead of in small containers.

✧ Grow them – Options like mint and rosemary grow easily from one plant and give all year round. Blend spare fresh herbs into oil and freeze in an ice cube tray for use another day.

Carbohydrates

✧ **Pasta** – Affordable and versatile, it can be used in many different dishes.

✧ **Rice** – Buy a larger bag, as this is always cheaper than microwave or smaller bagged options. Check the world-food aisle.

✧ **Potatoes** – Both fresh and frozen potatoes are budget-friendly and can be prepared in various ways.

✧ **Oats** – Great for breakfast or baking and can be used in both sweet and savoury dishes.

✧ **Bread** – Opt for budget loaves if needed, and freeze extras to avoid waste.

✧ **Couscous and bulgur wheat** – These grains cook quickly and can be bought in bulk for affordable, nutritious meals.

✧ **Polenta** – This is affordable and can be used as a side dish or in baking for a budget-friendly alternative to pasta or rice.

✧ **Flour** – Stock up on flour for homemade bread, pizza dough, pancakes and baking. Wholemeal or plain flour in larger quantities tends to be cheaper.

Protein-rich foods

✧ **Beans, pulses and legumes** – Dried or tinned are both cheap and versatile protein sources that can be added to a wide range of dishes.

✧ **Fish** – Fresh fish can be swapped for frozen fish fillets, or tinned fish, such as salmon or sardines.

✧ **Meat** – Opt for budget cuts of meat such as chicken thighs, beef mince or pork shoulder. Frozen options can also be cheaper. Consider buying in bulk or on sale to save money.

✧ **Soya** – Soya-based products like tofu and tempeh are great plant-based protein sources. Tofu can be bought fresh (but can be frozen), and dried soya mince is an inexpensive and shelf-stable alternative to meat in dishes like Bolognese or chilli.

✧ **Eggs** – Affordable, versatile and protein-packed, these are great for breakfasts, baking or quick meals like omelettes, frittatas or scrambled eggs.

✧ **Nuts and seeds** – Buy in bulk where possible for an affordable protein source, perfect for adding to dishes. Peanut butter is also a budget-friendly option rich in protein.

Dairy

✧ Buy larger blocks of cheese instead of individual cheeses or pre-grated. Hard cheese also freezes well.

✧ Buy milk in bulk or on offer, and freeze.

References

I have not listed all the references to the studies and research that I have mentioned throughout this book, as it's not been designed as an academic-style text. That said, if you would like more information or links to any scientific paper, report or research mentioned within the book, please do reach out via www.thechildrensdietitian.co.uk and I'd be happy to provide these.

Helpful resources and organisations

For many topics covered in this book the NHS website has accessible and first-line information. You can also find additional information from the resources below, depending on what area you'd like support with. I've largely listed bigger organisations, however, there are many fantastic health professionals, from doctors to dietitians, who are now accessible online. Please consider where and who you get your medical and nutritional advice online from very carefully, as there is a huge amount of noise and misinformation out there. Look into the credentials of any 'expert'.

Breastfeeding

✧ UNICEF – www.unicef.org.uk
✧ National Breastfeeding Helpline – 0300 100 0212, www.nationalbreastfeedinghelpline.org.uk
✧ La Leche League — 0345 120 2918, laleche.org.uk
✧ Association of Breastfeeding Mothers – 0300 330 5453, abm.me.uk
✧ NCT Infant Feeding Helpline – 0300 330 0700
✧ Lactation Consultants of Great Britain: lcgb.org/find–an–ibclc

Books:

✧ *A Judgement-free Guide to Feeding Your Baby: Boob, bottle and all*, Olivia Hinge (Yellow Kite, 2024)
✧ *You've Got it in You: A Positive Guide to Breastfeeding*, Emma Pickett (Matador, 2016)
✧ *Supporting Breastfeeding Past the First Six Months and Beyond: A Guide for Professionals and Parents*, Emma Pickett (Jessica Kingsley, 2022)

Bottle Feeding

✧ UNICEF – www.unicef.org.uk
✧ First Steps Nutrition Trust – www.firststepsnutrition.org
✧ NHS Start for Life –www.nhs.uk/start-for-life
✧ National Childbirth Trust – www.nct.org.uk

Baby and Child First Aid

✧ St John Ambulance – www.sja.org.uk

- British Red Cross – www.redcross.org.uk/first-aid/learn-first-aid-for-babies-and-children
- Mini First Aid – www.thefirstaidteam.co.uk
- Daisy First Aid –www.daisyfirstaid.com

Coeliac Disease
- Coeliac UK – www.coeliac.org.uk

Food Allergy
- Allergy UK – www.allergyuk.org
- Anaphylaxis UK – www.anaphylaxis.org.uk
- British Society for the (BSACI) – including the location of your closest allergy services – www.bsaci.org
- Sadie Bristow Foundation – www.sadiebristowfoundation.org.uk
- Natasha Allergy Research Foundation – www.narf.org.uk
- Available from Lucy's website for free – www.thechildrensdietitian.co.uk
  - o Allergen Tracker
  - o Food and Symptom Diary
  - o Two free allergy cookbooks (ebooks)

Plant-based nutrition
- The Vegan Society – www.vegansociety.com
- The Vegetarian Society – www.vegsoc.org
- Plant-based Professionals – www.plantbasedhealthprofessionals.com
- First Steps Nutrition, Eating well: vegan infants and under-5s – www.firststepsnutrition.org/vegan-infants

Books
- *Plant Powered Little People: A practical guide to plant-based nutrition for under-fives,* Paula Hallam (Meze Publishing, 2023)

Premature Babies

✧ Bliss Charity – For babies born premature or sick – www.bliss. org.uk

✧ Tommy's – The pregnancy and baby charity – www.tommys.org

General Nutrition and Feeding guidance for the early years

✧ First Steps Nutrition Trust – www.firststepsnutrition.org

✧ Infant and Toddler Forum – infantandtoddlerforum.org

✧ British Nutrition Foundation – www.nutrition.org.uk

✧ The British Dietetic Association – www.bda.uk.com

Children's Bowel and Bladder Troubles

✧ ERIC The Children's Bowel & Bladder Charity – eric.org.uk

✧ Guts UK – www.gutscharity.org.uk

Eating or children's feeding disorders organisations

✧ ARFID Awareness UK – www.arfidawarenessuk.org

✧ The Feeding Trust – www.feedingtrust.org

✧ Beat Eating Disorders – www.beateatingdisorders.org.uk

Government Support Schemes

✧ Healthy Start Scheme – www.healthystart.nhs.uk

✧ Scotland – Best Start Grant and Best Start Foods – www.mygov. scot

Weaning

✧ NHS Start for Life – www.nhs.uk/start-for-life

✧ First Steps Nutrition – www.firststepsnutrition.org

Glossary

ALLERGEN: A usually harmless thing that can make some people's bodies react with symptoms like itching, sneezing or swelling. Examples include dust mites, pollen or certain foods.

ANAPHYLAXIS: A very serious and fast reaction to <u>an allergen</u> that can make it hard to breathe and cause a rash or swelling. It needs immediate medical help.

ANTIOXIDANT: A substance that helps protect your body from damage caused by harmful molecules called 'free radicals'.

ATOPY: A tendency (inherited) to have hay fever, food allergy, asthma or eczema.

AUTONOMY: Being able to make your own choices and decisions without being told what to do by others. It's about having the freedom to do things in your own way and control your own actions.

AVOIDANT/RESTRICTIVE FOOD INTAKE DISORDER (ARFID): ARFID is characterised by a pattern of eating that avoids certain foods or food groups entirely and/or is restricted in quantity (eating small amounts). Avoidant and restrictive eating cannot be due to lack of available food, or cultural norms (such as someone who is fasting or chooses not to eat certain foods for religious or cultural reasons alone). It is not just 'picky' or 'fussy' eating.

BIOPSY: A medical procedure that involves removing a small sample of tissue or cells from the body to look for signs of disease or damage.

BOWEL: part of your digestive system. It helps break down the food you eat and moves it through your body. The bowel is divided into two main parts: the small intestine, where most digestion happens; and the large intestine, which absorbs water and gets rid of waste.

CARBOHYDRATE: A type of macronutrient that has many important roles, including providing energy, helping the brain function well and keeping the gut healthy. It is found in foods like bread, pasta, fruits and vegetables.

COELIAC DISEASE: A condition caused by the immune system attacking and damaging the gut when food containing gluten (a protein found in breads, pastas, cereals wheat, rye, barley and sauces) is eaten. It can cause difficulty digesting food, and tummy, gut and skin symptoms. People with coeliac disease have to avoid eating gluten for life.

COGNITION: The process of thinking, learning and understanding things.

COGNITIVE DEVELOPMENT: How a child's brain develops and learns to think, understand and solve problems.

CORRECTED AGE: This is the age a premature baby would be if they had been born on their due date, rather than when they were actually born.

DEFICIENCY: A lack or shortage of something. In the context of nutrition, this is often a lack or shortage of certain nutrients.

DERMATOLOGIST: A doctor who specialises in the management of skin conditions and differences.

ENZYME: Special proteins (often like tiny scissors) that help with many processes in the body like breaking down food into smaller pieces so it can be used for energy and growth, heal from cuts and bruises, fight illness and remove unhelpful things from your body.

FAT: a type of <u>macronutrient</u> with several important roles, including providing energy, helping regulate body temperature and assisting in the absorption of certain <u>vitamins</u>. Fat is found in foods such as meat, fish, nuts, seeds, butter and vegetable oils.

FATTY ACID: A small part of fat that helps the body do important things, including making energy, hormones and keeping the brain working well.

FERMENTATION: A process where tiny living things, like yeast or bacteria, break down sugars in food to make something new. For example, yeast helps turn sugar into bubbles and alcohol when making bread or juice into soda or alcohol. This process also makes foods like yoghurt taste different and last longer.

FREE SUGAR: A sugar that is added to foods and drinks like sweets and fizzy drinks or found in honey, syrup and fruit juice. It is called 'free' because it's not inside the food's cells, so your body can use it quickly for energy.

GENES: A tiny set of instructions inside the body made up of a special code called DNA. They tell your body how to do things, like deciding the colour of your eyes, your hair, how tall you may grow and many other things that make you who you are. We get our genes from our parents.

HORMONES: Tiny messengers that travel around the body and tell it how to grow, feel, work and keep it healthy.

INFANCY: A baby from birth to 12 months/one year of age.

INSOLUBLE FIBRE ('BULKING' FIBRE): Insoluble fibre doesn't dissolve in water. It adds bulk to the stool, helping it move through the digestive system more easily and preventing constipation. Sources include wholegrains (e.g. wheat bran, brown rice, quinoa), nuts (e.g. almonds, walnuts), seeds (e.g. sunflower, flaxseeds), potato skins, skins of fruits and vegetables (e.g. apples, cucumbers, tomatoes), dark leafy greens (e.g. spinach, kale).

LAXATIVE: A medicine or component of food that helps you poo and may be used if you're having trouble going to the bathroom; for example, if you are constipated.

MACRONUTRIENTS: The parts of food you need in large amounts to give you energy and help your body grow, work well and stay healthy. There are three macronutrients: carbohydrates, fats and proteins.

MECONIUM: A baby's first poo after birth. It's sticky, thick and dark green or black. This poo forms while the baby is still growing inside the mother. It's made up of things the baby swallowed in the womb, like skin cells and fluids.

MICROBIOME: The community of microorganisms (such as fungi, bacteria and viruses) that live in a particular environment. For example, those that live in the gut are the gut microbiome, those on the skin are the skin microbiome.

MICRONUTRIENTS: The parts of food that are needed in small amounts to provide energy and help your body grow, work well and stay healthy. There are three groups of micronutrients called vitamins, minerals and trace elements.

MINERALS: A type of <u>micronutrient</u> that your body requires in small amounts. They have many roles, including helping build strong bones and keeping your heart healthy.

MOTOR DEVELOPMENT: How babies and kids learn to use their muscles to move and do things, such as crawling, walking and throwing.

NEURODEVELOPMENT: This is how the brain and nervous system grow and change from birth to adulthood. It involves making new brain cells, connecting them and improving these connections.

NEURON: A cell in the brain or body that helps to send messages. Neurons talk to each other using tiny electrical signals. Think of them as messengers that help your brain communicate with the rest of your body.

PAEDIATRIC DIETITIAN: A healthcare professional who specialises in nutrition for babies, children and adolescents. They provide expert advice on managing dietary needs, supporting healthy growth and development, and addressing specific nutritional concerns or conditions in babies and children.

PHYTOESTROGEN: A naturally occurring compound found in plants and plant-based foods that has a similar chemical structure to oestrogen.

PREBIOTIC: non-digestible fibres that act as food for good gut bacteria, promoting their growth and activity.

PROBIOTIC: living microorganisms ('good bacteria') that, when consumed in adequate amounts, can provide health benefits.

PROTEIN: A type of macronutrient that has many important roles, including helping your muscles grow strong, healing from cuts and bruises, making important things for your body and helping you stay well. Protein is found in foods like meat, fish, beans, dairy and nuts.

RED BOOK: This is also known as the Personal Child Health Record (PCHR), and is the little red book that you're given after your baby is born. It contains information like growth charts, development questions and vaccination records.

REFERENCE NUTRIENT INTAKE (RNI): the amount of a nutrient that is enough to meet the needs of around 97.5 per cent of a group of people.

SOLUBLE FIBRE ('WATER HOLDING' FIBRE): Soluble fibre dissolves in water and forms a gel-like substance. It helps to absorb excess water in the stool, making it easier to pass. Sources include oats, apples, carrots, beans (e.g. kidney beans, black beans), lentils, citrus fruits (e.g. oranges, grapefruits), barley, peas, psyllium husk.

TRACE ELEMENT: A type of <u>micronutrient</u> which your body requires in very tiny amounts. They have many roles including making your blood, keeping your bones strong and helping your body work properly. Examples of trace elements include iron, zinc, iodine and selenium.

VITAMIN: A type of <u>micronutrient</u> that your body requires in small amounts. They have many roles including helping you grow, keep well and stay strong. Vitamins are grouped into water-soluble ones (vitamins B and C) and fat-soluble ones (vitamins A, D, E and K). You can find vitamins in many different foods like milk and dairy, fish, cereals, fruits and vegetables.

Index

B
babies: appetite regulation 62
  growth 283
  see also breast milk; formula milk;
    newborn babies
baby food, pre-prepared 112, 113–15
baby-led weaning 85, 86–8, 90, 209
bacteria: antibiotic-associated diarrhoea
    393–4
  in breast milk 11–12
  fermentation 445
  prebiotics 311
  see also gut microbiome; probiotics
bananas 436
beans 438
  for constipation 386
  fibre content 264, 265
  first foods 133
  for toddlers 182
  zinc content 300
beige foods 247–8
berries 436
beta-carotene 301
bibs 83–4
bilberry extract 196
biopsies 444
bitter flavours 91
blenders 84
blood, in poo 382, 383, 395, 396
blood-sugar levels 262, 263
body image 341, 343–4, 418
body language, and picky eaters 221
body mass index (BMI) 284–5, 413, 417, 418
bonding 19, 55–6
bottle feeding 3–4, 36–54
  and allergies 30–1
  and bonding 55–6
  bottle aversion 59–61
  checking milk intake 66–70
  combination feeding 55
  and constipation 56–8
  costs 44–5
  for Cow's Milk Protein Allergy 49–51
  DHA fortification 292
  follow-on formula 129
  how to feed 51–2
  introducing bottles 32–4
  making up feeds in advance 58–9
  nutrition 37–42
  other ingredients 40–2
  and poo 68, 396
  preparation of formula 42–4

professional help 426
quantities 52–3
and reflux 376
reheating milk 56
responsive feeding 61–4
safety 44
signs of fullness 66
sterilising bottles 43
supplements 54, 135
toddlers and 165–6
tracking apps 54
transitioning from 165–6
types of formula milk 37–8, 45–51
for vegan families 58
in warm weather 70–1
and weaning 127–9
bottled water 56, 129
botulism 102
bowel 444
  see also poo
bowls, for weaning 84
brain: brain-building nutrients 289–304
  fats and 104
  gut-brain axis 305, 307–8, 369–70
  neurodevelopment 446
  neurons 299, 301, 447
  neurotransmitters 210, 296, 299
  preschoolers 250
  toddlers 158
bran 149
bread 236, 438
breakfast 271–3
  brain-building nutrients 303
  gut-friendly foods 315
  and immune system 325
  iron-rich foods 403, 404
  toddlers 187–8
breastfeeding and breast milk 3, 4–35
  allergies 28–31
  benefits of 13–15
  bioactive factors 11–13
  boosting supply 31
  breast problems 28
  checking milk intake 27, 66–70
  combination feeding 55
  and constipation 31–2
  expressed breast milk 34–5, 71
  first feeds 19–20
  fluid in breast milk 10
  frequency of feeds 20–2
  and immune system 320
  introducing a bottle 32–4

Acknowledgements

Like raising a child, this book wouldn't be what it is without a village. I am incredibly grateful to my colleagues who have selflessly shared their own time, expertise and guidance with me to ensure this book is evidence-based, and who peer reviewed but also continue to be a source of inspiration and guidance to me in daily practice. Thank you!!

✦ Stacey Zimmels – IBCLC and Speech-and-Language Therapist. Thank you for being an exceptional ear, adviser, reasoner, supporter, friend and advocate for this book and me. Your expertise, no BS approach and honest feedback has been invaluable. As always.

✦ Emilia Fish – Registered Dietitian, who has supported this book from its infancy, been the key author behind the nutritional tables and glossary, and proofread for me many times!

✦ Karen Murphy, Clinical Psychologist. Your kind, empathetic and supportive eyes are so, so valued, especially for a book which parents may pick up at many a vulnerable time.

✦ Helen Howells – GP and specialist allergy doctor. The busiest woman I know and you still made time to medically review this for me – I'm always in awe of your energy, expertise and dedication – especially to allergy families.

- Natalia Stasenko – Paediatric Dietitian. Your bright, supportive, kind and honest feedback and support is invaluable.
- Lucy Jackman – Specialist Dietitian. I am forever in awe of your knowledge, kindness and enthusiasm. Thank you for giving the same to my book and me!
- Paula Hallam – Specialist Paediatric Dietitian (and wonderful friend). Your constant support, guidance, time, energy and effort to get this book where it is will never be forgotten.
- Deirdre Fagan – Specialist Dietitian and a wonderful friend. Thank you for looking after all our families who needed help and support while I was busy with this book. You have kept me going in some tricky times, so thank you for being such a cheerleader and all round wonderful person.

To Harry, thank you for all of the cups of coffee, wiping my tears, morale and parenting support, every day I worked on this book, and always. For proofing this book, and keeping me sane. You are my biggest cheerleader and I wouldn't and couldn't have done this without you.

To my friends who have also taken their precious time and energy to read this book, especially Alison – thank you.

For my literary agent, Jon, I think you believed I could do this far before I did. Thank you for investing in me and this book since day one. Your endless support, guidance and expertise have kept me going on tough days and been nothing short of invaluable.

To Yellow Kite, my editor, Carolyn, assistant editor, Zoe, and everyone else involved in bringing this book to life. An endless thank you for entrusting me with a resource I hope will help so many families. Your passion, expertise, energy and endless support behind the scenes has been inspiring. Thank you.

Thanks to Rebecca Wilson for being my first insight into the literary world, trusting me with her books, and sharing her time and energy to write a humbling foreword for mine.

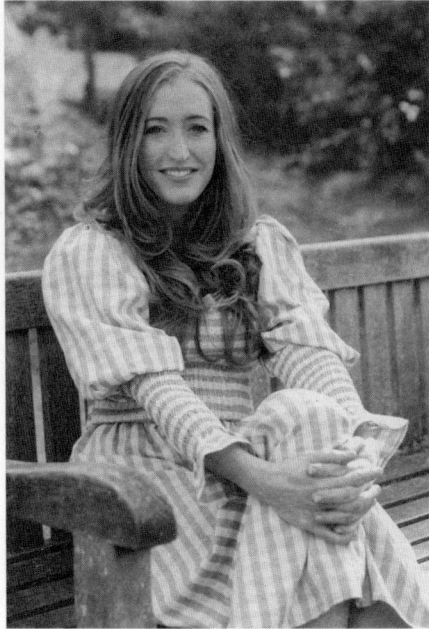

Lucy Upton, The Children's Dietitian, is a UK-leading paediatric dietitian and nutritionist with over 15 years of experience helping families navigate children's nutrition. From fussy eating to allergies and growth concerns, she makes food and mealtimes easier with evidence-based, practical advice. A trusted media expert, Lucy has been a guest on *BBC Breakfast*, collaborates with brands like What Mummy Makes, Pampers and Tilda Rice, and speaks at events including The Baby Show.

As a mum herself, Lucy understands the everyday challenges of feeding little ones and combines expert knowledge with genuine empathy for the realities of family life.

Her debut book, *The Ultimate Guide to Children's Nutrition*, is a must-read for parents feeding kids in the first five years, offering accessible advice and practical strategies on feeding from milk feeding through to weaning, fussy eating, and allergies.